ATLASES IN
DIAGNOSTIC SURGICAL PATHOLOGY

Consulting Editor
Gerald M. Bordin, M.D.
Department of Pathology
Scripps Clinic and Research Foundation

Published:

WOLD, McLEOD, SIM, AND UNNI:
ATLAS OF ORTHOPEDIC PATHOLOGY

COLBY, LOMBARD, YOUSEM, AND KITAICHI:
ATLAS OF PULMONARY SURGICAL PATHOLOGY

KANEL AND KORULA
ATLAS OF LIVER PATHOLOGY

Forthcoming Titles:

OWEN AND KELLY
ATLAS OF GASTROINTESTINAL PATHOLOGY

ATLAS OF HEAD AND NECK PATHOLOGY

Bruce M. Wenig, M.D.
Assistant Chairman
Department of Otolaryngic-Endocrine Pathology
Armed Forces Institute of Pathology
Washington, DC

W.B. SAUNDERS COMPANY
Harcourt Brace & Company
Philadelphia ■ London ■ Toronto ■ Montreal ■ Sydney ■ Tokyo

W.B. SAUNDERS COMPANY
A Division of
Harcourt Brace & Company
The Curtis Center
Independence Square West
Philadelphia, Pennsylvania 19106

Library of Congress Cataloging-in-Publication Data

Wenig, Bruce M.
    Atlas of head and neck pathology / Bruce M. Wenig.
       p.   cm.
    ISBN 0-7216-4032-X
    1. Head—Diseases—Atlases. 2. Neck—Diseases—Atlases.
  I. Title. II. Title: Atlas of head and neck pathology.
    [DNLM: 1. Head—pathology—atlases. 2. Neck—pathology—atlases.
WE 17 W475a]
  RC936.W38 1993   617.5′1′00222—dc20
DNLM/DLC   92-48904

Atlas of Head and Neck Pathology   ISBN 0-7216-4032-X

Printed in the United States of America.

Last digit is the print number: 9 8 7 6 5 4 3 2

This book is dedicated to my wife, Ana, for the resolve to maintain our love as "beginners," and for our mutual respect of one another's individual solitudes;

to the loves and joys of our lives, our children, Sarah Amelia and Eli Jonathan;

to my parents, Sidonia and Louis Wenig, who understood long before I did and for whom words are not nearly enough;

to the Urrutia clan for who they are

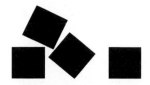

FOREWORD

We have been close associates of Dr. Bruce M. Wenig for over six years, and during this time his diligent work has been devoted virtually full time to surgical pathology of the head and neck. Through the consultation service of the Armed Forces Institute of Pathology, Dr. Wenig has had an opportunity to garner a broad and very intensive experience in head and neck pathology. It is a great pleasure to see how this experience has resulted in the very valuable contribution of the *Atlas of Head and Neck Pathology* for use by the pathology and otolaryngology communities. Certainly both groups should find this work extremely helpful.

Dr. Wenig has succeeded admirably in his intention to provide an atlas useful to a broad range of medical professionals. The pithy textual comments provide a ready reference for the busy clinician. The text and illustrations are organized to provide a maximum of pertinent information in a limited space, and this will be useful to students or residents initially learning about head and neck diseases. Yet the information is detailed and comprehensive enough to be of benefit to the experienced doctor. For example, it is quite unlikely that a surgeon or pathologist will encounter a patient with a sinonasal tumor that is not covered in this atlas. The abundant photomicrographs will be very helpful to the surgical pathologist for whom the well-chosen picture is, indeed, worth a thousand words.

The information in the atlas has a broad scope. The references are well chosen, mostly current, and, for an atlas, abundant. The space devoted to anatomy and normal histology is important. If pathologists do not have a firm grasp on normal histoanatomy, the efforts to diagnose the abnormal (i.e., disease) will surely result in errors in diagnosis. For example, the files of the Armed Forces Institute of Pathology contain numerous instances of normal turbinate vascular tissues being misdiagnosed as hemangiomas or angiofibromas. Essentially normal "transitional" mucosal epithelium at the edges of the true vocal cord (intermediate between the squamous epithelium of the cord and the respiratory lining of the ventricle) has been misdiagnosed many times as severe dysplasia or carcinoma in situ.

This atlas will help provide a substrate for fostering understanding and communication among the surgeons, radiologists, and pathologists who are involved in diagnosing and treating patients with diseases of the upper respiratory tract and related head and neck areas. It is an honor for us to be asked to make these forwarding comments.

Dennis K. Heffner, M.D., Chairman,
and Vincent J. Hyams, M.D., Chairman Emeritus,
Department of Otolaryngic-Endocrine Pathology
Armed Forces Institute of Pathology

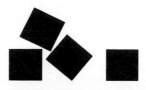

PREFACE

The head and neck, in relationship to the rest of the body, encompass a relatively small anatomic area. However, the anatomy and pathology of all the components of this region are extremely complex, with a rich array of disease processes. Within the limitations of an atlas attempting to detail the pathology of the diseases of the head and neck, *Atlas of Head and Neck Pathology* is intended to offer as much information with corresponding illustrations as possible. To this end and with the understanding that the pathologist practices his or her discipline as an integral member of the clinical team, I have attempted to make this atlas "usable" for a wide spectrum of individuals in the medical profession irrespective of their training status, level, or area of expertise.

Atlas of Head and Neck Pathology is organized into five major sections according to anatomic regions. Each section begins with brief textual highlights of the anatomy and histology of that specific region. Corresponding supplemental embryologic and anatomic facts are offered in the appendix portion of the book. Following the anatomy and histology, classifications of non-neoplastic and neoplastic lesions are listed for the specific regions. This in turn is followed by the pathologic states, beginning with non-neoplastic lesions and followed by benign neoplasms and malignant neoplasms, respectively. The final chapter in each section includes the TNM staging of neoplasms for the regions discussed. The format for each disease entity begins with its definition followed by its synonym(s) and then, in order, the clinical details (epidemiologic facts, signs and symptoms, etiology, etc.), major radiographic features (if pertinent), pathologic features (gross and microscopic), differential diagnoses, treatment and behavior, and additional facts. Within each of these segments, only the major features are listed. As this atlas is primarily intended to describe the pathology, an attempt was made to be as detailed as possible in describing the histopathology of each entity. The latter includes special stains (histochemistry and immunohistochemistry) and ultrastructural features when applicable. The differential diagnosis section is a histopathologic differential diagnosis. Because of the limitation in space, this section lists only those diseases included in the differential diagnosis; however, cross references are provided so that the reader can turn to other sections of the book to read about specific differentiating points in more detail. The additional facts sections contain information that I felt was of practical importance to the surgical pathologist and/or clinician but that did not neatly "fit" within the previously detailed subdivisions. The illustrations include clinical, radiographic, and gross pathology photographs when they significantly add to the description of the disease state; photomicrographs illustrating the essential pathologic features accompany each disease entity. When especially helpful or of major significance, special stains (histochemistry and/or immunocytochemistry) are illustrated. Finally, each disease has a limited number of references. I have attempted to list the key references. To this end, the references are as recent as possible but also include older articles that originally described the clinicopathologic features or significantly contributed to the understanding of the specific disease.

Some liberties I took in order to make the book more readable included the description of fibrous dysplasia, a non-neoplastic disease, within the section of fibro-osseous neoplasms. This would allow the reader to have at hand descriptions and illustrations of diseases with overlapping clinical and pathologic features rather than having to leaf back and forth between different sections of the book. Also, although necrotizing sialometaplasia, mucocele, and ranula are diseases of salivary glands, I included them within the section of the oral cavity because they are more often identified in those locations rather than in association with major salivary gland structures. Further, head and neck neoplasms are not necessarily limited to any one specific site of origin but may arise as a primary tumor in a variety of separate areas of the head and neck. With limited exceptions, neoplasms are discussed within the site/region where they are most frequently identified. For selected tumors, additional information is given relating to their occurrence in other anatomic regions. I have tried to maintain the continuity of discussing benign and malignant neoplasms of the same histogenesis in the same sections of the book. One notable exception is rhabdomyoma and rhabdomyosarcoma. Discussions of these entities occur in different sections of the book. The reason for this relates to the previous statement regarding discussing neoplasms within the anatomic areas in which they most commonly occur. Because of the unique clinical features related to jugulotympanic paragangliomas, discussions of extra-adrenal (carotid body and jugulotympanic) paragangliomas appear in two different sections of the atlas.

Atlas of Head and Neck Pathology is an attempt to be as complete as possible within the context of the atlas format. Given the breadth of anatomy and pathology of all components forming the nasal cavity, paranasal sinuses, oral cavity, pharynx (oro-, naso-, and hypopharnyx), neck, larynx, salivary glands (major and minor), and the ear (external, middle, and inner ear), I believe that this attempt has for the most part been successful. However, this atlas is by no means an all-inclusive text but should be utilized in conjunction with texts containing abundant information pertaining to the anatomy and pathology of the head and neck region.

BRUCE M. WENIG, M.D.

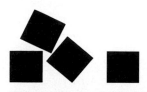

ACKNOWLEDGEMENTS

This book could not have been completed without the assistance and support of numerous individuals. First and foremost, I thank my brother, Barry L. Wenig, M.D., for his encouragement, expertise, and willingness to contribute the majority of the clinical illustrations utilized in this book (not to mention for our shared passion for sports, especially for the New York Football Giants).

Thanks also to my sister, Hally Frist, for her example of honesty, humility, and dedication in all aspects of life; to Drs. Jerome Kleinerman, Stephen A. Geller, and Mamuro Kaneko, who represent examples of physicians of unparalleled integrity and dedication, and who taught me to appreciate all aspects of pathology; to Drs. Dennis K. Heffner and Vincent J. Hyams, for their innumerable contributions and suggestions for this book but above all for teaching me the pathology of the head and neck; to Dr. James G. Smirniotopolous, for his friendship and camaraderie, as well as for his encouragement and assistance in this endeavor; to Drs. Franz J. Wippold, II, and Mahmood F. Mafee, for contributing most of the radiographs illustrated in this book; to Drs. Paul L. Auclair, Gary L. Ellis, John F. Fetsch, Clara S. Heffess, Theresa T. Holland, Silloo B. Kapadia, Harvey P. Kessler, Aileen M. Marty, Elizabeth A. Montgomery, and Ronald C. Neafie, in various departments at the Armed Forces Institute of Pathology (AFIP), for their willingness to contribute slides utilized for photomicrography; to the photographic staff at the AFIP, particularly Mr. George L. Jones (even if he is a Redskins' fan) and Zan Arnold, for their efforts to meet my needs and the quality of the photomicrographs in this book; and to the editorial staff of the W.B. Saunders Company, particularly Joan Meyer, Jennifer Mitchell, Linda Mills, Tina Rebane, Peter Faber, and Carolyn Naylor, for their assistance and professionalism.

BRUCE M. WENIG, M.D.

CONTENTS

Section 3
LARYNX AND HYPOPHARYNX

Section 4
MAJOR AND MINOR SALIVARY GLANDS

Section 5

EXTERNAL, MIDDLE, AND INTERNAL EAR

APPENDICES

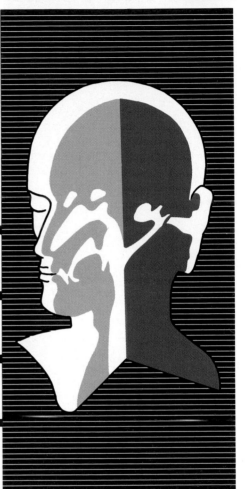

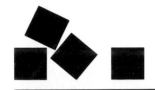

NASAL CAVITY

AND

PARANASAL

SINUSES

CHAPTER 1

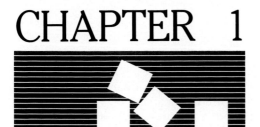

Anatomy and Histology

NASAL CAVITY

Anatomic Borders

■ The nasal cavity is divided into right and left halves by the septum; each half opens on the face via the nares or nostrils and communicates posteriorly with the nasopharynx through the posterior nasal apertures or the choanae.

■ Each half of the nasal cavity has the following borders (walls):
Superior (roof)—slopes downward in front and back, and is horizontal in its middle.
Frontal and nasal bones form the anterior sloping part.
The cribriform plate of the ethmoid bone forms the horizontal part and separates the nasal cavity from the anterior cranial fossa (medial part of floor); this area represents the deepest part of the cavity.
The body of the sphenoid bone forms the posterior sloping part.

■ Inferior (floor)—majority (75%) is formed by the palatine processes of the maxillary bone, thereby intervening between the oral and nasal cavities; the remainder is formed by the horizontal process of the palatine bone.

■ Lateral—formed in the most part by the nasal surface of the maxilla below and in front, posteriorly by the perpendicular plate of the palatine bone, and above by the nasal surface of the ethmoidal labyrinthe, separating the nasal cavity from the orbit.
Along the lateral wall of each nasal cavity, three horizontal bony projections are identified: the superior, middle, and inferior conchae. Occasionally, a small fourth concha is identified

above the superior concha and is called the supreme concha.

■ The air spaces or meatuses (superior, middle, and inferior) lie beneath and lateral to the conchae and are named according to the concha immediately above it.

■ Medial—formed by the bony nasal septum, entirely formed by the vomer and the perpendicular plate of the ethmoid; the anterior portion of the nasal septum represents the septal cartilage.

Histology

■ The nasal vestibule is a cutaneous structure, composed of keratinizing squamous epithelium and underlying subcutaneous tissue with cutaneous adnexal structures (hair follicles, sebaceous glands, and sweat glands).

■ The mucocutaneous junction (limen nasi) is approximately 1 to 2 cm posterior from the nares and represents the point at which the epithelial surface changes from keratinizing squamous epithelium to a ciliated pseudostratified columnar (respiratory) epithelium; the latter lines the entire nasal cavity.

■ The submucosa underlying the epithelium is thin, adherent to the periosteum and perichondrium, and noteworthy for the presence of seromucous (minor salivary) glands and a distinct vascular component, which consists of large, thick-walled blood vessels, referred to as erectile tissue. These vascular structures are particularly prominent along the inferior and middle turbinate and may be mistaken for a hemangioma.

■ The olfactory epithelium consists of:
Bipolar, spindle-shaped olfactory neural (receptor)

cells, composed of myelinated axons that penetrate the basal lamina to protrude from the mucosal surface, and nonmyelinated proximal processes, which traverse the cribriform plate.

Columnar sustentacular or supporting cells.

Rounded basal cells.

Olfactory or Bowman glands in the lamina propria, representing purely serous-type glands.

■ Nasal cartilage is of the hyaline type and has a bluish, translucent, homogenous appearance.

PARANASAL SINUSES

Anatomic Borders

Maxillary Sinuses

■ Largest of the paranasal sinuses and located in the body of the maxilla; from above, the maxillary sinus has a triangular shape, with the base formed by the lateral wall of the nasal cavity and the apex projecting into the zygomatic arch.

Superior (roof)—orbital surface of the maxilla (floor of the orbit).

Inferior (floor)—alveolar and palatine process of the maxilla.

Anterolateral—facial surface of the maxilla.

Posterior—infratemporal surface of the maxilla.

Medial—lateral wall of the nasal cavity.

■ The maxillary ostium (hiatus semilunaris) is on the highest part of the medial wall of the sinus; it does not open directly into the nasal cavity, but into the posterior ethmoid infundibulum (uncinate groove), which opens into the middle meatus of the nasal cavity.

Ethmoid Sinuses

■ Consist of thin-walled cavities in the ethmoidal labyrinth, completed by the frontal, maxillary, lacrimal, sphenoidal, and palatine bones; these cavities vary in size and number, usually consisting of two to eight anterior and middle ethmoid cells and two to eight posterior ethmoid cells.

■ Based on the relation to the ethmoid infundibulum, the ethmoid cells are grouped into:

Anterior group—ostia open directly in relation to the ethmoid infundibulum.

Middle or bullous group—ostia open on or above the ethmoid infundibulum.

Posterior group—ostia open into the superior meatus.

Frontal Sinuses

■ Roughly pyramid-shaped and located in the vertical part of the frontal bone; these sinuses are frequently asymmetric in size and often contain septa, subdividing the cavity.

■ The ostia of the frontal sinus opens into the anterior part of the middle meatus.

■ Important anatomic relations include proximity to the anterior cranial fossa and orbit separated only by a thin plate of bone from these structures.

Sphenoid Sinuses

■ Contained within the sphenoid bone situated posterior to the upper part of the nasal cavity.

■ Related above to the optic chiasm and the hypophysis cerebri.

■ Related on each side to the internal carotid artery and cavernous sinus.

■ Open into the sphenoethmoidal recess lying above and behind the superior nasal concha.

Histology

■ All of the sinuses are lined by ciliated, pseudostratified, columnar epithelium, and together with the nasal cavity, are called the schneiderian membrane; this epithelium is ectodermally derived, in contrast with the similar-appearing epithelium lining the nasopharynx, which is of endodermal derivation.

■ Although the epithelia are the same, the mucous membranes of the paranasal sinuses are thinner and less vascular than those of the nasal cavity and have a fibrous layer adjacent to the periosteum.

■ Seromucous glands are scattered throughout the paranasal sinus submucosae and particularly are seen in the ostial areas.

References

Embryology, Anatomy, and Histology

Fawcett DW: The nose and paranasal sinuses. *In*: Fawcett DW, ed. Bloom and Fawcett: a textbook of histology, 11th ed. Philadelphia: W.B. Saunders Co., 1986; pp 731–734.

Hollinshead WH: The nose and paranasal sinuses. *In*: Hollinshead WH, ed. Anatomy for surgeons, vol. 1, 3rd ed. Philadelphia: Harper & Row, 1982; pp 223–267.

Moore KL: The branchial apparatus and the head and neck. *In*: Moore ML, ed. The developing human: clinically oriented embryology, 4th ed. Philadelphia: W.B. Saunders Co., 1988; pp 170–206.

Moore KL: The respiratory system. *In*: Moore ML, ed. The developing human: clinically oriented embryology, 4th ed. Philadelphia: W.B. Saunders Co., 1988; pp 207–216.

Warwick R, Williams PL: The nasal cavity. *In*: Warwick R, Williams PL, eds. Gray's anatomy, 35th British ed. Philadelphia: W.B. Saunders Co., 1973; pp 279–280.

Warwick R, Williams PL: The olfactory apparatus. *In*: Warwick R, Williams PL, eds. Gray's anatomy, 35th British ed. Philadelphia: W.B. Saunders Co., 1973; pp 1086–1095.

CHAPTER 2

CLASSIFICATION OF NON-NEOPLASTIC LESIONS AND NEOPLASMS OF THE NASAL CAVITY AND PARANASAL SINUSES

CLASSIFICATION OF NASAL CAVITY AND PARANASAL SINUS NON-NEOPLASTIC LESIONS

Table 2-1
CLASSIFICATION OF NASAL CAVITY
AND PARANASAL SINUS
NON-NEOPLASTIC LESIONS

Nasal (inflammatory) polyps
Antrochoanal polyp
Cysts
Mucocele
Heterotopic central nervous system tissue and encephalocele
Hamartomas
Infectious diseases
   Allergic fungal sinusitis (inspissated mucus)
   Rhinoscleroma
   Rhinosporidiosis
   Tuberculosis
   Sarcoidosis
   Syphilis
   Leprosy
   Leishmaniasis
   Others
Myospherulosis
Extranodal sinus histiocytosis with massive lymphadenopathy
Wegener's granulomatosis
Fibro-osseous lesions (fibrous dysplasia)
Others

CLASSIFICATION OF NASAL CAVITY AND PARANASAL SINUS NEOPLASMS

Table 2-2
CLASSIFICATION OF NASAL CAVITY
AND PARANASAL SINUS NEOPLASMS

Benign
1. Epithelial
   Schneiderian papillomas
   Squamous papilloma (nasal vestibule)
2. Mesenchymal
   Lobular capillary hemangioma (pyogenic granuloma)
   Hemangiopericytoma
   Peripheral nerve sheath tumors
   Fibrous histiocytoma
   Fibromatosis (tumefactive fibroinflammatory lesion)
   Osteoma
   Fibro-osseous lesions (ossifying fibroma, juvenile active ossifying fibroma)
   Leiomyoma
   Myxoma/fibromyxoma/chondromyxoid fibroma
   Ameloblastoma
   Others
Malignant
1. Epithelial
   Squamous cell carcinoma
   Respiratory carcinoma
   Adenocarcinoma (mucosal)
   Minor salivary gland neoplasms
2. Mesenchymal/Neuroectodermal
   Malignant melanoma
   Olfactory (esthesio)neuroblastoma
   Midline malignant reticulosis
   Malignant fibrous histiocytoma
   Fibrosarcoma
   Malignant schwannoma
   Leiomyosarcoma
   Angiosarcoma
   Osteosarcoma
   Chondrosarcoma
   Teratocarcinosarcoma
   Others

CHAPTER 3

NON-NEOPLASTIC LESIONS OF THE NASAL CAVITY AND PARANASAL SINUSES

1. SINONASAL INFLAMMATORY POLYPS

Definition: Non-neoplastic inflammatory swellings of the sinonasal mucosa.

Clinical

- No sex predilection; occurs in all ages but commonly seen in adults over 20 years of age and rarely seen in children less than 5 years of age.
- Most arise from the lateral nasal wall or from the ethmoid recess.
- May be unilateral or bilateral, single or multiple.
- Symptoms vary and include nasal obstruction, rhinorrhea, and headaches.
- Etiology linked to multiple factors, including allergy, cystic fibrosis, infections, diabetes mellitus, aspirin intolerance.

Radiology

- Soft tissue densities, air–fluid levels, mucosal thickening, and opacification of the paranasal sinuses.
- When extensive, inflammatory polyps may expand and even destroy bone.

Pathology

Gross

- Soft, fleshy, polypoid, myxoid/mucoid, translucent gray to pink mass.
- Variation in size, ranging up to several centimeters in diameter.

Histology

- The surface epithelium is intact, composed of a respiratory epithelium, and often demonstrating squamous metaplasia; the basement membrane may be thickened.
- The stroma is markedly edematous with a myxomatous appearance and contains variable numbers of fibroblasts.
- Associated inflammatory infiltrate is predominantly composed of eosinophils, plasma cells, and lymphocytes; neutrophils may predominate in polyps of infectious origin.
- The vascularity varies but is a readily identifiable component.
- Absence of seromucous glands.
- Secondary changes seen in association with sinona-

sal polyps may include surface ulceration, fibrosis, infarction, granulation tissue, deposition of an amyloid-like stroma, osseous or cartilaginous metaplasia, glandular hyperplasia, granuloma formation, and stromal atypical cells.

■ Stromal atypical cells can be pleomorphic with hyperchromatic nuclei, but lack mitoses or cross striations; immunoreactivity may demonstrate actin, suggesting a myofibroblastic derivation.

Differential Diagnosis

■ Infectious diseases (tuberculosis, sarcoid) (Chapter 8, #7b,e).
■ Amyloidosis (Chapter 13, #4).
■ Nasopharyngeal angiofibroma (Chapter 9A, #2).
■ Wegener's granulomatosis (Chapter 3, #8).
■ Squamous epithelial lesions (dysplasia, carcinoma in situ) (Chapter 13, #6; Chapter 14, #1).
■ Rhabdomyosarcoma (Chapter 9B, #5).
■ Malignant fibrous histiocytoma (Chapter 4B, #6).

Treatment and Prognosis

■ Surgical excision.
■ Identification and treatment of etiologic factors.

Additional Facts

■ Stromal atypical cells may present diagnostic difficulties and may be misdiagnosed as a rhabdomyosarcoma.
■ Granulomas result from ruptured mucous cysts and cholesterol granulomas, and as a reaction to medicinal intranasal injections (steroids) or inhalants.

References

Barnes L: Nasal polyps. *In*: Barnes L, ed. Surgical pathology of the head and neck. New York: Marcel Dekker, 1985; pp 403–408.

Compagno J, Hyams VJ, Lepore ML: Nasal polyposis with stromal atypia: review and follow-up of 14 cases. Arch Pathol Lab Med 100:224–226, 1976.

Hyams VJ, Batsakis JG, Michaels L: Nasal and paranasal polyposis. *In*: Hyams VJ, Batsakis JG, Michaels L, ed. Tumors of the upper respiratory tract and ear. Fascicle 25, second series. Washington, DC: Armed Forces Institute of Pathology, 1988; pp 11–13.

Kindblom LG, Angervall L: Nasal polyps with atypical stromal cells: a pseudosarcomatous lesion. A light and electron microscopic and immunohistochemical investigation with implications on the type and nature of the mesenchymal cells. Acta Pathol Microbiol Immunol Scand [A] 92:65–72, 1984.

Maloney JR: Nasal polyps, nasal polypectomy, asthma and aspirin sensitivity: their association in 445 cases of nasal polyps. J Laryngol Otol 91:837–846, 1977.

Myers D, Myers EN: The medical and surgical treatment of nasal polyps. Laryngoscope 84:833–847, 1974.

Winestock DP, Bartlett PC, Sondheimer FK: Benign nasal polyps causing bone destruction in the nasal cavity and paranasal sinuses. Laryngoscope 88:675–679, 1978.

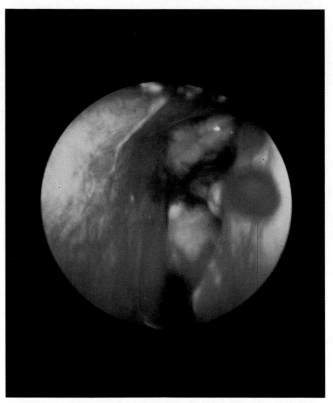

Figure 3–1. Endoscopic appearance of sinonasal inflammatory polyps, consisting of multiple polypoid masses with a glistening mucoid appearance.

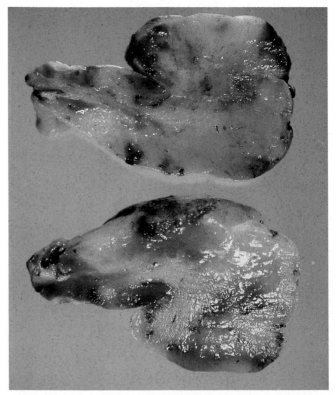

Figure 3–2. Transected sinonasal inflammatory polyp showing tan-white, polypoid-shaped tissue with a shiny, myxoid/mucoid appearance.

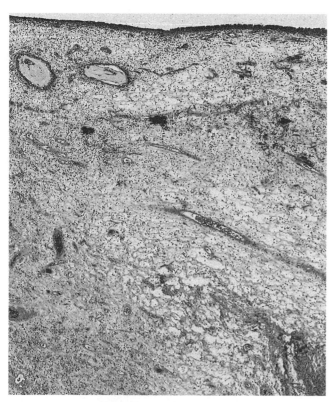

Figure 3-3. The histologic appearance of sinonasal polyps consists of an overlying intact respiratory epithelium with the underlying stroma characterized by edema, admixed inflammatory cell infiltrate, and variable vascularity; seromucous glands are typically absent.

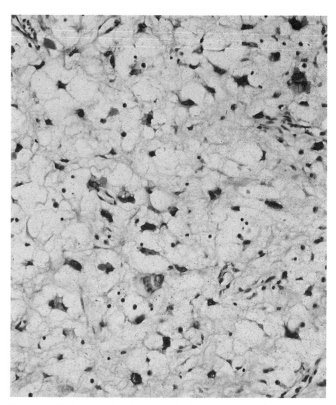

Figure 3-5. An associated finding in inflammatory polyps may be the presence of stromal atypical cells, which can be pleomorphic with hyperchromatic nuclei, thereby suggesting the presence of a malignant cellular infiltrate; these cells typically lack mitoses or the presence of cross striations.

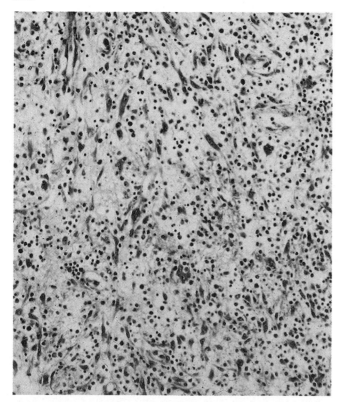

Figure 3-4. Mixed inflammatory cell infiltrate composed of eosinophils, plasma cells, and lymphocytes set in an edematous or myxoid background, which contains variable numbers of fibroblasts.

2. ANTROCHOANAL POLYP

Definition: Sinonasal inflammatory polyp, specifically arising from the maxillary sinus antrum.

Clinical

■ Represents approximately 3% to 6% of all sinonasal polyps.

■ Affects males more than females; occurs primarily in teenagers and young adults.

■ Generally presents as a single, unilateral polyp with nasal obstruction; however, extension from the maxillary sinus posteriorly to the nasopharynx may result in obstruction of the nasopharynx and clinical suspicion of a primary nasopharyngeal tumor.

■ Often associated with bilateral maxillary sinusitis and, despite correlation in up to 40% of cases of associated allergies, the antrochoanal polyp is believed to be of an inflammatory etiology.

■ May be associated with conventional sinonasal polyp.

Radiology

■ Soft-tissue density in the posterior choanal region or in the nasopharynx, with clouding or opacification of the maxillary sinus.

Pathology

Gross

■ Identical to other nasal polyps, except for the presence of a stalk with attachment to the maxillary sinus.

Histology

■ Similar to sinonasal polyps, except for a relative lack of mucous glands and an eosinophilic inflammatory infiltrate.

■ Similar to sinonasal polyps, reactive atypical stromal cells may be seen.

Differential Diagnosis

■ Nasopharyngeal angiofibroma (Chapter 9A, #2).

Treatment and Prognosis

■ Cured following complete surgical excision.

■ May recur if the polyp, including the stalk, is incompletely excised.

References

Hardy G: The choanal polyp. Ann Otol Rhinol Laryngol 66:306–326, 1957.

Heck WE, Hallberg O, Williams HL: Antrochoanal polyp. Arch Otolaryngol Head Neck Surg 52:538–548, 1950.

Sinha SN, Kumar A: Bilateral antrochoanal polyps. Ear Nose Throat J 59:63–64, 1980.

Sirola R: Choanal polyps. Acta Otolaryngol (Stockh) 61:42–48, 1966.

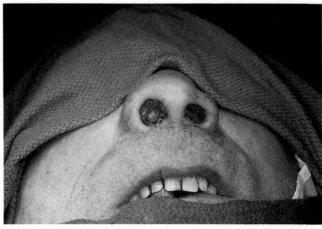

Figure 3–6. Antrochoanal polyp, appearing as polypoid, tan-pink mass filling the right nasal cavity. This polyp is clinically indistinguishable from other sinonasal inflammatory polyps.

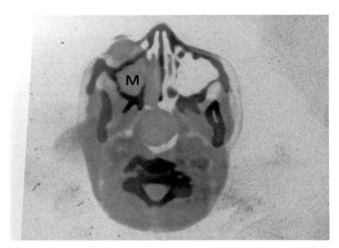

Figure 3–7. Axial CT section demonstrates a soft tissue mass (M; antrochoanal polyp) extending through an enlarged ostium of the right maxillary sinus and filling and extending into the nasal cavity and nasopharynx.

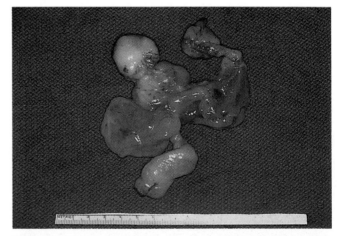

Figure 3–8. Resected antrochoanal polyps similar to other sinonasal inflammatory polyps, but characterized by the presence of a pedicle that is generally absent from nonchoanal-derived sinonasal inflammatory polyps.

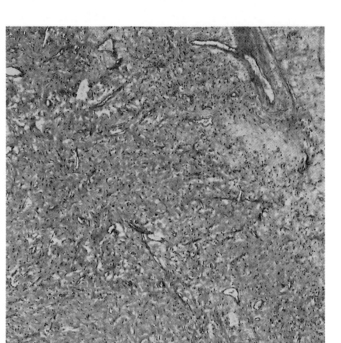

Figure 3–9. Histology of antrochoanal polyps consisting of an edematous and fibrous stroma associated with a predominantly lymphocytic cell infiltrate; the presence of fibroblasts and narrow vascular channels may simulate a nasopharyngeal angiofibroma, but the latter typically lacks an inflammatory cell infiltrate.

3. PARANASAL SINUS MUCOCELE

Definition: Chronic, cystic lesion of the paranasal sinuses, lined by a respiratory epithelium, and which occurs as a result of obstruction of the draining ostia.

Clinical

- No sex predilection; may occur in all age groups.
- Occurs most commonly in the frontal and ethmoid sinuses (>90%); the maxillary sinus may be involved but is uncommon (5% to 10%); sphenoid sinus involvement occurs but is considered rare.
- Symptoms depend on the site of involvement, as well as the direction and extent of expansion, and include pain, facial swelling or deformity, proptosis, enophthalmos, diplopia, rhinorrhea, nasal obstruction.
- Two types:
  Internal: herniation of the cyst into subucosal tissue adjacent to the bony wall of the sinus.
  External: herniation of the cyst through the bony wall of the sinus, with extension into subcutaneous tissue or into the cranial cavity.
- Expansion of a mucocele is in the direction of least resistance.

- Irrespective of the sinus involved, the pathogenesis of mucoceles is thought to occur as a result of an increase in pressure within a given sinus secondary to blockage of the sinus outlet (ostium), most often the result of an inflammatory or allergic process; additional factors implicated in the development of a mucocele include trauma, postsurgical state, or a neoplasm.
- The clinical picture may be mistaken for a neoplasm.

Radiology

- Opacification of the involved sinus; with time, there is increase in pressure, resulting in:
  Erosion or destruction of the sinus walls, with loss of the typical scalloped outline along the mucoperiosteum.
  Abnormal radiolucency due to loss of bone.
  Sclerosis of adjacent bone.

Pathology

Gross

- Cysts filled with thick mucoid or gelatinous secretions.

- Contents are sterile.
- Cases complicated by infection (pyocele) are filled with a purulent exudate.

Histology

- Cysts lined by a flattened, pseudostratified, ciliated columnar epithelium.
- Reactive bone formation lying in proximity to the cyst epithelium.
- In long-standing cases, the cyst epithelium may demonstrate squamous metaplasia.
- Additional reactive changes may include fibrosis, granulation tissue, hemorrhage, and cholesterol granuloma.

Differential Diagnosis

- Mucous retention cyst (Chapter 8, #3).

Treatment and Prognosis

- Prognosis is excellent after complete surgical excision.
- Complications include:
  Superimposed infection (pyocele).
  Meningitis.
  Brain abscess.

Additional Facts

- The diagnosis of a paranasal sinus mucocele is a correlation between clinical, radiographic, and pathologic findings; diagnosis of a paranasal sinus mucocele by histopathology alone may be extremely difficult, given the nonspecific histologic features, with the lining of (paranasal sinus) mucoceles being the same as that of the normal paranasal sinus or the lining associated with nonspecific sinusitis.

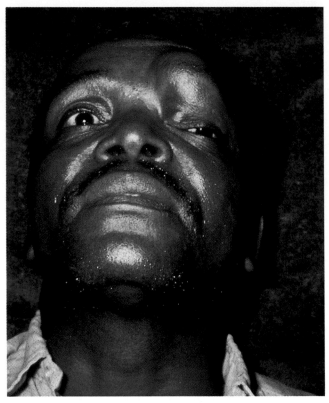

Figure 3–10. Supraorbital swelling and enophthalmos caused by a large mucocele.

References

Close LG, O'Conner WE: Sphenoethmoidal mucoceles with intracranial extension. Otolaryngol Head Neck Surg 91:350–357, 1983.

Evans C: Aetiology and treatment of fronto-ethmoidal mucocele. J Laryngol Otol 95:361–375, 1981.

Hall RE, Delbalso AM, Carter LC: Mucoceles. *In*: Delbalso AM, ed. Maxillofacial imaging. Philadelphia: W.B. Saunders Co.; 1990; pp 172–177.

van Nostrand AWP, Goodman WS: Pathologic aspects of mucosal lesions of the maxillary sinus. Otolaryngol Clin North Am 9:35–42, 1976.

Weber AL: Inflammatory diseases of the paranasal sinuses and mucoceles. Otolaryngol Clin North Am 21:421–437, 1988.

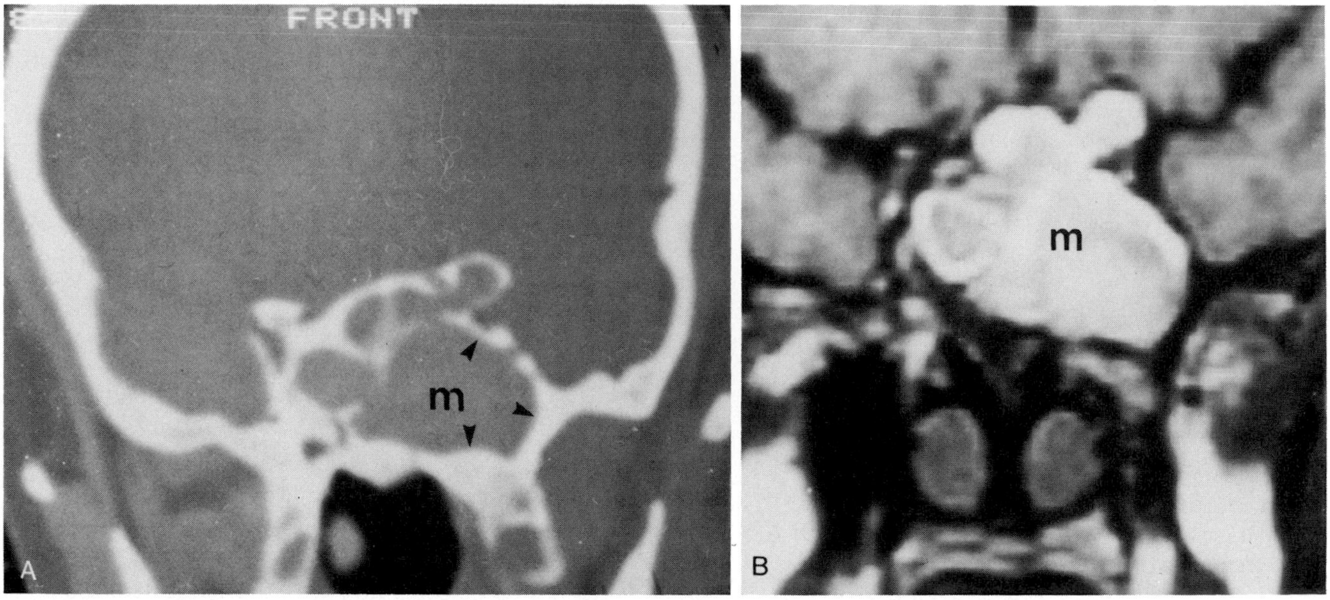

Figure 3–11. (*A*) Coronal CT bone windows of a sphenoid sinus mucocele with the mass (m) expanding the sinus (*arrowheads*). (*B*) Corresponding coronal T1-weighted MR image demonstrating the mass (m) within the sphenoid sinus. The high signal is caused by the protein content of the mucocele; the MR appearance of mucoceles can be variable, reflecting the composition of the contents. (Courtesy of Franz J. Wippold II, M.D., Mallinckrodt Institute of Radiology, St. Louis, MO.)

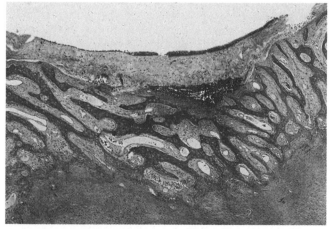

Figure 3–12. Internal mucocele with herniation of the cyst, lined by a respiratory epithelium, into submucosal tissue adjacent to the bony wall of the sinus.

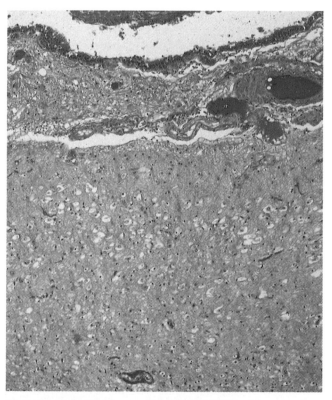

Figure 3–13. External mucocele with herniation of the cyst, lined by a respiratory epithelium (*top*), through the bony wall of the sinus with extension into the cranial cavity as seen by the presence of central nervous system tissue (*lower half*).

4. HETEROTOPIC CENTRAL NERVOUS SYSTEM TISSUE

Definition: Congenital non-neoplastic displacement of neuroglial tissue in extracranial sites, without connection to the cranial cavity.

Synonyms: Glioma; glial heterotopia.

Clinical

■ No sex predilection; generally presents at birth or within the first few years of life, but may affect any age group.

■ Most commonly occurs in and around the nasal cavity; other sites of involvement include the ethmoid sinus, palate, middle ear, tonsil, and pharyngeal area.

■ No evidence of familial predisposition.

■ Extranasal lesions:
Most common, making up approximately 60% of cases.
Present as a subcutaneous blue or red mass along the bridge of the nose.

■ Intranasal lesions:
Represent approximately 30% of cases.
Present with obstruction or septal deviation.
Clinically confused with nasal polyps.
Nasal attachment occurs high within the nasal vault, along the lateral wall of the nasal fossa or middle turbinate.

■ Mixed extra- and intranasal lesions.
Represent approximately 10% of cases.
Communication occurs through a defect in the nasal bone.

■ Negative Furstenberg test (swelling or pulsating lesion following pressure on the ipsilateral jugular vein—typically positive in an encephalocele).

Radiology

■ Radiographic studies are indicated in order to rule out a bony defect that may identify communication to the cranial cavity (encephalocele).

Pathology

Gross

■ Firm, smooth mass measuring from 1 to 3 cm in diameter.

■ Rarely described or recognized as brain tissue.

Histology

■ Composed of astrocytes and neuroglial fibers asso-ciated with a fibrous, vascularized connective tissue.

■ May identify multinucleated or gemistocytic astrocytes.

■ Neurons are sparse.

■ In long-standing clinically undetected cases, a fibrous stroma may predominate and obscure the astrocytes and neuroglial fibers.

■ Immunohistochemistry: glial fibrillary acidic protein (GFAP) and S-100 protein positive.

Differential Diagnosis

■ Encephalocele (congenital or acquired).
■ Nasal polyps (Chapter 3, #1).
■ Teratoma (Chapter 8, #2).

Treatment and Prognosis

■ Surgery is the treatment of choice and results in the cure of the patient.

■ Ten percent recurrence or persistence rate after incomplete excision.

Additional Facts

■ Glial heterotopias are generally considered to represent a variant of encephalocele in which the communication to the central nervous system has closed, remains undetected, or has become fibrotic.

■ The glial heterotopias are non-neoplastic, and therefore the term glioma is a misnomer.

■ Prior to biopsy of a lesion in the superior portion of the nasal cavity or base of the nose, detailed clinical and radiographic evaluation of possible continuity with the central nervous system (CNS) is indicated; CNS involvement may be clinically apparent by evidence of meningitis, cerebrospinal fluid rhinorrhea, and anosmia.

■ Communication with the CNS necessitates craniotomy, followed by surgical removal of the mass.

References

Karma P, Räsänen O, Kärjä J: Nasal gliomas: a review and report of two cases. Laryngoscope 87:1169–1179, 1977.

Pashley NRT: Nasal glioma and encephalocele. *In:* Cummings CW, Frederickson JM, Harker LA, Krause CJ, Schuller DE, eds. Otolaryngology—head and neck surgery. St. Louis: C.V. Mosby Co.; 1986; pp 578–582.

Strauss RB, Collicott JH, Hargett IR: Intranasal neuroglial heterotopia: so-called nasal glioma. Am J Dis Child 111:317–320, 1966.

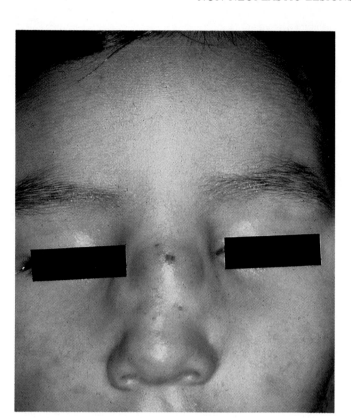

Figure 3–14. Extranasal heterotopic central nervous system tissue manifesting as a subcutaneous mass along the bridge of the nose.

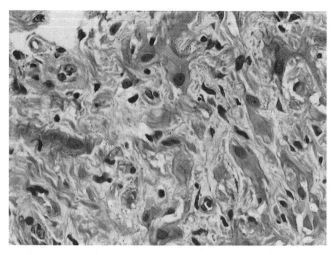

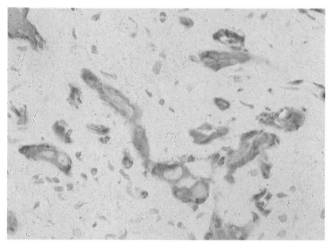

Figure 3–16. (*Top*) Irregularly shaped neuroglial cells composed of round to oval nuclei, eosinophilic nucleoli, and abundant granular-appearing cytoplasm. (*Bottom*) Confirmation of neuroglial origin can be seen by the presence of glial fibrillary acidic protein (GFAP) immunoreactivity.

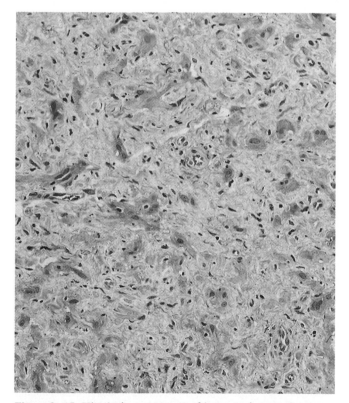

Figure 3–15. Histologic appearance of heterotopic central nervous system tissue composed of astrocytes and neuroglial fibers, which are associated with a fibrous and vascularized connective tissue.

5. INFECTIOUS-RELATED DISEASES OF THE NASAL AND PARANASAL SINUSES

a. Allergic Fungal Sinusitis

Definition: Noninvasive benign collection of impacted mucus and cellular debris.

Synonyms: Inspissated mucus; allergic sinonasal aspergillosis; snotoma.

Clinical

■ No sex predilection; may occur in all ages but is most commonly seen in children or young adults.

■ Primarily involves the maxillary and ethmoid sinuses but may involve any sinus.

■ Clinical presentation includes headaches and airway obstruction.

■ Related to history of chronic sinusitis and thought to be an allergic response to fungi.

■ Fungi implicated in the pathogenesis include *Aspergillus* (represents the most frequent organism seen), and dematiaceous fungi—Culvularia, Dreshella, Bipolaris and Exserohilum species.

Radiology

■ Sinus opacity.

■ On rare occasions, may be associated with bone destruction.

Pathology

Gross

■ Rubbery to firm, translucent mass.

■ Can attain large size, completely filling a sinus.

Histology

■ Amorphous collection of homogenous, chondroid-like material associated with a prominent acute and chronic inflammatory cell infiltrate; the inflammatory component is most often composed of eosinophils and neutrophils, and scattered plasma cells, lymphocytes, and histiocytes may also be seen.

■ Charcot-Leyden crystals may be seen among the eosinophilic infiltrate.

■ Desquamated respiratory cells can be identified within this amorphous material.

■ Histochemistry: scattered fungal hyphae may be seen by Gomori methenamine silver (GMS) stain; chondroid-like material is mucin positive.

Differential Diagnosis

■ Fungus ball or invasive fungal sinusitis (see below).

■ Benign mixed tumor (Chapter 19, #1).

■ Rhabdomyosarcoma (Chapter 9B, #5).

Treatment and Prognosis

■ Surgical evacuation of involved sinus.

■ Antifungal agents are not used unless there is invasion into the tissue.

Additional Facts

■ Similar pathogenesis to allergic bronchopulmonary aspergillosis.

■ Given the specific histopathologic findings, a diagnosis of allergic fungal sinusitis can be made even in the absence of fungal identification by special stains; fungal cultures are an important diagnostic tool in the identification of a fungal organism.

■ The histologic picture is the same, irrespective of the fungal organism involved.

■ *Invasive fungal sinusitis* results in destruction of the involved sinus within days, is often identified in immunocompromised patients, and requires surgical intervention with antifungal chemotherapy.

References

Friedman GC, Hartwick WJ, Ro JY, Saleh GY, Tarrand JT, Ayala AG: Allergic fungal sinusitis: report of three cases associated with dematiaceous fungi. Am J Clin Pathol 96:368–372, 1991.

Hartwick RW, Batsakis JG: Sinus aspergillosis and allergic fungal sinusitis. Ann Otol Rhinol Laryngol 100:427–430, 1991.

Katzenstein ALA, Sale SR, Greenberger PA: Pathologic findings in allergic aspergillus sinusitis: a newly recognized form of sinusitis. Am J Surg Pathol 7:439–443, 1983.

Macmillan RH, Cooper PH, Body BA, Mills AS: Allergic fungal sinusitis due to curvularia lunata. Hum Pathol 18:960–964, 1987.

Morgan MA, Wilson WR, Neel HB, Roberts GD: Fungal sinusitis in healthy and immunocompromis.d individuals. Am J Clin Pathol 82:597601, 1984.

Rinaldi MG, Phillips P, Schwartz JG, et al: Human curvularia infections: report of five cases and review of the literature. Diagn Microbiol Infect Dis 6:27–39, 1987.

Zieske LA, Kopke RD, Hamill R: Dematiaceous fungal sinusitis. Otolaryngol Head Neck Surg 105:567–577, 1991.

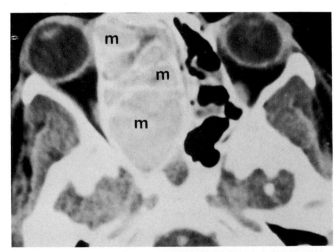

Figure 3–17. Axial CT demonstrating a polypoid ethmoid sinus mucocele with superimposed inspissated mucus. The polypoid dense soft tissue masses (m) expand the right ethmoid sinus air cells; the increased attenuation can be attributed to the mineral content of the mycocetoma. (Courtesy of Franz J. Wippold II, M.D., Mallinckrodt Institute of Radiology, St. Louis, MO.)

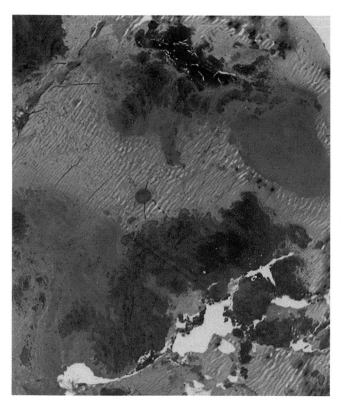

Figure 3–18. Inspissated mucus composed of amorphous collection of eosinophilic material associated with nests of inflammatory cells.

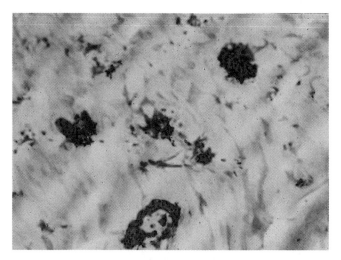

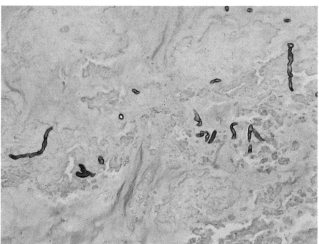

Figure 3–20. (*Top*) Eosinophilic cell infiltrate set within a chondroid-like stroma and associated with crystal-like material (Charcot-Leyden crystals); (*Bottom*) Fungal organisms characteristic of *Aspergillus* species, with septated hyphae and acute angle branching (GMS stain).

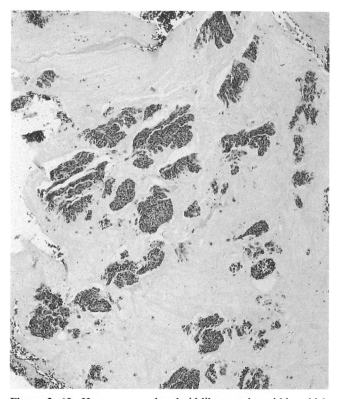

Figure 3–19. Homogenous chondroid-like matrix, within which the inflammatory cells nests (predominantly eosinophils) are seen.

b. Rhinoscleroma

Definition: Chronic granulomatous infectious disease, primarily occurring in the upper respiratory tract (nasal cavity and nasopharynx) and caused by *Klebsiella rhinoscleromatis,* a gram-negative bacterium.

Clinical

- Sex predisposition is equal; occurs in young age groups during the first three decades of life.
- Disease of lower socioeconomic class, in which poor living conditions and malnutrition foster the growth and spread of disease.
- Endemic in Egypt, parts of Central and South America, North and Central Africa, and Eastern Europe.
- Occurs but considered uncommon in the United States.
- Infection manifests initially in the nasal cavity (nasal septum) and spreads posteriorly to the nasopharynx; other sites of involvement include the paranasal sinuses, orbit, larynx, tracheobronchial tree, and middle ear.
- Three clinical phases:
  1. Rhinitic—characterized by mucopurulent nasal discharge.
  2. Florid—marked by mucosal thickening, which may result in nasal obstruction; diagnosis is usually made in this phase.
  3. Fibrotic—represents resolution of disease.

Pathology

Gross

- Typically, in the florid phase the infected mucosa is pale in appearance and demonstrates diffuse nodular thickening.

Histology

- Characteristic lesion seen in the florid phase con-

sists of a submucosal granulomatous infiltrate composed of macrophages with clear to foamy cytoplasm (Mikulicz cells) intimately associated with an admixture of lymphocytes and plasma cells.
- Overlying epithelium may demonstrate a pseudo-epitheliomatous hyperplasia; rarely, ulceration is seen.
- Macrophages harbor the bacteria, which are best seen by silver stain (Warthin-Starry stain); tissue Gram stain also reveals the organisms.
- Characteristic Mikulicz cells may be difficult to identify in the fibrotic phase.

Differential Diagnosis

- Syphilis (Chapter 8, #7f).
- Extranodal sinus histiocytosis with massive lymphadenopathy (Chapter 3, #7).

Treatment and Prognosis

- Treatment of choice is with tetracycline; surgical resection may be necessary where airway obstruction is life threatening.
- CO_2 laser surgery may represent an alternative means of therapy.
- Prognosis is good after initiation of antibiotic therapy.

References

Goldman SN, Canalis RF: Rhinoscleroma as a cause of airway obstruction. Ear Nose Throat J 59:6–14, 1980.

Hyams VJ, Batsakis JG, Michaels L: Rhinoscleroma. *In*: Hyams VJ, Batsakis JG, Michaels L, eds. Tumors of the upper respiratory tract and ear. Fascicle 25, second series. Washington DC: Armed Forces Institute of Pathology, 1988; pp 24–26.

Maher AI, El-Kashlan HK, Soliman Y, Galal R: Rhinoscleroma: management by carbon dioxide laser therapy. Laryngoscope 100:783–788, 1990.

Myerowitz RL: Rhinoscleroma. *In*: Barnes L, ed. Surgical pathology of the head and neck. New York: Marcel Dekker, 1985; pp 1778–1780.

Stiernberg CM, Clark WD: Rhinoscleroma—a diagnostic challenge. Laryngoscope 93:866–870, 1983.

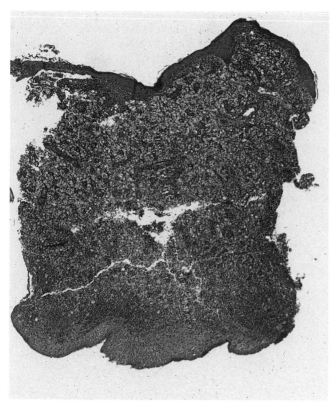

Figure 3–21. Sinonasal rhinoscleroma showing a diffuse submucosal infiltrate that replaces seromucous glands; the overlying epithelium demonstrates squamous metaplasia.

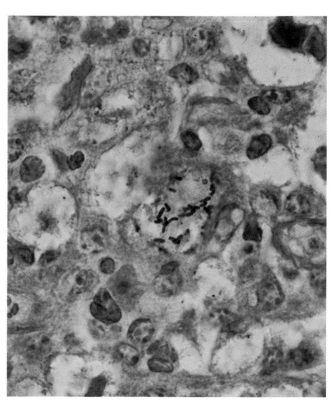

Figure 3–23. Warthin-Starry silver stain demonstrates the presence of the *Klebsiella rhinoscleromatis,* gram-negative bacteria, within the macrophages.

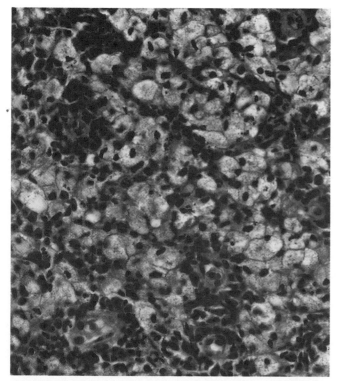

Figure 3–22. Cellular infiltrate seen in association with rhinoscleroma is mixed, including lymphocytes, plasma cells, scattered eosinophils, and neutrophils; the predominant cell type is macrophages with clear to foamy cytoplasm (Mikulicz cells).

c. Rhinosporidiosis

Definition: Chronic infectious disease of the upper respiratory tract (nose and nasopharynx), characterized by formation of polypoid masses and caused by the fungus *Rhinosporidium seeberi.*

Clinical

- Affects males more than females, affects all ages, but most common in the third and fourth decades of life.
- Endemic in India, Sri Lanka, and Brazil, with only sporadic occurrences in the United States.
- Thought to be a zoonotic organism, because rhinosporidiosis is seen in cattle, horses, and mules.
- Mode of transmission is thought to occur via water or dust, from which the endospore penetrates the nasal cavity mucosa, matures into sporangium within the submucosal compartment and, after maturation, the sporangia burst, with release of endospores into surrounding tissue.
- The most common sites of involvement are the nasal cavity (inferior turbinate along the lateral nasal wall) and the nasopharynx; infection may involve the larynx, tracheobronchial tree, esophagus, conjunctiva, and ears.
- Most common symptoms include nasal obstruction, epistaxis, and rhinorrhea.

Pathology

Gross

- Single or multiple polypoid, pedunculated, or sessile masses.

Histology

- Submucosal cysts (sporangia) ranging in size from 10 to 300 microns in diameter.
- Sporangia contain innumerable endospores, seen by hematoxylin and eosin stain; organisms also stain with periodic acid-Schiff (PAS) and mucicarmine.
- A chronic inflammatory response consisting of lymphocytes, plasma cells, and eosinophils accompanies the organisms.
- Rupture of the cysts induces an acute inflammatory response; however, a granulomatous reaction is not seen.
- Overlying epithelium may be hyperplastic or demonstrate squamous metaplasia.

Differential Diagnosis

- Coccidioidomycosis infection (*Coccidioides immitis*).
- Schneiderian papilloma, cylindrical cell type (Chapter 4A, #1).

Treatment and Prognosis

- Surgical excision of the lesion.
- Recurrences, necessitating additional surgical excision, may occur in up to 10% of cases.
- No antibiotic therapy is effective.

Additional Facts

- In contrast to cylindrical cell papilloma, the cysts in rhinosporidiosis are essentially limited to the submucosa but, infrequently, may also be identified in the epithelium.

References

Lasser A, Smith HW: Rhinosporidiosis. Arch Otolaryngol Head Neck Surg 102:308–310, 1976.

Myerowitz RL: Rhinosporidiosis. *In*: Barnes L, ed. Surgical pathology of the head and neck. New York: Marcel Dekker, 1985; pp 1793–1795.

Satyanarayana C: Rhinosporidiosis with a record of 225 cases. Acta Otolaryngol (Stockh) 51:348–356, 1960.

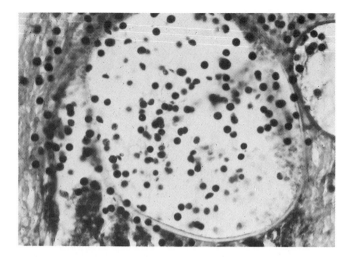

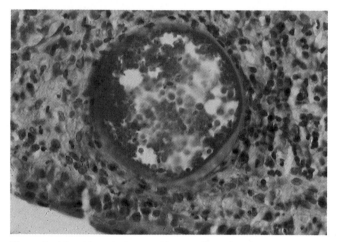

Figure 3–24. Sinonasal rhinosporidiosis showing a polypoid fragment of tissue characterized by the presence of multiple submucosal cysts (sporangia); the overlying epithelium is hyperplastic, with associated squamous metaplasia.

Figure 3–26. Although the organisms (*Rhinosporidium seeberi*) are readily identifiable by hematoxylin-eosin staining, additional stains may be used to detail these fungi. (*Top*) Periodic acid-Schiff (PAS) stain. (*Bottom*) Mucicarmine stain.

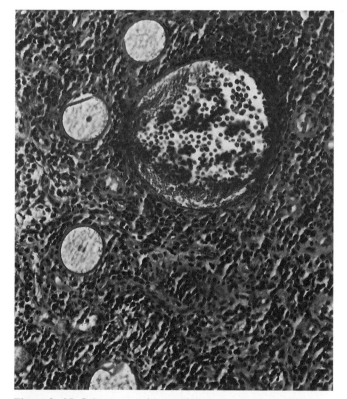

Figure 3–25. Submucosa with multiple and variably sized sporangia, which contain innumerable endospores; an associated chronic inflammatory response, consisting of lymphocytes, plasma cells, and eosinophils, accompanies the organisms.

6. MYOSPHERULOSIS

Definition: Innocuous, iatrogenically induced pseudo-mycotic disease, resulting from the interaction of red blood cells and petrolatum-based ointments.

Clinical

■ Typically, prior to the development of a nasal cavity or paranasal sinus mass, patients had prior surgery for a variety of disease processes (inflammatory or neoplastic lesions), followed by packing of the area with a petrolatum-based ointment.

■ Similar lesions have been seen after surgery involving the ear.

■ Similar lesions reported in soft-tissue areas of the extremities.

■ In the nose and paranasal sinuses, symptoms generally relate to a mass lesion with or without airway obstruction.

Pathology

Gross

■ No specific macroscopic findings, other than a nondescript mass.

Histology

■ Pseudocysts embedded within fibrotic tissue, with an associated chronic inflammatory infiltrate composed of lymphocytes, histiocytes, giant cells, and plasma cells.

■ Pseudocysts contain round, saclike structures called "parent bodies"; these parent bodies in turn contain numerous spherules or endobodies.

■ Fungal stains are negative.

Differential Diagnosis

■ Fungal infections (rhinosporidiosis, coccidioidomycosis) (Chapter 3, #5c).

Treatment and Prognosis

■ Symptomatic.

Additional Facts

■ Origin of the myospherules are from red blood cells that react with petrolatum or lanolin found in ointment used in "packing" the nasal cavity after surgery.

■ Emulsified fat may also induce the formation of myospherules, so that fat necrosis may result in myospherulosis.

References

Barnes L: Myospherulosis. *In:* Barnes L, ed. Surgical pathology of the head and neck. New York: Marcel Dekker, 1985; pp 1795–1796.

Kyriakos M: Myospherulosis of the paranasal sinuses, nose and middle ear: a possible iatrogenic disease. Am J Clin Pathol 67:118–130, 1977.

Rosai J. The nature of myospherulosis of the upper respiratory tract. Am J Clin Pathol 69:475–481, 1978.

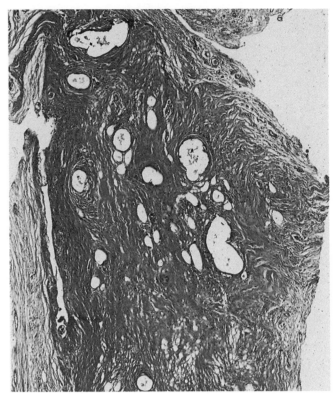

Figure 3–27. Myospherulosis of the sinonasal tract, consisting of multiple, irregularly shaped cystic spaces embedded within fibrotic tissue.

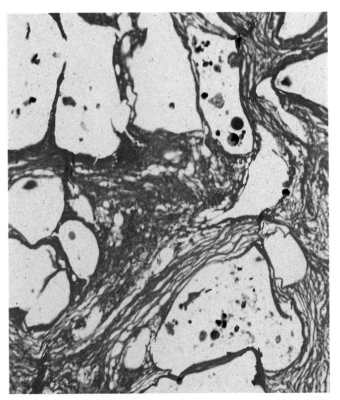

Figure 3–28. Myospherulosis pseudocystic spaces contain round, saclike structures ("parent bodies").

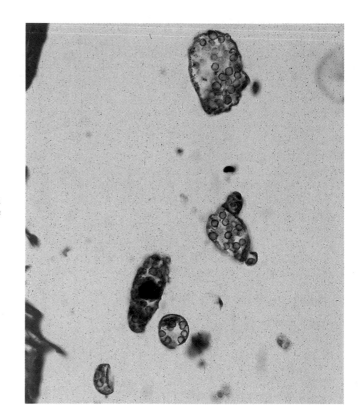

Figure 3–29. The "parent bodies" are brown staining and contain numerous spherules or endobodies; stains for microorganisms are absent.

7. SINONASAL CAVITY EXTRANODAL SINUS HISTIOCYTOSIS WITH MASSIVE LYMPHADENOPATHY (SHML)

Definition: Rare, idiopathic histiocytic proliferative disorder, generally characterized by lymph node–based disease and an indolent behavior; extranodal manifestations occur, with the upper respiratory tract being among the more common sites of involvement.

Synonyms: Rosai-Dorfman disease.

Clinical

- Slight female predominance; occurs over a wide age range.
- May be identified in virtually all extranodal head and neck sites, including sinonasal cavity > orbit > salivary gland > oral cavity > lower respiratory tract > nasopharynx and tonsil > middle ear and temporal bone.
- Symptoms depend on the site of occurrence, and in the sinonasal tract predominantly relate to nasal obstruction; non-sinonasal tract–related symptoms include proptosis, ptosis, decreased visual acuity, pain, stridor, cranial nerve deficits, or a mass lesion.

- Presentation often includes multiple concurrent sites of involvement; may occur without evidence of lymph node involvement.
- Hematologic and immunologic status generally intact, but may be associated with polyclonal elevations in serum protein levels and raised erythrocyte sedimentation rates.
- To date, etiology remains unknown, but an infectious origin is suspected.

Pathology

Gross

- Mucosal thickening or polypoid, rubbery to firm, pink to tan-gray lesions with variation in the size of the lesions.

Histology

- Polymorphous cellular infiltrate, predominantly composed of an admixture of mature lymphocytes and plasma cells.
- Histiocytes are seen in sheets or clusters and have vesicular nuclei and abundant, clear cytoplasm.
- Phagocytized mononuclear cells (emperipolesis) can be seen and are a valuable aid in diagnosis; however, in the upper respiratory tract, emperipo-

lesis may be less apparent as compared to nodal disease.

- Lymphoid aggregates often seen and, together with the polymorphic cellular infiltrate, give the affected extranodal tissue an architectural appearance similar to that of nodal parenchyma.
- Plasma cell component is mature, with identification of Russell bodies; plasma cells may predominate and obscure the diagnostic histiocytes.
- Fibrosis may be a prominent feature.
- Special stains for infectious organisms are negative but are required for differential diagnosis.
- Immunophenotypic profile consistent with a macrophage/histiocyte histogenesis: positive reactivity with S-100 protein, KP-1, MAC387, Ki-1, lysozyme, α-1-antitrypsin, α-1-antichymotrypsin; the plasma cell component is polyclonal, with positive reactivity for κ and λ light chains.

Differential Diagnosis

- Rhinoscleroma (Chapter 3, #5b).
- Leprosy.
- Lipid storage diseases.
- Histiocytosis X (eosinophilic granuloma) (Chapter 24B, #4).
- Midline destructive disease (Wegener's granulomatosis; midline malignant reticulosis) (Chapter 3, #8; Chapter 4B, #4).

Treatment and Prognosis

- In general, SHML is a self-limited disease that remits spontaneously.
- Upper and lower respiratory tract involvement usually requires surgical intervention in order to alleviate the cause of airway obstruction; however, surgical eradication of disease may prove difficult in cases with craniofacial bone or cranial cavity involvement.
- Steroids, radiotherapy, and chemotherapy have been used with some beneficial results but have not been proven to be completely effective.
- Extension of disease to vital structures, particularly to the cranial cavity, may result in the death of the patient; however, mortalities related to SHML are rare occurrences.
- No specific therapies have been used and therapy may be empirical to the clinical picture.

Additional Facts

- In general, the diagnosis of extranodal sinus histiocytosis with massive lymphadenopathy is a pathologic diagnosis, rarely suspected by clinical evaluation.
- Diagnosis can often be suspected based on the architectural and cytologic features; however, this is a diagnosis of exclusion and, even in the face of the characteristic light microscopic findings, special stains for the presence of an infectious agent should be performed before rendering the diagnosis.

References

Eisen RN, Buckley PJ, Rosai J: Immunophenotypic characterization of sinus histiocytosis with massive lymphadenopathy (Rosai-Dorfman disease). Semin Diagn Pathol 7:74–82, 1990.

Foucar E, Rosai J, Dorfman RF: Sinus histiocytosis with massive lymphadenopathy: ear, nose and throat manifestations. Arch Otolaryngol Head Neck Surg 104:687–693, 1978.

Foucar E, Rosai J, Dorfman R: Sinus histiocytosis with massive lymphadenopathy (Rosai-Dorfman disease): review of the entity. Semin Diagn Pathol 7:19–73, 1990.

Komp DM: The treatment of sinus histiocytosis with massive lymphadenopathy (Rosai-Dorfman disease). Semin Diagn Pathol 7:83–86, 1990.

Lopez P, Estes ML: Immunohistochemical characterization of the histiocytes in sinus histiocytosis with massive lymphadenopathy: analysis of an extranodal case. Hum Pathol 20:711–715, 1989.

Paulli M, Rosso R, Kindl S, et al: Immunophenotypic characterization of the cell infiltrate in five cases of sinus histiocytosis with massive lymphadenopathy (Rosai-Dorfman disease). Hum Pathol 23:647–654, 1992.

Rosai J, Dorfman RF: Sinus histiocytosis with massive lymphadenopathy: a newly recognized benign clinicopathological entity. Arch Pathol Lab Med 87:63–70, 1969.

Rosai J, Dorfman RF: Sinus histiocytosis with massive lymphadenopathy: a pseudolymphomatous benign disorder. Analysis of 34 cases. Cancer 30:1174–1188, 1972.

Wenig BM, Abbondanzo SL, Childers EL, Kapadia SB, Heffner DK: Extranodal sinus histiocytosis with massive lymphadenopathy (Rosai-Dorfman Disease) of the head and neck. Hum Pathol (in press).

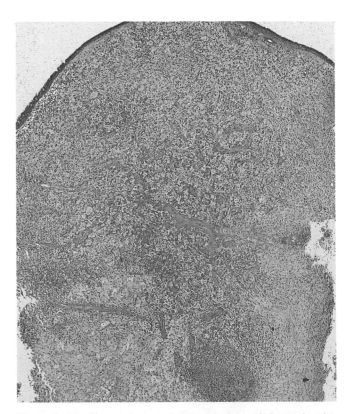

Figure 3–30. Sinonasal tract extranodal sinus histiocytosis with massive lymphadenopathy (SHML) demonstrating replacement of normal submucosal structures by a diffuse polymorphic inflammatory cell infiltrate; a lymphoid aggregate is seen at the lower portion of the illustration.

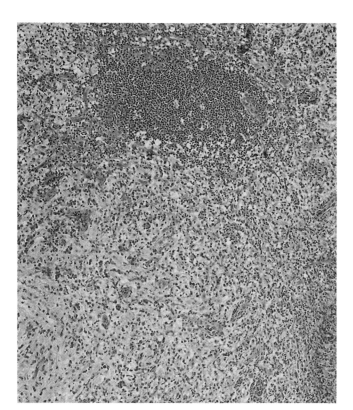

Figure 3–31. SHML involving the sinonasal tract submucosa is characterized by the presence of a lymphoid aggregate seen at the top of the field associated with a mixed cellular infiltrate composed of histiocytes admixed with lymphocytes, plasma cells, and scattered eosinophils.

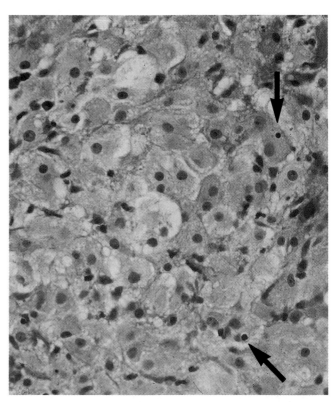

Figure 3–33. Clusters of histiocytes (SHML cells) predominate in this field and are composed of round nuclei with abundant clear to lightly eosinophilic cytoplasm. Within the cytoplasm of these histiocytes an occasional mononuclear cell can be seen (emperipolesis; *arrows*).

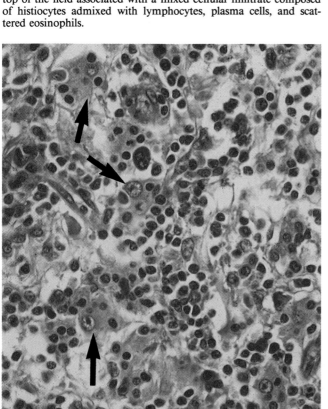

Figure 3–32. Lymphocytes and plasma cells predominate in this field, obscuring the characteristic histiocytic cell infiltrate. The SHML cells are large with round to oval nuclei, one or more prominent eosinophilic nucleoli, and abundant foamy to granular appearing cytoplasm within which mononuclear cells are engulfed (emperipolesis; *arrows*).

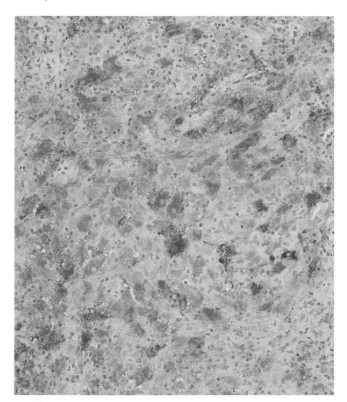

Figure 3–34. The histiocytes in SHML demonstrate diffuse immunoreactivity with S-100 protein.

8. WEGENER'S GRANULOMATOSIS

Definition: Non-neoplastic, idiopathic aseptic necrotizing disease with predilection for the upper/lower respiratory tract and the genitourinary system, characterized by the presence of vasculitis and destructive properties.

Clinical

■ May be systemic or localized:
Extent of disease reflected in the clinical manifestations, such that limited or localized disease may be asymptomatic, whereas in systemic involvement the patient is always sick.
Disease may progress from localized to systemic involvement.
■ Affects males more than females (except in laryngeal Wegener's granulomatosis, which is seen predominantly in women); occurs over a wide age range, with the average age of occurrence in the fourth and fifth decades of life.
■ In the head and neck (upper respiratory tract) the most common site of occurrence is the sinonasal region with the nasal cavity > maxillary > ethmoid > frontal > sphenoid; other sites of involvement include nasopharynx, larynx (subglottis), oral cavity, ear (external and middle ear, including the mastoid), and salivary glands.
■ Symptoms vary according to the site of involvement and include:
Sinonasal and nasopharyngeal: sinusitis with or without a purulent rhinorrhea, obstruction, pain, epistaxis, anosmia, headaches.
Laryngeal: dyspnea, hoarseness, voice changes.
Oral: ulcerative lesion, gingivitis.
Ear: hearing loss, pain.
■ Useful laboratory studies include elevated erythrocyte sedimentation rate (ESR) and, in renal disease, elevated serum creatinine and abnormal urinary sediment.
■ An important laboratory finding is an elevated antineutrophil cytoplasmic antibody (ANCA), with a reported specificity for the diagnosis of Wegener's granulomatosis from 85% to 98% of cases; sensitivity is equally high.
■ No known etiologic factors.

Radiology

■ Sinus opacification, bone destruction, ossification of the sinus walls, and soft-tissue destruction.

Pathology

Gross

■ Sinonasal area: diffuse ulcerative and crusted lesions with tissue destruction; in advanced cases, septal perforation may be seen, resulting in a "saddle nose" deformity.
■ Laryngeal area: subglottic stenosis with associated ulcerative lesions.

■ Oral cavity: ulcerative, destructive lesions often seen along the palate and alveolar region.

Histology

■ Vasculitis, involving small to medium-sized arteries and consisting of a polymorphous inflammatory infiltrate composed of lymphocytes and histiocytes and, less frequently, eosinophils and polymorphonuclear leukocytes.
■ "Ischemic" or "geographic" type necrosis, with a basophilic, smudgy appearance.
■ Multinucleated giant cells or non-necrotizing granulomas are almost invariably seen; well-formed granulomas may be seen but are generally not a common feature.
■ Parenchymal chronic inflammatory infiltrate, predominantly composed of lymphocytes, histiocytes, and plasma cells, is seen; microabscesses with or without granuloma formation may be identified; eosinophils although generally uncommon, may be numerous on occasion.
■ Histochemistry: elastic stains may assist in the identification of vasculitis.
■ Immunohistochemistry: polymorphous cellular population demonstrating immunoreactivity with both B-cell (L-26) and T-cell (UCHL) markers.

Differential Diagnosis

■ Infectious disease: fungal, mycobacterial, parasitic.
■ Nonspecific sinusitis/rhinitis.
■ Collagen vascular disease.
■ Churg-Strauss syndrome.
■ Non-Hodgkin's malignant lymphoma (malignant reticulosis) (Chapter 4B, #4; Table 4.3).

Treatment and Prognosis

■ Patients with limited disease are treated with cyclophosphamide.
■ Patients with fulminating disease, especially with renal failure, are treated with high doses of prednisone; this treatment is maintained until the disease is under control (as evidenced by improved ESR, serum creatinine, or ANCA titer), at which time cyclophosphamide therapy is begun. **Note:** Prednisone is continued until the cyclophosphamide can take effect, which occurs approximately 2 to 3 weeks after initiation of therapy.
■ Limited Wegener's granulomatosis responds well to cyclophosphamide or steroid therapy and has a good prognosis.
■ The major source of morbidity and mortality is chronic renal failure or sepsis.
■ Occasional spontaneous remissions may be seen with milder forms of disease when only one or a few organs are involved (but not the kidneys).

Additional Facts

■ Diagnosis may be suggested by the clinical signs and symptoms; however, the most important part of diagnosis is tissue biopsy with histomorphologic confirmation.

■ Histomorphologic diagnosis may be limited based on the tissue sampling; therefore, it is imperative that the clinician obtain multiple biopsy specimens, especially from areas of the ulcer bed as well as in areas of more viable-appearing tissue.

■ In general, Wegener's granulomatosis is a disease of exclusion once other, more common causes of associated symptoms are ruled out.

■ Vasculitis is not limited to Wegener's granulomatosis and also can be seen in infectious diseases.

■ Bacterial superinfection of the diseased mucosa, particularly *Staphylococcus aureus,* may complicate the clinical picture.

■ Despite limited clinical manifestastions of disease, detailed evaluation of other organ systems (chest radiograph and renal function) is indicated.

References

Devaney KO, Travis WD, Hoffman G, Leavitt R, Lebovics R, Fauci AS: Interpretation of head and neck biopsies in Wegener's granulomatosis: a pathologic study of 126 biopsies in 70 patients. Am J Surg Pathol 14:555–564, 1990.

Fauci AS, Haynes BF, Katz P, Wolff SM: Wegener's granulomatosis: prospective clinical and therapeutic experience with 85 patients for 21 years (review). Ann Intern Med 98:76–85, 1983.

Haynes BF: Wegener's granulomatosis and midline granuloma. *In*: Wyngaarden JB, Smith LH, eds. Cecil textbook of medicine. Philadelphia: W.B. Saunders Co., 1988; pp 2030–2033.

McDonald TJ, Neel HB, DeRemee RA: Wegener's granulomatosis of the subglottis and the upper portions of the trachea. Ann Otol Rhinol Laryngol 91:588–592, 1982.

McDonald TJ, DeRemee RA: Wegener's gramulomatosis. Laryngoscope 93:220–231, 1983.

Nolle B, Specks U, Ludemann J, Rohrbach MS, DeRemee RA, Gross WL: Anticytoplasmic autoantibodies: their immunodiagnostic value in Wegener's granulomatosis. Ann Intern Med 111:28–40, 1989.

Specks U, Wheatley CL, McDonald TJ, Rohrbach MS, DeRemee RA: Anticytoplasmic autoantibodies in the diagnosis and follow-up of Wegener's granulomatosis. Mayo Clin Proc 64:28–36, 1989.

Wegener F: Wegener's granulomatosis: thoughts and observations of a pathologist. Eur Arch Otorhinolaryngol 247:133–142, 1990.

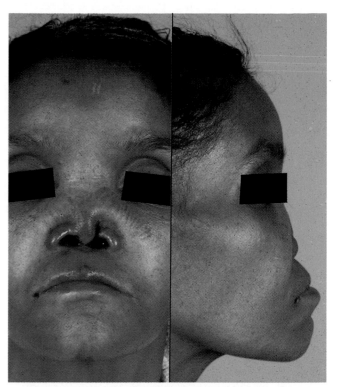

Figure 3–36. Severe nasal deformity including nasal septal destruction is seen in this adult with Wegener's granulomatosis.

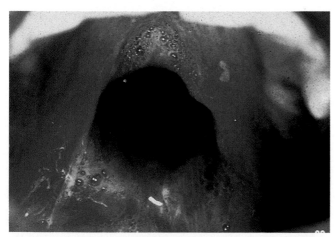

Figure 3–35. Wegener's granulomatosis of the floor of the nasal cavity resulting in complete erosion through the palate. Palatal destruction is considered an unusual occurrence in association with Wegener's granulomatosis and is a finding more commonly identified in association with midline malignant reticulosis.

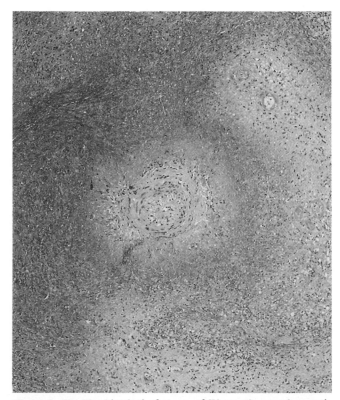

Figure 3–37. The histologic features of Wegener's granulomatosis include vasculitis that involves small- to medium-sized vessels and an "ischemic" or "geographic" type of necrosis with a basophilic, smudgy appearance.

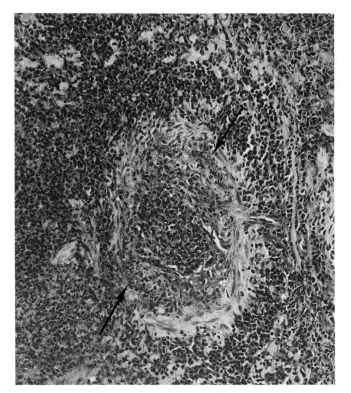

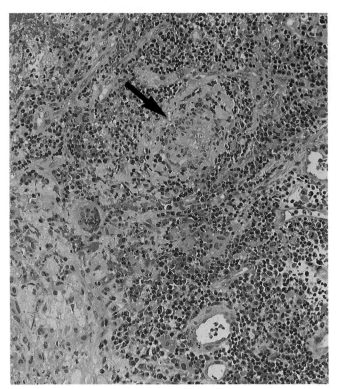

Figure 3–38. The vasculitic component of Wegener's granulomatosis may be difficult to identify and is aided by elastic stains (Movat). The lumen of this medium-sized vessel is obliterated by the inflammatory infiltrate, which has penetrated through the vessel wall, disrupting the external elastic membrane along the peripheral aspect of the vessel (*arrow*).

Figure 3–39. The cellular component seen in Wegener's granulomatosis is polymorphous, typically composed of lymphocytes, histiocytes, and plasma cells, and does not demonstrate atypical features; a multinucleated giant cell is seen to the left of center. Infiltration and obliteration of a medium-sized blood vessel is seen (*arrow*).

CHAPTER 4

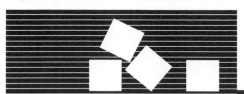

Neoplasms of the Nasal Cavity and Paranasal Sinuses

A. BENIGN NEOPLASMS
 1. Sinonasal or Schneiderian Papillomas
 2. Lobular Capillary Hemangioma
 3. Sinonasal Hemangiopericytoma
 4. Benign Fibrous Histiocytoma
 5. Fibromatosis
 6. Leiomyoma
 7. Benign Fibro-osseous and Osseous Lesions
 a. Fibrous Dysplasia
 b. Ossifying Fibroma
 c. Juvenile Active Ossifying Fibroma
 8. Osteoma
 9. Sinonasal Myxoma and Fibromyxoma
 10. Ameloblastoma

B. MALIGNANT NEOPLASMS
 1. Squamous Cell Carcinoma
 2. Sinonasal (Mucosal) Adenocarcinoma
 3. Mucosal Malignant Melanoma
 4. Midline Malignant Reticulosis
 5. Olfactory Neuroblastoma
 6. Malignant Fibrous Histiocytoma
 7. Fibrosarcoma
 8. Leiomyosarcoma
 9. Angiosarcoma
 10. Osteosarcoma
 11. Teratocarcinosarcoma

A. BENIGN NEOPLASMS

1. Sinonasal or Schneiderian Papillomas

Definition: Benign neoplasm arising from the sinonasal tract (Schneiderian) mucosa composed of a squamous or columnar epithelial proliferation with associated mucous cells or pools, and a myxomatous stroma.

Clinical (Table 4–1)

■ Histologically divided into three types: septal, inverted, and cylindrical cell.
■ Biologic behavior essentially the same for all types; however, clinical findings may differ.
■ Occur over a wide age range but generally are not seen in children; septal papillomas tend to occur in a younger age group.
■ Symptoms vary according to site of occurrence and include airway obstruction, epistaxis, and pain.
■ Septal (exophytic or fungiform) papillomas almost invariably are seen limited to the nasal septum; inverted and cylindrical cell papillomas occur along the lateral nasal wall (middle turbinate) and, less frequently, in the paranasal sinuses; rarely, if ever, are the inverted and cylindrical cell subtypes identified on the nasal septum.
■ Tendency to spread along the mucosa into adjacent areas.
■ In general, papillomas are unilateral, but bilateral papillomas occur infrequently.
■ Etiology remains unproven; however, human papillomavirus (HPV) types 6/11 have been identified in sinonasal papillomas.
■ May occur simultaneously with nasal inflammatory polyps.
■ Not associated with an increased risk or with the development of additional papillomas elsewhere in the upper respiratory tract.

Radiology

■ Unilateral mass in the nasal cavity.
■ Opacification and mucosal thickening of a paranasal sinus.
■ Pressure erosion of bone.

Table 4-1.
SINONASAL (SCHNEIDERIAN) PAPILLOMAS

	Septal	Inverted	Cylindrical
Percentage	50%	47%	3%
Age (Years)	20-50	40-70	40-70
Sex	♂ > ♀	♂ > ♀	♂ > ♀
Symptoms	Epistaxis, mass	Obstruction, epistaxis, pain	Similar to inverted type
Location	Nasal septum	Lateral nasal wall and paranasal sinuses	Lateral nasal wall and paranasal sinuses
Biology	Recurs if incompletely excised	Recurs if incompletely excised	Recurs if incompletely excised
Malignant degeneration	Rare	Approximately 10%	< 10%

Pathology

SEPTAL PAPILLOMA

Gross

■ Papillary, exophytic, verrucoid, cauliflower-like lesion with a pink to tan appearance and a firm to rubbery consistency.
■ Attached to mucosa by a narrow or broad-based stalk.

Histology

■ Papillary fronds, composed of a thick epithelium and predominantly squamous (epidermoid) and less frequently respiratory in type.
■ Mucocytes (goblet cells) and intraepithelial mucous cysts are seen.
■ Stromal component composed of delicate, fibrovascular cores.
■ Surface keratinization is uncommon.
■ Seromucous glands, mitoses, and an associated inflammatory infiltrate are usually not present.

Differential Diagnosis

■ Verruca vulgaris (Chapter 14A, #1).
■ Squamous papilloma (Chapter 9A, #1).

INVERTED PAPILLOMA

Gross

■ Large, bulky, translucent mass with a red to gray color and varying from firm to friable in consistency.

Histology

■ Endophytic or "inverted" growth pattern, consisting of markedly thickened squamous epithelial proliferation admixed with mucocytes and intraepithelial mucous cysts.
■ Surface component may be composed of a respiratory epithelium.
■ Epidermoid component may demonstrate extensive clear cell features, indicative of abundant glycogen content.
■ Epithelial proliferation, noted for uniformity of nuclei maintaining a consistency in polarity; nuclei are round with uniform, dark-appearing chromatin.
■ Mitoses may be seen in the basal and parabasal layers, but atypical mitotic figures are not seen.
■ Surface keratinization may be present.
■ Stromal component varies from myxomatous to fibrous, admixed with chronic inflammatory cells and variable vascularity.

Differential Diagnosis

■ Inflammatory polyps (Chapter 3, #1).
■ Nonkeratinizing respiratory ("transitional") carcinoma (Chapter 4B, #1).
■ Verrucous carcinoma (Chapter 14B, #3).

CYLINDRICAL CELL PAPILLOMA

Gross

■ Dark red to brown papillary lesion.

Histology

■ Multilayered epithelial proliferation, composed of cells with an eosinophilic to granular cytoplasm with uniform, round nuclei.
■ Intraepithelial mucin cysts, often containing polymorphonuclear leukocytes, are seen; cysts are not identified in the submucosa.
■ Outer surface of the epithelial proliferation may demonstrate cilia.

Differential Diagnosis

■ Rhinosporidiosis (Chapter 3, #5c).
■ Low-grade papillary adenocarcinoma (Chapter 4B, #2).

Treatment and Prognosis

■ Complete surgical excision of the neoplasm, including adjacent uninvolved mucosa; aggressive surgery including a lateral rhinotomy or medial maxillectomy may be necessary to allow for adequate exposure for total removal.
■ Adjuvant therapy (chemo- and radiotherapy) has not been shown to be of benefit for the treatment of sinonasal papilloma.

- In general, prognosis is good after complete surgical excision; however, if left unchecked, these neoplasms have the capability of continued growth with extension along the mucosal surface and with destruction of bone and invasion of vital structures.
- Complications associated with schneiderian papillomas include recurrence and malignant transformation; the septal papilloma rarely, if ever, undergoes malignant transformation.

Additional Facts

- The derivation of the sinonasal papillomas is from the schneiderian mucosa, which is ectodermally derived; in comparison, the nasopharyngeal mucosa is of endodermal derivation.
- This group of neoplasms recurs if incompletely resected; recurrence probably represents persistence of disease, rather than multicentricity of the neoplasm.
- Growth and extension along the mucosa results from the induction of squamous metaplasia in the adjacent sinonasal mucosa.
- No histologic features that prospectively predict the development of malignancy in the papilloma.
- In the presence of surface keratinization or dyskeratosis, increased cellularity with pleomorphism and the presence of atypical mitoses, the surgical pathologist should be wary of the presence of a carcinoma and submit additional tissue specimens for sectioning.
- The majority of the malignancies associated with sinonasal papillomas are squamous cell carcinomas.
- Treatment for malignant transformation of a sinonasal papilloma includes surgery and radiotherapy.

References

Barnes L: Papillomas of the nose and paranasal sinuses. *In*: Barnes L, ed. Surgical pathology of the head and neck. New York: Marcel Dekker, 1985; pp 408–416.

Brandwein M, Steinberg B, Thung S, Biller H, Dilorenzo T, Galli R: Human papillomavirus 6/11 and 16/18 in schneiderian inverted papillomas: in situ hybridization with human papillomavirus RNA probes. Cancer 63:1708–1713, 1989.

Christensen WN, Smith RRL: Schneiderian papillomas: a clinicopathologic study of 67 cases. Hum Pathol 17:393–400, 1986.

Hyams VJ: Papillomas of the nasal cavity and paranasal sinuses: a clinicopathologic study of 315 cases. Ann Otol Rhinol Laryngol 80:192–206, 1971.

Hyams VJ, Batsakis JG, Michaels L: Papilloma of the sinonasal tract. *In*: Hyams VJ, Batsakis JG, Michaels L, eds. Tumors of the upper respiratory tract and ear. Fascicle 25, second series. Washington, DC: Armed Forces Institute of Pathology, 1988; pp 34–44.

Judd R, Zaki SR, Coffield LM, Evatt BL: Sinonasal papilloma and human papillomavirus: human papillomavirus 11 detected in fungiform schneiderian papillomas by in situ hybridization and polymerase chain reaction. Hum Pathol 22:550–556, 1991.

Lawson W, Le Benger J, Som P, Bernard PJ, Biller HF: Inverted papilloma: an analysis of 87 cases. Laryngoscope 99:1117–1124, 1989.

Myers EN, Fernau JL, Johnson JT, Tabet JC, Barnes EL: Management of inverted papilloma. Laryngoscope 100:481–490, 1990.

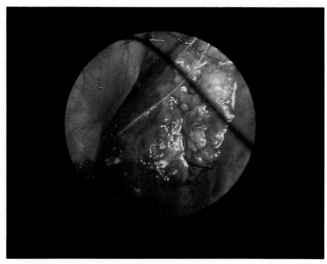

Figure 4–1. Sinonasal septal papilloma consisting of an exophytic, tan-white lesion with a cauliflower-like appearance.

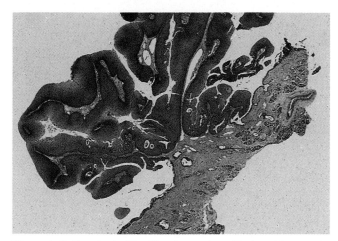

Figure 4–2. Exophytic (fungiform) septal papilloma with a papillary growth protruding from the surface respiratory epithelium and composed of a thickened, nonkeratinized squamous (epidermoid) epithelium.

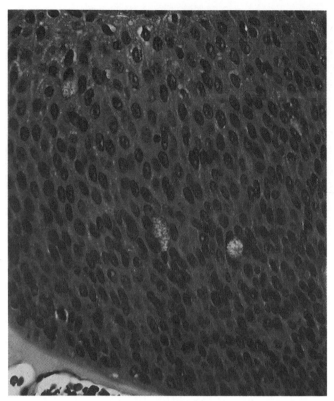

Figure 4–3. The epithelium is cytologically bland, with uniform cells of even polarity and normal maturation with intraepithelial mucocytes (goblet cells); mitoses can be seen and are generally confined to the basal areas.

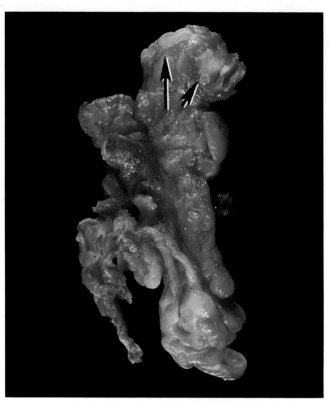

Figure 4–5. Resected inverted papilloma. The tumor can be seen arising along the surface of the resected specimen as a flat, tan-white thickened area (*arrow*) with an endophytic or inverted growth within the submucosal compartment (*arrowhead*).

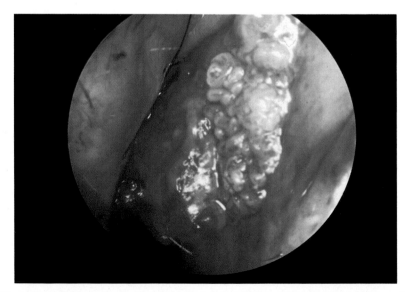

Figure 4–4. Endoscopic appearance of inverted papilloma along the floor and lateral wall of the nasal cavity; the tumor appears as a sessile, tan-white mucosal lesion.

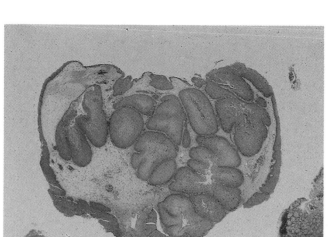

Figure 4–6. Endophytic or "inverted" growth pattern, consisting of thickened squamous epithelial nests growing down into the stroma, which is made up of myxomatous to fibrous tissue admixed with chronic inflammatory cells and variable vascularity.

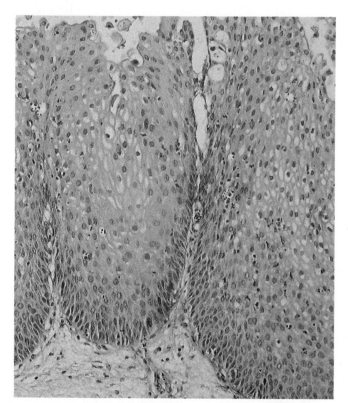

Figure 4–7. Epithelial proliferation, noted for uniformity of nuclei maintaining a consistency in polarity, normal maturation toward the surface, scattered mucous cysts, and the presence of neutrophils throughout the epithelium; clear cell features indicative of abundant glycogen content can be seen.

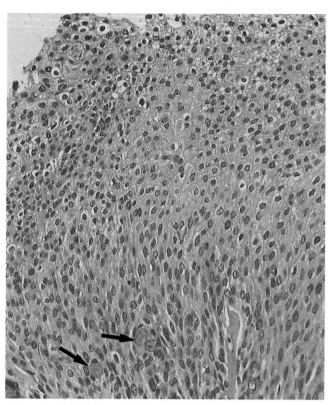

Figure 4–8. This inverted-type papilloma demonstrates increased cellularity but maintains polarity and nuclear uniformity; intraepithelial mucocytes are seen (*arrows*).

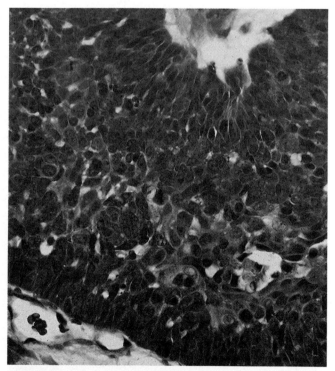

Figure 4–9. Inverted-type papilloma that has undergone malignant transformation, as demonstrated by marked increase in cellularity, absence of cellular maturation, loss of nuclear polarity, presence of pleomorphic nuclei, increase in the nuclear–cytoplasmic ratio, and mitotic figures at all epithelial layers.

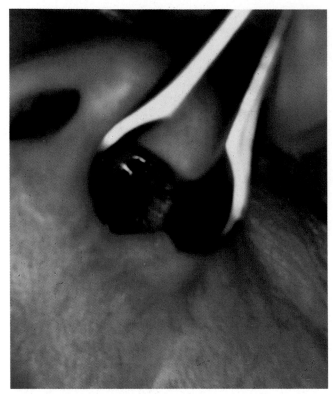

Figure 4–10. Cylindrical cell papilloma within the nasal cavity, appearing as a dark red to brown mass.

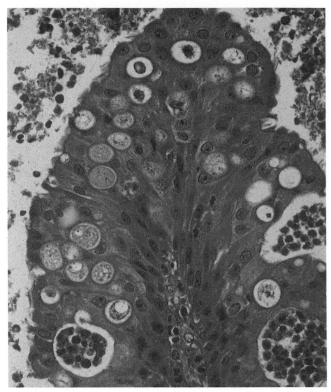

Figure 4–12. Cellular composition seen in cylindrical cell papilloma, consisting of cells with an eosinophilic to granular cytoplasm, uniform, round nuclei, and intraepithelial mucin cysts containing amorphous pink material or polymorphonuclear leukocytes. Cilia can be seen at the outer surface of the epithelial proliferation.

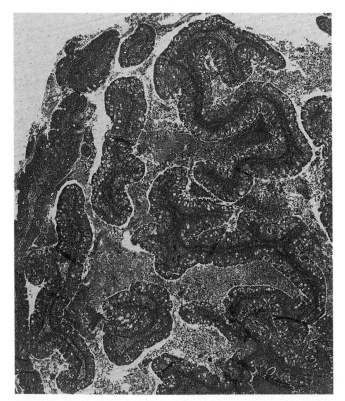

Figure 4–11. Cylindrical cell papilloma is histologically characterized by a multilayered papillary epithelial proliferation with multiple intraepithelial mucin cysts; cysts are not identified in the submucosal compartment.

2. Lobular Capillary Hemangioma

Definition: Benign polypoid form of capillary hemangioma, primarily occurring on skin and mucous membranes.

Synonyms: Pyogenic granuloma; pregnancy tumor.

Clinical

- No sex predilection; wide age range, commonly seen in the fourth to fifth decades of life, but uncommon under 16 years of age.
- Most often identified in the anterior portion of the nasal septum referred to as Little's area or Kisselbach's triangle; next most common sinonasal location is the tip of the turbinates.
- Etiology remains unclear but is associated with prior trauma and with pregnancy ("pregnancy" tumor).
- The most common complaint is epistaxis.

Pathology

Gross

- Smooth, lobulated, polypoid mass measuring up to 1.5 cm in diameter.

Histology

- Vascular component arranged in lobules or clusters composed of central capillaries that give off smaller ramifying tributaries.
- Vascular component surrounded by granulation tissue and a chronic inflammatory cell infiltrate.
- Endothelial cell lining may be prominent and may display endothelial tufting as well as mitoses.
- Surface epithelium often ulcerated.
- "Active" cases may become quite cellular, with increased mitotic activity.

Differential Diagnosis

- Hemangiopericytoma (Chapter 4A, #3).
- Angiosarcoma (Chapter 4B, #9).

Treatment and Prognosis

- Local surgical excision.
- Recurrences rarely occur.

Additional Facts

- This lesion has been synonymously referred to as pyogenic granuloma; however, the latter term is a misnomer in that this lesion is neither an infectious process nor granulomatous.
- "Pregnancy" tumor is a lobular capillary hemangioma that occurs in the gravid state and that regresses after parturition.
- Cavernous hemangiomas occur less frequently in the upper respiratory tract, as compared with the

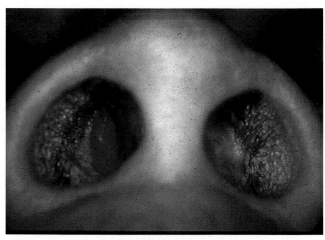

Figure 4-13. Intranasal lobular capillary hemangioma, characterized by a smooth, lobulated, polypoid red mass.

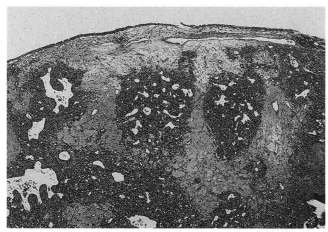

Figure 4-14. Submucosal cellular lobules consisting of dilated vascular spaces with ramification and "staghorn" appearance, surrounded by granulation tissue and a chronic inflammatory cell infiltrate.

capillary hemangioma; in general, cavernous hemangiomas have a similar clinical presentation as the capillary hemangiomas but are more often identified on the turbinates rather than on the nasal septum.

References

Kerr DA: Granuloma pyogenicum. Oral Surg Oral Med Oral Pathol 4:158–176, 1951.

Mills SE, Cooper PH, Fechner RE: Lobular capillary hemangioma: the underlying lesion of pyogenic granuloma: a study of 73 cases from the oral and nasal membranes. Am J Surg Pathol 4:471–479, 1980.

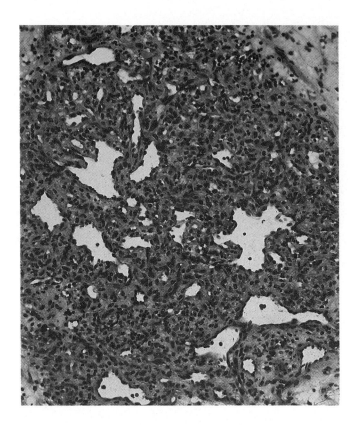

Figure 4–15. Vessels vary in caliber from slit-like to widely dilated, with irregular configurations lined by plump endothelial cells; vascular tufting may be seen, and the surrounding cellular component may be "active," with increased cellularity and with mitotic figures.

3. Sinonasal Hemangiopericytoma

Definition: Vascular neoplasm of varying biologic behavior, arising from pericytic cells that function as baroreceptors and are identified within the outer portion of the capillary wall.

Clinical

■ Uncommon neoplasm, predominantly identified in the lower extremities, pelvis, and retroperitoneum.
■ From 15% to 25% of all hemangiopericytomas occur in the head and neck region.
■ No sex predilection; seen over a wide age range, but most commonly occurs in the sixth to seventh decades of life.
■ In the head and neck, hemangiopericytomas can be identified in virtually any site, but the most common site of occurrence is the nasal cavity and paranasal sinuses (>50% of cases); other common sites of involvement include the orbital region, parotid gland, and the neck (approximately 20% of cases).
■ Most common presenting symptoms are nasal obstruction and epistaxis.
■ No known etiologic factors.

Radiology

■ Opacification of involved sinus.
■ Bone erosion may be seen.
■ Arteriographic findings reveal a richly vascular neoplasm.

Pathology

Gross

■ Red to tan-gray, soft to firm polypoid mass of varying size.

Histology

■ Circumscribed cellular tumor, composed of tightly packed small cells situated around endothelial-lined vascular spaces.
■ Tumor cells are uniform and have round to oval nuclei with vesicular to hyperchromatic chromatin and an indistinct cytoplasm; occasionally, spindle-shaped cells are seen.
■ Vascular channels range from capillary size to large sinusoidal spaces that have a "'staghorn" or "antlerlike" configuration.
■ Cellular proliferation may compress and obscure vessels of smaller size.

- Fibrosis or a myxoid stroma may be seen, especially in tumors undergoing degenerative change.
- Occasional mitoses are seen, but significant mitotic activity and necrosis are generally not found.
- Heterologous metaplastic elements, including bone and cartilage, may occasionally be seen.
- Histochemistry: reticulin stain reveals a distinctive pattern, characterized by envelopment of individual pericytes by reticulin fibers.
- Immunohistochemistry: noncontributory; tumor cells do not react with endothelial markers (factor VIII–related antigen, *Ulex europaeus*).
- Criteria for malignancy include:
  Mitoses (> 1 mitosis/10 high-power fields).
  Increased cellularity with cellular pleomorphism.
  Invasive or destructive growth.
  Necrosis.
  Metastasis.

Differential Diagnosis

- Lobular capillary hemangioma (Chapter 4A, #2).
- Nasopharyngeal angiofibroma (Chapter 9A, #2).
- Glomus tumor (glomangioma).
- Benign and malignant fibrohistiocytic neoplasms (Chapter 4A, #4; Chapter 4B, #6).
- Synovial sarcoma (Chapter 14B, #8).
- Mesenchymal chondrosarcoma.

Treatment and Prognosis

- Surgery is the treatment of choice.
- In contrast to soft-tissue hemangiopericytoma, those occurring in the upper aerodigestive tract generally behave in an indolent manner amenable to surgical resection and are notable for the absence of malignant behavior (metastases).
- Up to 60% of tumors will recur locally following inadequate excision; only 10% metastasize and metastases are usually preceded by recurrent tumor; metastatic disease usually involves the lungs and rarely involves regional lymph nodes.
- Hemangiopericytomas are considered radioresistant neoplasms.

Additional Facts

- Given the absence of definitive, identifiable light microscopic, ultrastructural, or immunocytochemical features, the diagnosis of hemangiopericytoma rests on architectural features.
- Cell of origin is considered the pericyte, originally described by Zimmermann, which is a normal structure identified in the capillary wall external to the reticulin fiber network and which functions in regulating the caliber of the capillary lumen.
- Sinonasal hemangiopericytomas have been considered a related but separate entity, as compared with their soft-tissue counterparts, based on differences in the biologic behavior; however, despite the appellation of "hemangiopericytoma-like," the sinonasal hemangiopericytoma probably is a pericytic-derived tumor that has a favorable biology due to location and earlier presentation.

References

Compagno J, Hyams VJ: Hemangiopericytoma-like intranasal tumors. Am J Clin Pathol 66:672–683, 1976.

Compagno J: Hemangiopericytoma-like tumors of the nasal cavity: a comparison with hemangiopericytoma of soft tissues. J Laryngoscop 88:460–469, 1978.

Eichorn JH, Dickersin GR, Bhan AK, Goodman ML: Sinonasal hemangiopericytoma: a reassessment with electron microscopy, immunohistochemistry, and long-term follow-up. Am J Surg Pathol 14:856–866, 1990.

Enzinger FM, Smith BH: Hemangiopericytoma: an analysis of 106 cases. Hum Pathol 7:61–82, 1976.

McMaster MJ, Soule EH, Irvins JC: Hemangiopericytoma: a clinicopathologic study and long-term follow-up of 60 patients. Cancer 36:2232–2244, 1975.

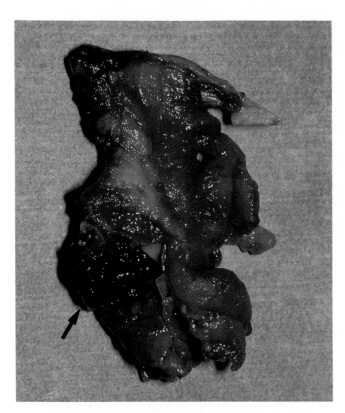

Figure 4–16. Sinonasal hemangiopericytoma (HPC): a red to tan-gray polypoid mass (*arrow*).

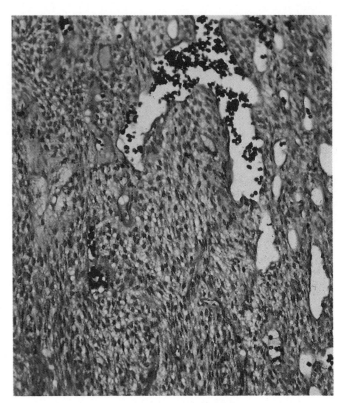

Figure 4–18. HPC typified by dilated, ramifying endothelial-lined vascular channels surrounded by the pericytic cell component, which consists of uniform cells with round to oval to spindle-shaped nuclei, vesicular to hyperchromatic chromatin, and an indistinct cytoplasm.

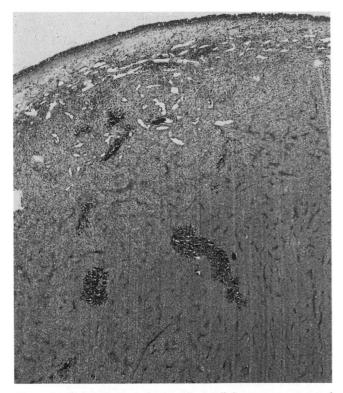

Figure 4–17. Submucosal circumscribed cellular tumor, composed of tightly packed small cells situated around endothelial-lined vascular spaces; the more superficial aspect of this HPC demonstrates dilated, irregularly shaped vascular channels, as compared with the deeper portion of the tumor, where the dense cellular component compresses the vessels, which appear as slit-like spaces.

4. Benign Fibrous Histiocytoma

Definition: Benign neoplasms composed of an admixture of fibroblastic and histiocytic cells.

Synonyms: Sclerosing hemangioma; cutaneous-derived are called dermatofibromas.

Clinical

- Relatively uncommon neoplasm in the head and neck, accounting for <5% of all fibrous histiocytomas.
- Affects men more than women; occurs over a wide age range, with a median age in the fifth decade of life.
- Excluding cutaneous sites, the most common location in the head and neck is the nasal cavity and paranasal sinuses; other more common sites of occurrence include neck, larynx, and trachea.
- Symptoms vary according to site and include: painless mass, nasal obstruction, epistaxis, pain, facial asymmetry, proptosis, loosening of teeth, hemoptysis, dyspnea, and stridor.

Pathology

Gross

- Polypoid or nodular, tan-white to yellow lesion varying in size.

Histology

- Submucosal lesion composed of an admixture of spindle-shaped cells (fibroblasts) and epithelioid cells (histiocytes) in a fascicular or storiform growth pattern.
- In addition, multinucleated giant cells, an inflammatory cell infiltrate (lymphocytes, plasma cells, and eosinophils), and foam cells are seen scattered throughout the tumor.
- Stroma varies and may consist of collagen production, myxoid change, and hyalinization.
- Vascularity varies from relatively inconspicuous vessels to prominent vascular pattern with striking hyalinization.
- Pleomorphism and mitoses may be seen, but these features in excess or in the presence of abnormal mitotic figures suggest malignancy.
- Special stains are of little or no contribution to the diagnosis.

Differential Diagnosis

- Nodular fasciitis (Chapter 8, #5).
- Benign peripheral nerve sheath tumor (neurofibroma or schwannoma) (Chapter 9A, #6).
- Leiomyoma (Chapter 4, #6).
- Dermatofibrosarcoma protuberans (see below).
- Malignant fibrous histiocytoma (Chapter 4B, #6).

Treatment and Prognosis

- Complete surgical excision is generally curative.

Additional Facts

- *Dermatofibrosarcoma protuberans (DFSP):*
  Fibrohistiocytic tumor of intermediate-grade malignancy (between that of benign and malignant fibrous histiocytomas) based on its infiltrative growth, capacity for local recurrence, and infrequent potential to metastasize.
  Affects men more than women; tumor of adult life.
  Most frequent on the trunk and extremities.
  Histologically, DFSP infiltrates the dermis and subcutis; in its central aspect, it is composed of plump fibroblasts arranged in a distinct storiform pattern; cellular pleomorphism is mild and variable mitotic activity is seen.
  Wide local excision is the treatment of choice.

References

Blitzer A, Lawson W, Biller HF: Malignant fibrous histiocytoma of the head and neck. Laryngoscope 87:1479–1499, 1977.

Del-Ray E, De-la-Torre FE: Fibrous histiocytoma of the nasal cavity. Laryngoscope 90:1686–1693, 1980.

Gonzalez-Campora R, Matilla A, Sanchez-Carrillo JJ, Navarro A, Galera H: "Benign" fibrous histiocytoma of the trachea. J Laryngol Otol 95:1287–1292, 1981.

Perzin KH, Fu YS: Non-epithelial tumors of the nasal cavity, paranasal sinuses, and nasopharynx: a clinicopathologic study. XI: fibrous histiocytomas. Cancer 45:2616–2626, 1980.

Rice DH, Batsakis JG, Headington JT, Boles R: Fibrous histiocytoma of the nose and paranasal sinuses. Arch Otolaryngol Head Neck Surg 100:398–401, 1974.

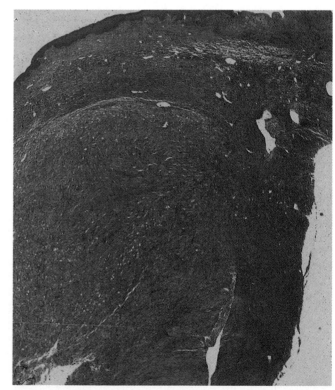

Figure 4–19. Benign fibrous histiocytoma, consisting of a submucosal cellular lesion with a fascicular or storiform growth pattern.

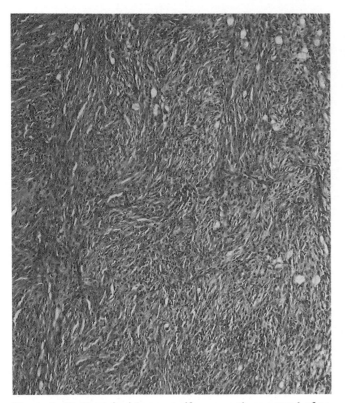

Figure 4–20. Short fascicles or storiform growth composed of an admixture of spindle-shaped cells (fibroblasts) and epithelioid cells (histiocytes).

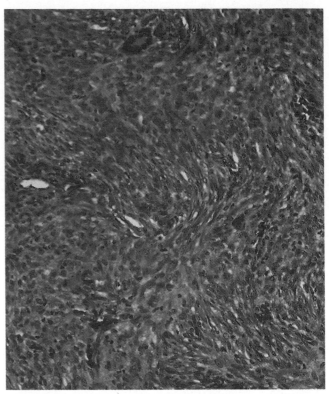

Figure 4–21. In addition to the fibroblasts and histiocytes, multinucleated giant cells and scattered chronic inflammatory cells can be seen. Benign fibrous histiocytomas may be quite cellular, with mild cellular pleomorphism and scattered mitoses, but these features are not seen in excess, nor are there abnormal mitotic figures.

5. Fibromatosis

Definition: "Infiltrating" or aggressive fibroblastic proliferation lacking histologic features of either an inflammatory process or a neoplasm.

Synonyms: Desmoid tumor; aggressive fibromatosis; tumefactive fibroinflammatory tumor; inflammatory pseudotumor.

Clinical

- Identified in the head and neck in 10% to 15% of cases; in children, this area of the body may be affected in up to 30% of cases.
- No sex preference; seen in both children and adults, but most commonly occurs in the third and fourth decades of life.
- Excluding the neck, the common sites of occurrence are nasal cavity and paranasal sinuses, nasopharynx, tongue, and oral cavity.
- Symptoms vary according to site, but usually present as a painless enlarging mass; other symptoms include pain, facial deformity, nasal obstruction, epistaxis, proptosis, dysphagia, dyspnea, hoarseness, and trismus.
- Lesions may be localized or multicentric.
- No known etiology; may be familial.

Pathology

Gross

- Firm, tan-white, poorly delineated or infiltrating lesion of varying size.
- On cut section, the lesion has a trabecular or whorled appearance.

Histology

- Poorly circumscribed lesion, composed of uniform-appearing spindle-shaped cells with sharply defined, pale-staining nuclei associated and separated by abundant collagen production.
- Cellularity varies, but in general is only moderately cellular.
- Mild pleomorphism and rare mitotic figures.
- Chronic inflammatory infiltrate composed of lymphocytes, plasma cells, and eosinophils may accompany the lesion and varies from being scant to dense in appearance.

- A myxoid or mucoid-appearing stroma may be seen; vascularity varies, but is generally not a prominent feature.
- Ill-defined margins with infiltration into surrounding soft-tissue structures (muscle, fat); erosion of bone may be seen.
- Special stains of little contribution to the diagnosis.

Differential Diagnosis

- Reactive fibrosis.
- Myxoma (Chapter 4A, #9).
- Peripheral nerve sheath tumor (neurofibroma, schwannoma) (Chapter 9A, #6).
- Fibro-osseous lesion (fibrous dysplasia, ossifying fibroma) (Chapter 4A, #7).
- Fibrosarcoma (Chapter 4B, #7).

Treatment and Prognosis

- The treatment of choice is complete surgical excision, including several centimeters beyond the apparent macroscopic extent of the lesion.
- Typically, the lesion is difficult to manage, because it insinuates into adjacent structures without clear demarcation, making complete excision difficult.
- Adjuvant therapies, including irradiation, chemotherapy, and steroid treatment, have been used with variable success and remain unproven.
- Recurrent disease is common, appearing within the first few postoperative years, and correlates with positive margins and not to the histologic appearance.
- Death may occur and relates to uncontrolled local disease with invasion into vital structures or to airway compromise.

Additional Facts

- Spontaneous regression of the lesion may occur.
- In extremely rare cases, transformation to an overt malignancy (fibrosarcoma) may occur and possibly relates to prior radiation therapy.

References

Ayala AG, Ro JY, Goepfert H, Cangir A, Khorsand J, Flake G: Desmoid fibromatosis: a clinicopathologic study of 25 children. Semin Diagn Pathol 3:138–150, 1986.

Fu YS, Perzin KH: Non-epithelial tumors of the nasal cavity, paranasal sinuses, and nasopharynx: a clinicopathologic study. VI: fibrous tissue tumors (fibroma, fibromatosis, and fibrosarcoma). Cancer 37:2912–2928, 1976.

Masson JK, Soule EH: Desmoid tumors of the head and neck. Am J Surg 112:615–622, 1966.

Olsen KD, DeSanto LW, Wold LE, Weiland LH: Tumefactive fibroinflammatory lesions of the head and neck. Laryngoscope 96:940–944, 1986.

Wara WM, Phillips TL, Hill DR, Borill E, Luk KH, Lichter AS, Leibel SA: Desmoid tumors—treatment and prognosis. Radiology 124:225–226, 1977.

Wold LE, Weiland LH: Tumefactive fibroinflammatory lesions of the head and neck. Am J Surg Pathol 7:477–482, 1983.

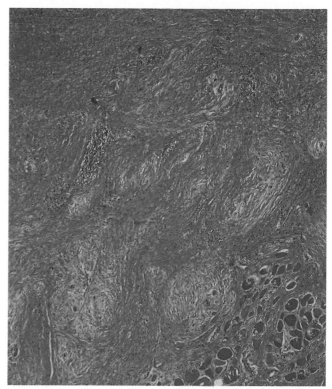

Figure 4–22. Fibromatosis, consisting of a poorly circumscribed, hypocellular lesion composed of spindle-shaped cells, collagen production, focal myxoid-appearing stroma, scattered inflammatory cells, and an infiltrative growth into surrounding muscle.

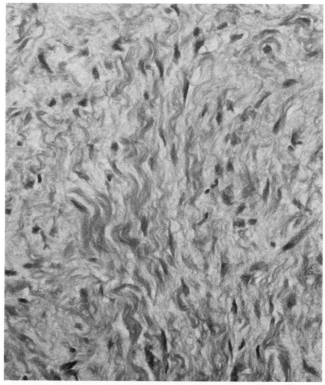

Figure 4–23. The spindle-shaped cellular infiltrate of fibromatosis is bland and uniform-appearing, with pale-staining nuclei that are associated with and separated by collagen production.

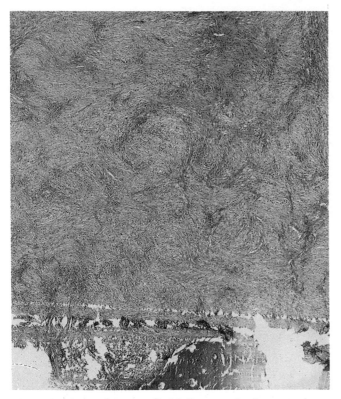

Figure 4–24. Another example of fibromatosis, demonstrating a vague, lobular pattern with a prominent inflammatory cell infiltrate; the lesion extends into adjacent bone.

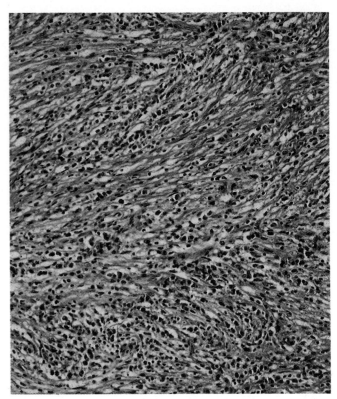

Figure 4–25. Fibromatosis with an associated, marked inflammatory component composed of lymphocytes, plasma cells, and eosinophils that obscure the bland-appearing fibroblasts.

6. Leiomyoma

Definition: Benign tumor of smooth muscle.

Clinical

■ In general, one of the least common mesenchymal tumors in the head and neck area, due to the relative absence of smooth muscle in this region.
■ Affects men more than women; may occur in all ages, but generally is a tumor of adult life.
■ Most common sites of occurrence in the head and neck are skin and oral cavity (lips, tongue, and palate); other sites that may be affected include the nasal cavity and paranasal sinuses, and the larynx.
■ A painless mass is the most common presenting complaint; other symptoms include dysphagia, airway obstruction, voice changes, and pain.
■ Origination thought to be from the smooth muscle within vascular structures or cutaneous appendages.

Pathology

Gross

■ Solitary, well-demarcated, sessile, tan-white submucosal lesion, usually measuring <3 cm in diameter, but may attain larger sizes.
■ On cut section, the tumor is homogeneous, with a whorled appearance.

Histology

■ Interlacing bundles or fascicles of cells composed of blunt-ended or "cigar-shaped" nuclei with abundant eosinophilic cytoplasm.
■ No significant pleomorphism or mitotic activity.
■ Vascularity is always seen and varies from being limited to marked (angiomyoma) in extent.
■ Nuclear palisading and perinuclear vacuolization may be seen.
■ Myxoid stroma, fibrosis, calcification, and ossification may occur.

- On rare occasions, the nuclei may appear epithelioid.
- Histochemistry: cytoplasmic myofibrils can be demonstrated by special stains, appearing red with Masson trichrome and blue with phosphotungstic acid-hematoxylin (PTAH).
- Immunohistochemistry: actin (smooth muscle and muscle-specific) positive; variably desmin positive.
- Electronmicroscopy: myofilaments, pinocytotic vesicles, investing basal laminae.

Differential Diagnosis

- Peripheral nerve sheath tumor (neurofibroma, schwannoma) (Chapter 9A, #6).

Treatment and Prognosis

- Complete surgical excision is curative.
- Rarely recurs.

References

Barnes L: Leiomyoma. *In*: Barnes L, ed. Surgical pathology of the head and neck. New York: Marcel Dekker, 1985; pp 742–746.

Cherrick HM, Dunlap CL, King OH: Leiomyomas of the oral cavity: review of the literature and clinicopathologic study of seven new cases. Oral Surg Oral Med Oral Pathol 35:54–66, 1973.

Farman AG: Benign smooth muscle tumours. S Afr Med J 49:1333–1340, 1975.

Fu YS, Perzin KH: Non-epithelial tumors of the nasal cavity, paranasal sinuses, and nasopharynx: a clinicopathologic study. IV: smooth muscle tumors (leiomyoma, leiomyosarcoma). Cancer 35:1300–1308, 1975.

Kleinsasser O, Glanz H: Myogenic tumors of the larynx. Arch Otorhinolaryngol 225:107–119, 1978.

Shibata K, Komune S: Laryngeal angioma (vascular leiomyoma): clinicopathological findings. Laryngoscope 90:1880–1886, 1980.

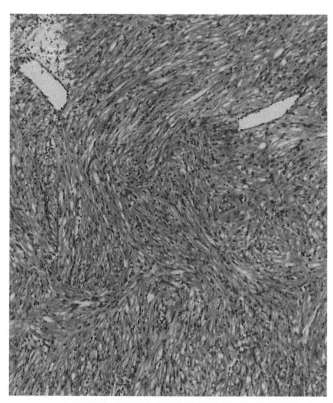

Figure 4–27. Portion of a submucosal (sinonasal) leiomyoma with a fascicular growth composed of interlacing cellular bundles and associated vascular spaces.

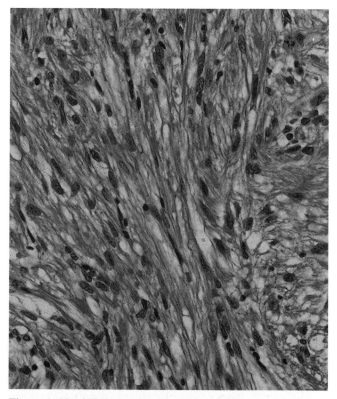

Figure 4–28. Cellular component of the leiomyoma consists of cells with blunt-ended or "cigar-shaped" nuclei, abundant eosinophilic cytoplasm, and perinuclear vacuolization; no significant pleomorphism or mitotic activity is seen.

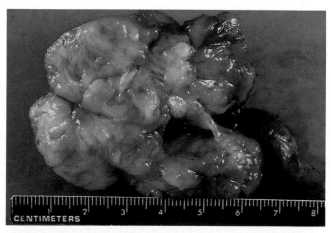

Figure 4–26. Large, sinonasal tract leiomyoma, characterized by a tan-white and whorled appearance.

7. Benign Fibro-Osseous and Osseous Lesions

a. Fibrous Dysplasia

Definition: Idiopathic, non-neoplastic bone disease, in which normal medullary bone is replaced by structurally weak fibrous and osseous tissue.

Clinical

■ Three variants: monostotic, polyostotic, McCune-Albright syndrome.

(1) MONOSTOTIC FIBROUS DYSPLASIA

Only a single osseous site is involved.

Represents >70% of all cases of fibrous dysplasia.

Frequently occurs in older children and young adults.

Most commonly affects the ribs, femur, and tibia, but involves head and neck sites in up to 25% of cases.

In the head and neck, the most common sites of involvement include maxilla (zygomatic process) > mandible (region of premolar and molar teeth) > frontal bone > ethmoid and sphenoid bones > temporal bone.

(2) POLYOSTOTIC FIBROUS DYSPLASIA

Involvement of two or more bones.

Represents approximately 25% of all cases of fibrous dysplasia.

May be limited to a few bones in one anatomic region, or may be diffuse, affecting virtually every bone in the skeleton.

In greater than half the cases, osseous involvement includes the long bones of the extremities, pelvic bones, ribs, metacarpals, metatarsals, and the humerus.

The bones of the head and neck are involved in up to 50% of cases.

(3) MCCUNE-ALBRIGHT SYNDROME

Triad identified in this syndrome includes:
1. Polyostotic fibrous dysplasia.
2. Endocrine dysfunction (hyperthyroidism or sexual precocity, the latter predominantly identified in females).
3. Cutaneous hyperpigmentation.

Least common variant of fibrous dysplasia, representing approximately 3% of cases.

■ Regardless of type, the majority of patients affected by fibrous dysplasia are under 30 years of age, although older individuals may be affected.

■ No sex predilection in the monostotic variant, but affects females more than males in the polyostotic type.

■ Head and neck symptoms of fibrous dysplasia include painless, asymmetric swelling associated with functional disturbances; displacement or malocclusion of teeth, failure of tooth eruption in children; headaches, proptosis, nasal obstruction, and hearing loss (conductive).

■ Serum calcium and phosphorous levels are normal; alkaline phosphatase may be elevated.

Radiology

■ Poorly defined expansile osseous lesion with a thin, intact cortex.

■ Predominantly fibrous lesions are radiolucent.

■ Predominantly osseous lesions are radiodense.

■ Equal admixture of fibrous and osseous components results in a ground-glass appearance.

■ Usually no periosteal reaction is seen unless there is an associated fracture.

Pathology

Gross

■ Tan-white to yellow, soft, rubbery, gritty, or firm tissue.

■ Thin cortex.

Histology

■ Fibrous tissue component is nondescript, without pattern and of variable cellularity.

■ Osseous component is immature (woven) bone that arises metaplastically from the fibrous stroma and is poorly oriented, with misshapen bony trabeculae, increased cellularity, and irregular margins, and forms odd geometric patterns, including "C"- or "S"-shaped configurations (Chinese characters).

■ Trabeculae typically lack osteoblastic rimming.

■ Multinucleated giant cells, macrophages, increased vascularity, and calcification may be seen.

■ Under polarized light, bone appears woven rather than lamellar; however, lamellar bone can be seen in fibrous dysplasia, and its presence does not exclude the diagnosis.

Differential Diagnosis

■ Ossifying fibroma (see below).

Treatment and Prognosis

■ Conservative surgical excision is the preferred treatment and is indicated only in cases with compromise of function, progression of deformity, pain, associated pathologic fracture, or the development of a malignancy.

■ Disease may stabilize at puberty and, in children, therapy should be delayed if possible until after puberty.

■ Recurrence rates are low, and death due to extension into vital structures rarely occurs.

■ Risk of malignant transformation occurs in <1% of cases and is identified more often in association with the polyostotic type; malignant transformation most often is an osteosarcoma.

■ Radiation treatment is not used because of the risk of inducing malignant transformation.

b. Ossifying Fibroma

Definition: Encapsulated, slow-growing benign fibro-osseous neoplasm, composed of fibrous tissue admixed with varying amounts of mature bone.
Synonyms: Fibrous osteoma; osteofibroma.

Clinical

■ In craniofacial bones, ossifying fibromas affect women more frequently than men; can occur over a wide age range, but are most frequently seen in the third and fourth decades of life.
■ The most common site of occurrence is the mandible (molar area), followed by the maxilla (antrum).
■ Generally asymptomatic, unassociated with pain or swelling and often diagnosed incidentally after radiographic examination; symptomatic tumors are manifested by displacement of teeth or as an expansile mass.

Radiology

■ Well-circumscribed lesion, with smooth contours having a variation in appearance based on the maturity of the tumor, including:
Completely radiolucent—immature lesion.
Completely radiopaque —mature lesion.
Mixed—increased mineralization with age results in radiopaque foci admixed with radiolucent areas.

Pathology

Gross

■ Tan/gray to white, gritty, and firm lesions, varying in size from 0.5 to 10 cm.

Histology

■ Encapsulated lesion, with randomly distributed mature (lamellar) bone spicules rimmed by osteoblasts admixed with a fibrous stroma.
■ Although the osseous component is generally described as mature, the central portions may be woven bone with lamellar bone at the periphery; complete bone maturation is seldom seen.
■ Fibrous stroma may be densely cellular; hemorrhage, inflammation, and giant cells may be seen.

Differential Diagnosis

■ Fibrous dysplasia (see above).

Treatment and Prognosis

■ Surgical excision is the treatment of choice, and the well-circumscribed nature of this lesion allows for relatively easy removal.

■ Prognosis is excellent after complete excision.
■ Recurrences rarely occur.

Additional Facts

■ Gnathic fibro-osseous lesions (fibrous dysplasia and ossifying fibromas) may be histologically indistinguishable; therefore, the diagnosis and differentiation rests on the clinical–radiologic–histopathologic correlation.
■ Differentiation of ossifying fibromas from fibrous dysplasia is important, because the therapeutic rationale differs for these lesions.
■ Ossifying fibroma has been suggested as arising from the mesenchyme of the periodontal ligament and as such is related to the cementifying fibroma and cemento-ossifying fibroma.

c. Juvenile Active Ossifying Fibroma

Definition: Variant of ossifying fibroma that may potentially behave aggressively, with locally destructive capabilities.
Synonym: Psammomatoid ossifying fibroma.

Clinical

■ No sex predilection; although identified in association with younger age groups (first and second decades), this lesion can occur over a wide age range, including older individuals.
■ May involve single or multiple sinuses, as well as the orbit (ethmoid > nasal cavity > maxillary sinus > frontal sinus).
■ Presenting symptoms include facial swelling, nasal obstruction, pain, sinusitis, headache, and proptosis.

Radiology

■ Lytic or mixed lytic/radiopaque osseous or soft-tissue mass, varying from well-demarcated to invasive with bone erosion.

Pathology

Histology

Variable admixture of:
■ Numerous small ovoid, calcified, or mineralized bony spicules with a psammomatoid appearance.
■ A cellular (active) stroma composed of spindle cells with hyperchromatic nuclei and indistinct cytoplasmic borders.
■ The presence of myxomatous material, which may become cystic.
■ A prominent vascular component may be seen within the stroma.

Differential Diagnosis

■ Osteoblastoma.
■ Osteosarcoma (Chapter 4B, #10).

Table 4–2.

CLINICOPATHOLOGIC COMPARISON OF FIBROUS DYSPLASIA, OSSIFYING
FIBROMA, AND JUVENILE OSSIFYING FIBROMA

	Fibrous Dysplasia	Ossifying Fibroma	Juvenile Active Ossifying Fibroma
Sex/age	♂ = ♀; 1st + 2nd decades	♀ > ♂; 3rd + 4th decades	♂ = ♀; 1st + 2nd decades
Site	Maxilla	Mandible	Maxilla; paranasal sinuses
Presentation	Painless swelling	Asymptomatic; expansile mass	Mass or swelling; facial asymmetry
Radiographic features	Ill-defined, expansile	Well-defined, circumscribed	Ill-defined, invasive
Histologic features	Immature (woven), odd-shaped bony trabeculae lacking osteoblastic rimming admixed with a fibrous stroma	Mature (lamellar) bone spicules rimmed by osteoblasts admixed with a fibrous stroma	Variable admixture of small mineralized (psammomatoid) bodies, a cellular (active) stroma, and the presence of myxomatous material that may become cystic
Treatment	Surgery	Surgery	Surgery
Prognosis	Good	Excellent	Generally good, but may have increased morbidity due to invasiveness
Malignant degeneration	Rare, if ever	Approximately 0.5% of cases	Rare, if ever

Treatment and Prognosis

■ Complete surgical excision, which may necessitate radical procedures.

■ Prognosis is good after complete excision, but recurrences may occur and the tumors may behave in an aggressive manner, with local destruction and potential invasion into vital structures.

References

Fibrous Dysplasia

Barnes L: Fibrous dysplasia. *In*: Barnes L, ed. Surgical pathology of the head and neck. New York: Marcel Dekker, 1985; pp 920–926.

Dahlgren SE, Lind PO, Linbom A, Martensson G: Fibrous dysplasia of the jaw bones: a clinical, roentgenographic and histopathologic study. Acta Otolaryngol (Stockh) 68:257–270, 1969.

Eversole LR, Sabes WR, Rovin S: Fibrous dysplasia: a nosologic problem in the diagnosis of fibro-osseous lesions of the jaws. J Oral Pathol Med 1:180–220, 1972.

Feldman MD, Vijay MR, Lowry LD, Kelly M: Fibrous dysplasia of the paranasal sinuses. Otolaryngol Head Neck Surg 95:222–225, 1986.

Mills SE, Fechner RE: Fibro-osseous lesions. *In*: Gnepp DR, ed. Pathology of the head and neck. New York: Churchill Livingstone, 1988; pp 382–391.

Waldron CA: Fibro-osseous lesions of the jaw. J Oral Maxillofac Surg 43:249–262, 1985.

Ossifying Fibroma

Fu YS, Perzin KH: Non-epithelial tumors of the nasal cavity, paranasal sinuses, and nasopharynx: a clinicopathologic study. II: osseous and fibro-osseous lesions including osteoma, fibrous dysplasia, ossifying fibroma, osteoblastoma, giant cell tumor, and osteosarcoma. Cancer 33:1289–1305, 1974.

Mills SE, Fechner RE: Fibro-osseous lesions. *In*: Gnepp DR, ed. Pathology of the head and neck. New York: Churchill Livingstone, 1988; pp 382–391.

Juvenile Active Ossifying Fibroma

Johnson LC, Yousefi M, Vinh TN, Heffner DK, Hyams VJ, Hartman KS: Juvenile active ossifying fibroma: its nature, dynamics and origin. Acta Otolaryngol (Stockh) Suppl 488:1–40, 1991.

Margo CE, Ragsdale BD, Perman KI, Zimmerman LE, Sweet DE: Psammomatoid (juvenile) ossifying fibroma of the orbit. Ophthalmology 92:150–159, 1985.

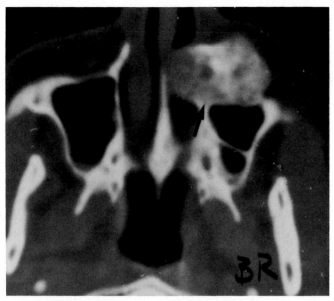

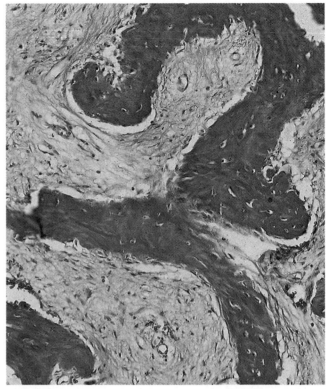

Figure 4–29. Axial CT of fibrous dysplasia, demonstrating an expansile enlargement of the alveolar ridge of the left maxilla with involvement of the anterior wall of the left maxillary sinus (*arrows*); the mass demonstrates an inhomogeneous osseous architecture with some regions displaying a ground-glass appearance. (Courtesy of Franz J. Wippold II, M.D., Mallinckrodt Institute of Radiology, St. Louis, MO.)

Figure 4–31. The fibrous tissue component of fibrous dysplasia is nondescript, without pattern, and of variable cellularity; the osseous component is immature (woven) bone, the trabeculae of which typically lack osteoblastic rimming.

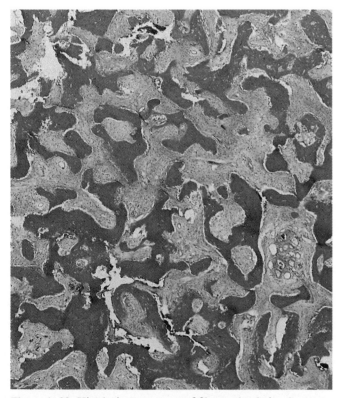

Figure 4–30. Histologic appearance of fibrous dysplasia, characterized by proliferation of fibrous tissue and osseous components; the latter have misshapen bony trabeculae and form odd geometric patterns, referred to as "Chinese" characters.

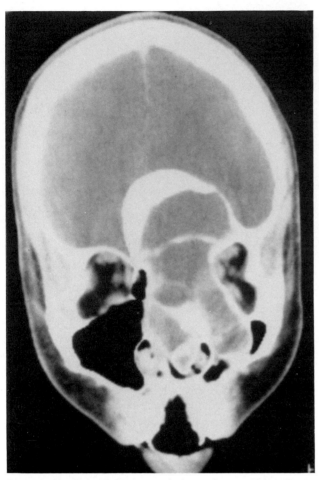

Figure 4-32. Coronal CT bone windows of an ossifying fibroma demonstrating an expansile lesion involving the floor of the anterior fossae and the underlying ethmoid sinus. The lesion encroaches on the left orbit. The intracranial portion is "capped" by thick hyperostosis. (Case courtesy of Mahmood F. Mafee, M.D., Department of Radiology, The University of Illinois College of Medicine, Chicago, IL.)

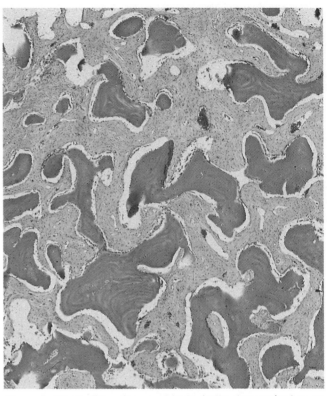

Figure 4-33. Ossifying fibroma, histologically characterized as an admixture of mature (lamellar) bone and a fibrous stroma.

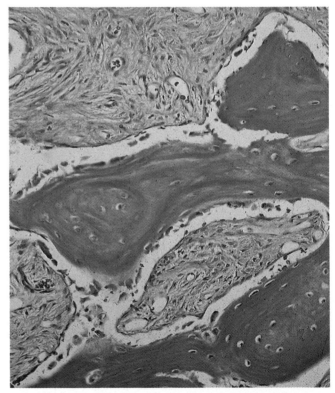

Figure 4-34. In contrast to fibrous dysplasia, the osseous component of ossifying fibroma is composed of mature (lamellar) bone with the spicules rimmed by osteoblasts; fibrous stroma is similar to that seen in fibrous dysplasia.

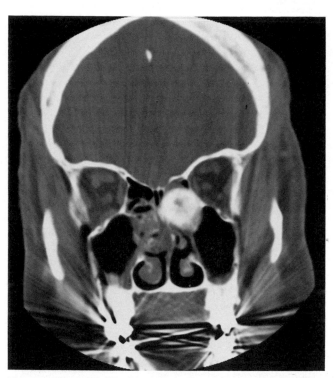

Figure 4–35. Axial CT of juvenile active ossifying fibroma (JAOF) demonstrating an inhomogenous, radiodense mass in the left ethmoid and maxillary sinuses that causes bowing outward of the medial wall of the left orbit and displacement but not destruction of the nasal septum.

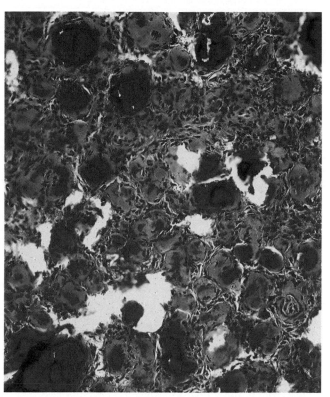

Figure 4–37. JAOF, composed of psammomatoid bony spicules with associated spindle cell stromal component with hyperchromatic nuclei and indistinct cytoplasmic borders.

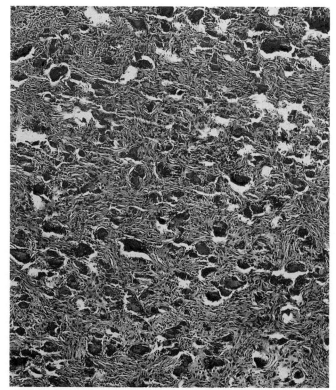

Figure 4–36. JAOF, characterized by the presence of numerous, small ovoid, calcified or mineralized bony spicules with a psammomatoid appearance, admixed and surrounded by a cellular (active) stroma.

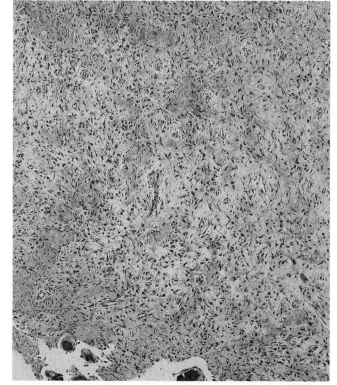

Figure 4–38. A myxomatous stroma can be seen in JAOF, which may result in the production of cystic spaces (not depicted); psammomatoid bony spicules can be seen at the lower portion of the illustration.

8. Osteoma

Definition: Benign bone-forming tumor.

Clinical

- Almost exclusively identified in the craniofacial skeleton.
- Affects men more than women; occurs over a wide age range, from the second to sixth decades.
- Most common sites of involvement are the paranasal sinuses, with the frontal sinus most often involved (frontal > ethmoid > maxillary > sphenoid); other areas of involvement include temporal bone (osseous external auditory canal), skull, mandible, maxilla.
- Usually asymptomatic, but may be associated with headaches, facial swelling or asymmetry, erosion of bone, meningitis secondary to cranial cavity extension, and sinus or aural obstruction.
- Etiology linked to trauma, infection (sinusitis), and development.
- Usually occurs as a single lesion, but may be associated with Gardner's syndrome, an inherited autosomal dominant trait characterized by intestinal (colorectal) polyposis, soft-tissue lesions (fibromatosis, cutaneous epidermoid cysts, lipomas, leiomyomas), and multiple craniofacial osteomas.

Radiology

- Sharply delineated, radiopaque lesion arising and confined to bone or protruding into a sinus.

Pathology

Histology

- Dense, mature, predominantly lamellar bone.

- Interosseous spaces may be composed of fibrous, fibrovascular, or fatty tissue.

Differential Diagnosis

- Exostosis.

Treatment and Prognosis

- Unless symptomatic, osteomas require no treatment.
- Symptomatic osteomas require complete surgical excision, which is curative.

Additional Facts

- Controversy exists as to whether the osteoma represents a true neoplasm or possibly the end-stage of a fibro-osseous lesion.
- No link to the development of osteosarcoma.

References

Atallah N, Jay MM: Osteomas of the paranasal sinuses. J Laryngol Otol 95: 291–304, 1981.

Fu YS, Perzin KH: Non-epithelial tumors of the nasal cavity, paranasal sinuses, and nasopharynx: a clinicopathologic study. II: osseous and fibro-osseous lesions including osteoma, fibrous dysplasia, ossifying fibroma, osteoblastoma, giant cell tumor, and osteosarcoma. Cancer 33:1289–1305, 1974.

Samy LL, Mostafa H: Osteomata of the nose and paranasal sinuses with a report of twenty-one cases. J Laryngol Otol 85:449–469, 1971.

Spjut HJ, Dorfman HD, Fechner RE, Ackerman LV: Tumors of the bone and cartilage. Atlas of tumor pathology. Fascicle 5, second series. Washington, DC: Armed Forces Institute of Pathology, 1971; pp 117–119.

Smith ME, Calcaterra TC: Frontal sinus osteoma. Ann Otol Rhinol Laryngol 98:896–900, 1989.

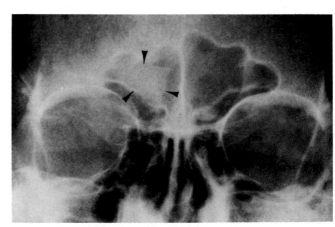

Figure 4–39. Plain frontal film of a frontal sinus osteoma demonstrating a well-defined bony density (*arrowheads*) within an otherwise aerated frontal sinus. (Case courtesy of Franz J. Wippold II, M.D., Mallinckrodt Institute of Radiology, St. Louis, MO.

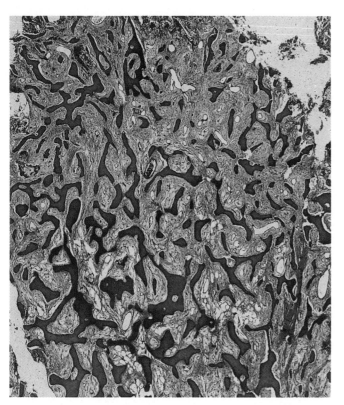

Figure 4–40. Osteoma composed of dense, mature, predominantly lamellar bone, which is associated with interosseous spaces composed of a loose fibrovascular stroma.

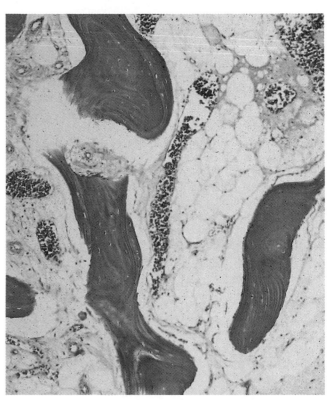

Figure 4–41. Portion of an osteoma with mature bony spicules, which are associated with an interosseous fatty tissue component.

9. Sinonasal Myxoma and Fibromyxoma

Definition: Benign neoplasm of uncertain histogenesis with a characteristic histologic appearance, often behaving in an aggressive (infiltrating) manner.

Clinical

■ In the head and neck, two forms of myxomas/fibromyxomas are identified: facial skeleton–derived and soft tissue–derived.

FACIAL SKELETON–DERIVED

■ No sex predilection; occurs over a wide age range but is most frequently seen in the second and third decades of life.
■ In general, this is a tumor of the jaw bones and is uncommon in extragnathic locations; the mandible (posterior and condylar regions) is affected more often than the maxilla (zygomatic process and alveolar bone); extragnathic involvement includes paranasal sinuses, primarily the maxillary sinus (antrum), often associated with extension into the nasal cavity, and the middle ear.
■ Presentation usually is as a painless swelling of the affected area.
■ Localization to the jaw bones has led to the belief that these tumors take origin from the primordial odontogenic mesenchyme or from an osteogenic embryonic connective tissue.

MYXOMA OF SOFT TISSUES

■ Primarily a tumor involving the extremities.
■ No sex predilection; is seen over a wide age range and is not specific to any decade of life.
■ In the head and neck, common sites include the paraoral soft tissues, pharynx, larynx, parotid gland, tonsil, and ear.
■ Presents as an asymptomatic mass.
■ Association between multiple myxomas and fibrous dysplasia has been noted.

Radiology

■ Unilocular or multilocular radiolucency with a "honeycomb" or "soap bubble" appearance.

Pathology

Gross

■ Well-delineated but unencapsulated multinodular, rubbery to firm, tan-yellow to gray-white lesion with a gelatinous appearance.

Histology

■ Scant, loosely cellular proliferation, consisting of spindle-shaped or stellate-appearing cells embedded in an abundant mucinous stroma.

■ Amount of collagenous fibrillary material varies for each case and, depending on the extent of its presence, may confer the term fibromyxoma on the tumor.

■ Limited or poorly vascularized but apparent vascular component can be identified.

■ Mitoses, cellular pleomorphism, and necrosis are absent.

■ Odontogenic epithelium may or may not be seen.

■ The periphery of the tumor appears circumscribed, but local infiltration with replacement of bone can be seen.

■ Mucinous stroma stains positive for mucopolysaccharides.

■ Special stains are of limited utility in the diagnosis.

Differential Diagnosis

■ Dental papillae.
■ Nasal (inflammatory) polyps (Chapter 3, #1).
■ Vocal cord polyps (Chapter 13, #1).
■ Peripheral nerve sheath tumors (Chapter 9A, #6).
■ Myxoid variants of malignant fibrous histiocytoma (Chapter 4B, #6), liposarcoma (Chapter 9B, #8), and rhabdomyosarcoma (Chapter 9B, #5).

Treatment and Prognosis

■ Conservative but adequate local excision.
■ These tumors tend to be slow growing and usually follow a benign course; they may have the potential for local destruction but, after adequate excision, rarely recur or metastasize.

Additional Facts

■ Metastases from a presumptive myxoma/fibromyxoma should seriously place that diagnosis in doubt and, in fact, may represent a myxoid variant of a sarcoma (liposarcoma, malignant fibrous histiocytoma, or rhabdomyosarcoma).

■ A separate and distinct benign tumor of cartilaginous origin that may involve the craniofacial and paranasal sinus bones is the *chondromyxoid fibroma:*

Affects men more than women; most common in the second to third decades of life.

The mandible is the most common site (symphysis or molar-retromolar area); symptoms include pain, loosening of the teeth, difficulties in opening the jaws, and headaches.

Radiographic appearance varies, depending on the involved bone, from round or oval, well-demarcated, radiolucent lesions, usually measuring <5 cm in long bones, to large, irregularly outlined lesions in flat bones.

Histology is characterized by a lobular appearance, with lobules separated by vascularized connective tissue and a zonal arrangement of the cellular component: centers of the lobules are predominantly myxoid, with scattered, stellate-appearing cells; peripheries of the lobules are more cellular, composed of cells with round to oval to spindle-shaped nuclei and an eosinophilic to amphophilic cytoplasm, often with multipolar, stellate extensions.

With time, the myxoid areas may become fibrotic; presence of cartilage varies but never exceeds 75% of the total tumor volume; osteoclastic giant cells and calcifications may be seen.

Surgery (en bloc resection) is the treatment of choice; local recurrences may occur if incompletely excised (curettage); malignant transformation in the absence of prior irradiation rarely occurs.

References

Barnes L: Chondromyxoid fibroma. *In*: Barnes L, ed. Surgical pathology of the head and neck. New York: Marcel Dekker, 1985; pp 962–965.

Barros RE, Dominguez FV, Cabrini RL: Myxoma of the jaws. Oral Surg Oral Med Oral Pathol 27:225–236, 1969.

Bochetta J, Minkowitz F, Minkowitz S, et al: Antral fibromyxoma presenting as a giant nasal polyp. Oral Surg Oral Med Oral Pathol 23:201–206, 1967.

Canalis RF, Smith GA, Konrad HR: Myxomas of the head and neck. Arch Otolaryngol Head Neck Surg 102:300–305, 1976.

Fu YS, Perzin KH: Non-epithelial tumors of the nasal cavity, paranasal sinuses, and nasopharynx: a clinicopathologic study. VII: Myxomas. Cancer 39:195–203, 1977.

Rahimi A, Beabout JW, Ivins JC, Dahlin DC: Chondromyxoid fibroma: a clinicopathologic study of 76 cases. Cancer 30:726–736, 1972.

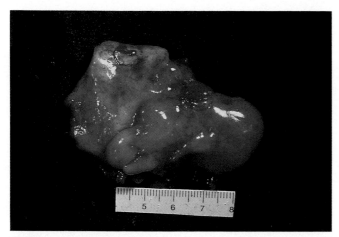

Figure 4–42. Large, multinodular sinonasal fibromyxoma with a glistening, tan-yellow appearance.

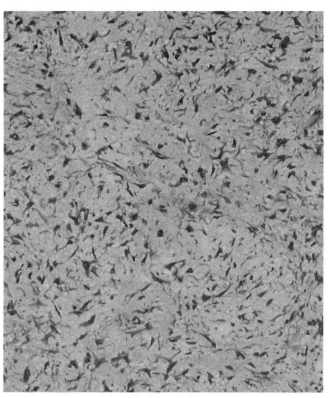

Figure 4–44. Loosely cellular proliferation, consisting of spindle-shaped or stellate-appearing cells embedded in an abundant mucinous stroma.

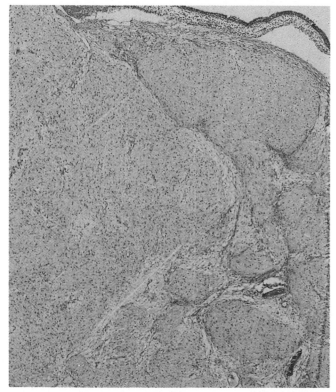

Figure 4–43. Fibromyxoma characterized by a lobular growth, which is composed of spindle-shaped, cellular proliferation associated with a mucinous stroma; a compressed, slit-like vascular component can be identified.

Figure 4–45. Sinonasal myxoma with predominantly myxoid stroma and a relatively hypocellular, spindle-shaped cellular proliferation; vascular component is scant but is readily identifiable.

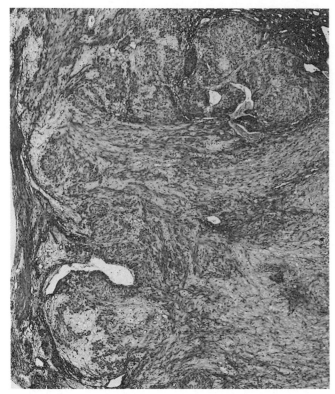

Figure 4–46. Chondromyxoid fibroma, characterized by a lobular appearance with lobules separated by vascularized connective tissue; the lobules demonstrate a zonal arrangement of the cellular component, with the center of the lobules being predominantly composed of a chondromyxoid matrix with scattered, stellate-appearing cells and the periphery of the lobules being more cellular.

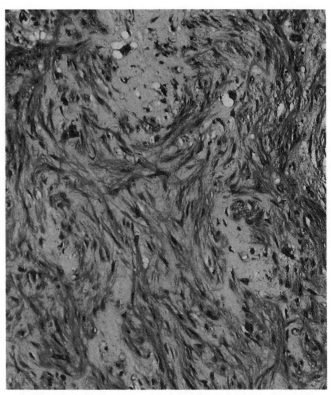

Figure 4–47. Cellular components of the chondromyxoid fibroma, which is composed of cells with round to oval to spindle-shaped nuclei and an eosinophilic to amphophilic cytoplasm, often with multipolar, stellate extensions set in a chondroid to mucinous-appearing matrix.

10. Ameloblastoma

Definition: Benign but locally invasive tumor, originating centrally in bone and arising from odontogenic epithelium.

Synonyms: Adamantinoma; adamantoblastoma.

Clinical

- The most common odontogenic tumor, but represents approximately 1% of all lesions of the jaws.
- No sex predilection; may occur at any age, but is most common in the third to fourth decades of life.
- May involve the sinonasal tract; in particular, the maxillary sinus.
- More than 80% involve the mandible (molar-ramus area > premolar area > symphysis); often associated with unerupted third molar teeth.
- Maxillary ameloblastomas primarily occur in the molar region, but the antrum and floor of the nasal cavity are often involved.
- The most common clinical presentation is a painless swelling of the affected area; maxillary sinus or nasal cavity involvement results in nasal obstruction.

Radiology

- Unilocular or multilocular radiolucent lesion, with a honeycomb appearance and scalloped borders.
- Extensive thinning of cortical bone can often be seen.
- Sinus involvement causes cloudiness or opacification and erosion or destruction of the antral walls.
- Completely osteolytic lesion, because ameloblastomas do not produce a mineralized component.
- Radiolucency often associated with an unerupted tooth, making it indistinguishable from a dentigerous cyst.

Pathology

Histology

- Unencapsulated proliferating nests, islands, or sheets of odontogenic epithelium that resemble the enamel organ.

- The epithelium is composed of:
  Central area of loosely arranged cells, similar to the stellate reticulum of the enamel organ.
  Peripheral area of palisading columnar or cuboidal cells, with hyperchromatic small nuclei oriented away from the basement membrane.
- Areas of hyalinization are often seen surrounding nests or follicles.
- Histologic subtypes of ameloblastoma include:
  Follicular (solid and cystic).
  Plexiform.
  Acanthomatous.
  Basal cell.
  Granular cell.

Differential Diagnosis

- Dentigerous cyst.
- Odontogenic keratocyst.
- Ameloblastic fibroma.
- Basal cell carcinoma (Chapter 25C, #1).
- Adenoid cystic carcinoma (Chapter 19B, #3).

Treatment and Prognosis

- Complete surgical excision, which may be conservative if the tumor is small and well delineated; en bloc surgical excision may be required for those tumors that have spread to adjacent bone.
- Curettement of the tumor is not an acceptable form of therapy.
- Hemi- and total mandibulectomies are seldom required.
- Ameloblastomas are considered radioresistant, and chemotherapy has no proven efficacy.
- In general, ameloblastomas are slow-growing, indolent tumors; however, recurrence of tumor is not uncommon and may lead to extensive local destruction with facial disfigurement or may pose life-threatening complications as a result of extension into vital structures.
- Metastases are rare and are generally related to long-standing tumors associated with multiple surgical procedures or radiation treatment; these are referred to as malignant ameloblastomas when the histologic features in both the primary and metastatic tumors are benign.

Additional Facts

- The histologic subtypes of ameloblastoma can be:
  Identified within the same tumor.
  Have no bearing on treatment or prognosis, except for the granular cell variant, which appears to be associated with an increased recurrence rate.
- Prognosis is dependent on size, extent, and location of the tumor:
  Mandibular ameloblastomas tend to be confined tumors, due to the inherently thick cortical bone of the mandible.
  Maxillary ameloblastomas are more likely to demonstrate extension beyond the bone, due to the maxilla's lacking a thick cortical bone and the intimate association with the sinonasal cavity.
- Histologic malignant transformation of an ameloblastoma is referred to as *ameloblastic carcinoma,* which is noteworthy for:
  Predilection for the mandible.
  Morphologically similar to squamous cell carcinoma.
  Metastasizes to the lungs, lymph nodes, bone, and liver.
  Treated by surgical excision.

References

Hoffman S, Jacoway JR, Krolls SO: Ameloblastoma. *In*: Hoffman S, Jacoway JR, Krolls SO, eds. Intraosseous and paraosteal tumors of the jaws. Atlas of tumor pathology. Fascicle 24, second series. Washington, DC: Armed Forces Institute of Pathology, 1985; pp 94–101.

Tsaknis PJ, Nelson JF: The maxillary ameloblastoma: an analysis of 24 cases. J Oral Surg 38:336–342, 1980.

Verbin RS: Ameloblastoma and related lesions. *In*: Barnes L, ed. Surgical pathology of the head and neck. New York: Marcel Dekker, 1985; pp 1331–1346.

Waldron CA: Ameloblastoma. *In*: Gnepp DR, ed. Pathology of the head and neck. New York: Churchill Livingstone, 1988, pp 403–416.

Figure 4–48. Ameloblastoma, right maxillary antrum. (*A*) Axial MR, T1-weighted; inhomogeneous soft tissue mass (m) expanding the right maxillary antrum and destroying the anterior wall. (*B*) Axial MR, T1-weighted, enhanced; following administration of intravenous gadopentate dimeglumine, the mass (m) contrast enhances. (Courtesy of Franz J. Wippold II, M.D., Mallinckrodt Institute of Radiology, St. Louis, MO.)

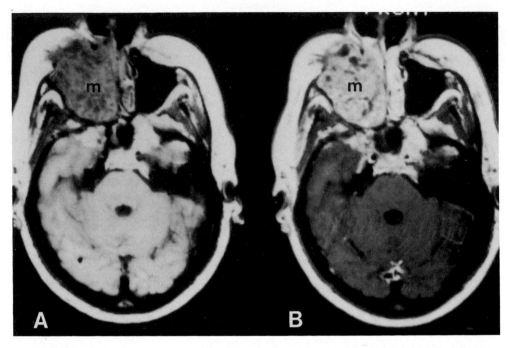

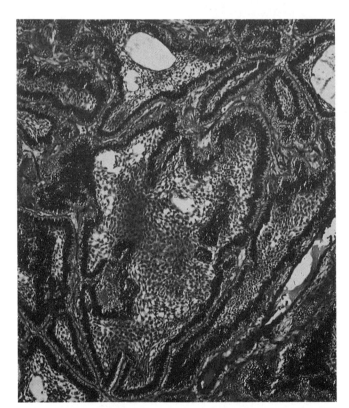

Figure 4–49. Ameloblastoma, composed of unencapsulated proliferating nests or islands of odontogenic epithelium.

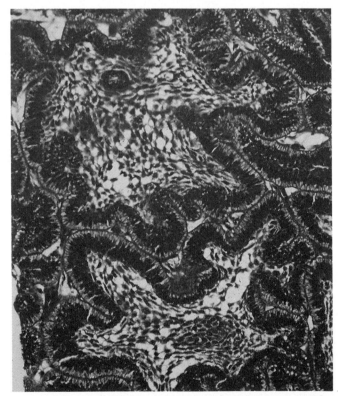

Figure 4–50. Ameloblastic epithelium, composed of a central area of loosely arranged cells, similar to the stellate reticulum of the enamel organ, and a peripheral area of palisading columnar or cuboidal cells with hyperchromatic small nuclei oriented away from the basement membrane.

B. MALIGNANT NEOPLASMS

1. Squamous Cell Carcinoma

Definition: Malignant epithelial neoplasms arising from the surface epithelium with squamous cell or epidermoid differentiation.

Synonyms: Epidermoid carcinoma; nonkeratinizing carcinoma; transitional carcinoma; respiratory mucosal carcinoma; Ringertz carcinoma.

Clinical

- Represents approximately 3% of head and neck malignant neoplasms and <1% of all malignant neoplasms.
- Represents the most common type of malignant epithelial neoplasm affecting this region.
- Affects men more than women; most frequently seen in the sixth and seventh decades of life, with 95% of cases arising in patients older than 40 years.
- Most common site of occurrence is the antrum of the maxillary sinus > nasal cavity > ethmoid sinus > sphenoid and frontal sinuses.
- The diagnosis of carcinoma of the paranasal sinuses is often delayed, because signs and symptoms often are identical to those of chronic sinusitis.
- The diagnosis of carcinoma of the nasal cavity is usually recognized relatively early in the course of disease, because symptoms prompt earlier clinical detection.
- Clinical presentations include asymmetry of the face, unilateral nasal obstruction, epistaxis, tumor mass palpable or visible in the nasal or oral cavity, pain, persistent purulent rhinorrhea, nonhealing sore or ulcer, exophthalmos.
- Risk factors include nickel and thorotrast exposure.

Radiology

- Nonexpansile mass causing sinus opacification with erosion or destruction of the sinus bony confines and extension to adjacent soft-tissue structures.

Pathology

Gross

- Variation in appearance, including friable polypoid, papillary, or fungating growth, with a tan/white to red/pink color.

Histology

KERATINIZING SUBTYPE (represents 80% to 85% of all cases)

- Architectural patterns include papillary, exophytic, or inverted.
- Surface keratinization and individual cell keratinization are generally readily identifiable.
- Varies from well differentiated to poorly differentiated.
- Dyskeratosis may be prominent.

NONKERATINIZING SUBTYPE (represents 15% to 20% of all cases)

- Papillary or exophytic growth pattern is often associated with an inverted growth phase.
- Typically, broad interconnecting bands of the neoplastic epithelium are seen.
- Hypercellular tumor, composed of elongated cells with a cylindrical or columnar appearance, oriented perpendicular to the surface and lacking evidence of keratinization.
- Cells vary from being fairly uniform to having marked pleomorphism with loss of polarity and with increased mitotic activity.
- Stroma composed of fibrovascular cores.
- In both histologic types, mucus-producing cells may be seen within the neoplastic epithelium and represent residual normal epithelial components.
- A spindle-cell component may be seen in association with either histologic type and may also occur independently.

Differential Diagnosis

- Schneiderian papillomas (Chapter 4A, #1).

Treatment and Prognosis

- Therapy and prognosis are related to clinical stage.
- Therapeutic modalities include surgery and radiotherapy.
- Recurrence of tumor occurs frequently.
- Metastases are uncommon if the tumor is confined to the involved sinus; however, extension beyond the sinus wall results in higher incidence of regional lymph node metastatic disease.
- In general, the overall 5-year survival rate is approximately 60%.
- Factors portending a poorer prognosis include:
  Involvement of more than one area.
  Extension beyond the nasal cavity or paranasal sinuses.
  Regional lymph node metastasis.
  Large size.
- Histomorphology has no bearing on the prognosis.

Additional Facts

- Carcinoma of the nasal septum is extremely rare.
- The nasal vestibule represents cutaneous tissue, and carcinomas arising in this region correlate pathologically and biologically to cutaneous-derived cancers.
- Although the frontal and sphenoid sinuses may be the sites of a primary carcinoma, most of the neoplasms involving these sinuses arise from the ethmoid sinus or from the nasopharynx.
- The respiratory ciliated columnar epithelium is capable of differentiating along various cell lines, ac-

counting for the morphologic variety of carcinomas arising from this surface (squamous cell carcinoma, adenocarcinoma, adenosquamous carcinoma).

■ The TNM staging (tumor, nodes, and metastases) of sinonasal tract mucosal carcinomas applies only to the maxillary sinus.

References

Batsakis JG, Rice DH, Solomon AR: The pathology of head and neck tumors: squamous and mucous-gland carcinomas of the nasal cavity, paranasal sinuses and larynx, part 6. Head Neck Surg 2:497–508, 1980.

Chaudhry AP, Gorlin RJ, Mosser DG: Carcinoma of the antrum: a clinical and histopathologic study. Oral Surg Oral Med Oral Pathol 13:269–281, 1960.

Hyams VJ, Batsakis JG, Michaels L: Squamous cell carcinoma of the sinonasal tract mucosa. *In*: Hyams VJ, Batsakis JG, Michaels L, eds. Tumors of the upper respiratory tract and ear. Fascicle 25, second series. Washington, DC: Armed Forces Institute of Pathology, 1988; pp 58–62.

Lavertu P, Roberts JK, Kraus DH, Levine HL, Wood BG, Medendorp SV, Tucker HM: Squamous cell carcinoma of the paranasal sinuses: the Cleveland Clinic experience. Laryngoscope 99:1130–1136, 1989.

Shidnia H, Hartsough AB, Weisberger E, Hornback NB: Epithelial carcinoma of the nasal fossa. Laryngoscope 97:717–723, 1987.

Sisson GA, Toriumi DM, Atiyah RA: Paranasal sinus malignancy: a comprehensive update. Laryngoscope 99:143–150, 1989.

Verbin RS: Squamous cell carcinoma of the maxillary sinus. *In*: Barnes L, ed. Surgical pathology of the head and neck. New York: Marcel Dekker, 1985; pp 423–430.

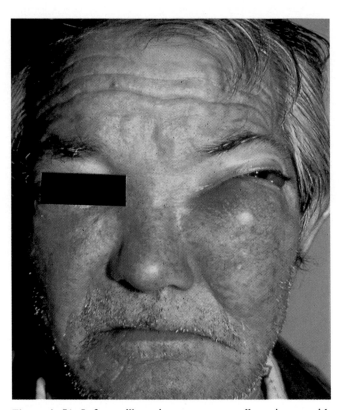

Figure 4–51. Left maxillary sinus squamous cell carcinoma with marked facial deformity, evidence of facial nerve paralysis, and orbital involvement.

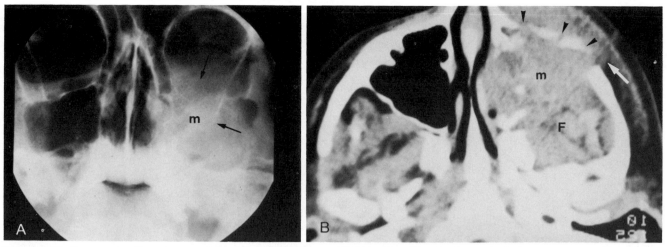

Figure 4–52. Squamous cell carcinoma of the left maxillary sinus. (*A*) Plain film, Water's view; soft tissue mass (m) opacifies the left maxillary antrum and destroys the bony lateral wall and roof (*arrows*). (*B*) Axial CT of the same patient, showing a soft tissue mass (m) extending to the soft tissues of the face (*white arrow*) through the partially destroyed anterior sinus wall (*arrowheads*). The mass also invades the infratemporal fossa (F) through the destroyed lateral wall. (Courtesy of Franz J. Wippold II, M.D., Mallinckrodt Institute of Radiology, St. Louis, MO.)

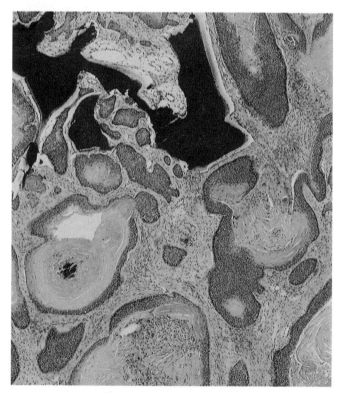

Figure 4–53. Histologic section from the tumor previously illustrated (Fig. 4–51), showing a well-differentiated squamous cell carcinoma with osseous invasion.

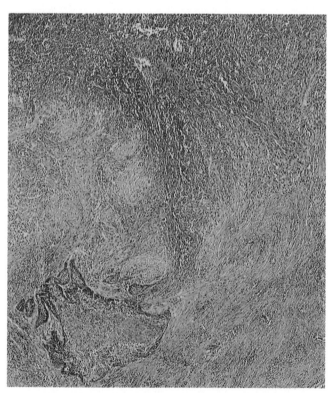

Figure 4–54. Another example of sinonasal squamous cell carcinoma; in contrast to the previous example, this neoplasm is an invasive, poorly differentiated squamous cell carcinoma.

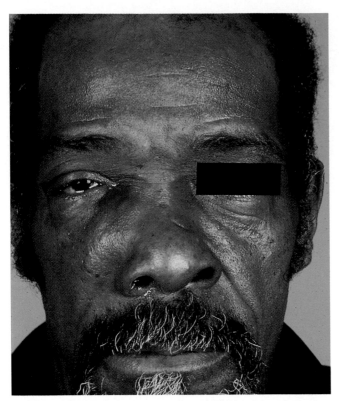

Figure 4–55. Right maxillary sinus squamous cell carcinoma, causing facial deformity with deviation of the nose to the left of midline and slight closure of the right eye.

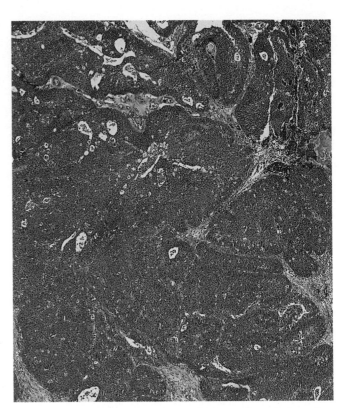

Figure 4–57. The histologic subtype of this neoplasm is that of an invasive, nonkeratinizing squamous carcinoma characterized by broad, interconnecting bands of the neoplastic epithelium, which grow down ("inverted") into the stroma.

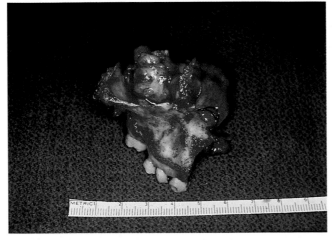

Figure 4–56. Portion of resected specimen, showing a bulging, tan-white mass in the maxillary sinus.

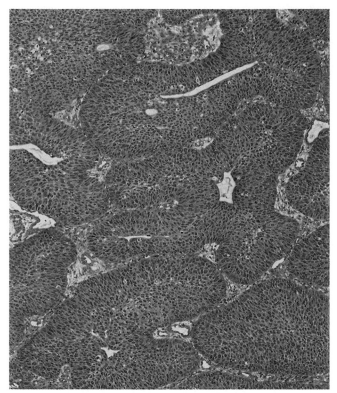

Figure 4–58. Broad, interconnecting hypercellular bands of nonkeratinizing squamous carcinoma with a growth pattern similar to transitional cell carcinoma of the urinary bladder; cells are elongated with a cylindrical or columnar appearance, oriented perpendicular to the surface, and lack evidence of keratinization.

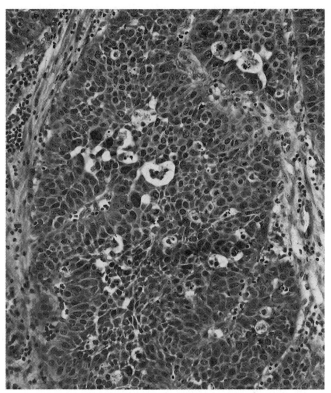

Figure 4–59. Marked cellular pleomorphism, with loss of polarity, increased nuclear–cytoplasmic ratio, and many mitotic figures characterize this nonkeratinizing squamous cell carcinoma of the maxillary sinus.

2. Sinonasal (Mucosal) Adenocarcinoma

Definition: Malignant epithelial neoplasm, arising from the surface epithelium or seromucous glands, with glandular differentiation.

Clinical

- Excluding the classic types of (minor) salivary gland adenocarcinomas, glandular neoplasms of the sinonasal tract are uncommon.
- Affects men more than women; wide age range, but most common in the sixth decade of life.
- All sites of the sinonasal cavity may be affected, with multiple sinus involvement in any one neoplasm; the intestinal type of adenocarcinomas frequently involve the ethmoid sinuses.
- Early symptoms tend to be nonspecific, varying from nasal stuffiness to obstruction that, with persistence, may have associated epistaxis, thereby prompting further clinical evaluation.
- Due to delay in diagnosis as a result of early symptoms similar to a chronic sinusitis, tumors may reach a large size with extensive invasion at the time of definitive diagnosis.
- Well-differentiated (low-grade) tumors tend to present in younger people, have a longer duration of symptoms, a minimal incidence of pain, and an absence of deformity as compared to poorly differentiated (high-grade) neoplasms.
- Etiologic factors associated with the development of certain histologic types of sinonasal adenocarcinoma have been established and include exposure to hardwood dust, leather, and softwood, with increased incidences of adenocarcinoma seen in woodworkers and workers in the shoe and furniture industries.

Pathology

Gross

- Variable appearance, ranging from tan/white to pink, flat to exophytic or papillary, friable to firm lesion of various sizes.

■ May be well demarcated or poorly defined and invasive.
■ Mucinous or gelatinous quality may be readily identifiable.

Histology

A variety of morphologic types are identified, which can be divided into well-differentiated (glandular, papillary), poorly differentiated (solid, glandular and papillary), and "colonic" or "intestinal" types.

WELL-DIFFERENTIATED SINONASAL ADENOCARCINOMA

■ May be circumscribed, but these are unencapsulated tumors arising from the surface, with transition from normal surface epithelium to neoplasm.
■ Numerous, uniform small glands or acini are seen, often with a back-to-back growth pattern without an intervening stroma; occasionally, large, irregular cystic spaces can be seen.
■ Glands are lined by a single layer of nonciliated, cuboidal to columnar cells with uniform, round nuclei, which may be limited to the basal aspect of the cell or may demonstrate stratification with loss of nuclear polarity and an eosinophilic cytoplasm.
■ A papillary variant may be seen, composed of complex papillary formations with fibrovascular cores; papillations are lined by columnar cells with vesicular to hyperchromatic nuclei with loss of cellular polarity.
■ Cellular pleomorphism is mild to moderate; occasional mitotic figures are seen, and necrosis is absent.
■ Cytomorphologic variants include clear cell and oncocytic cell types of adenocarcinoma.
■ Multiple morphologic patterns may be seen in any one neoplasm.
■ Despite the relatively bland histology, the complexity of growth, absence of two cell layers, absence of encapsulation, and presence of invasion into the submucosa confer a diagnosis of adenocarcinoma.

POORLY DIFFERENTIATED SINONASAL ADENOCARCINOMA

■ Invasive tumors that may demonstrate glandular and papillary growth but often have a predominantly solid growth pattern.
■ Moderate to marked cellular pleomorphism, increased mitotic activity, and necrosis are commonly seen.

COLONIC OR INTESTINAL-TYPE SINONASAL ADENOCARCINOMA

■ Invasive tumors with various growth patterns, including papillary-tubular, alveolar-mucoid or alveolar-goblet, signet ring, and mixed.

■ Papillary-tubular type is divided into grades I and II:

Grade I

■ Characterized by a predominant papillary growth, composed of fibrovascular cores with occasional tubular glands.
■ A single layer of pseudostratified columnar epithelial cells is seen, with oval, mildly hyperchromatic nuclei and eosinophilic cytoplasm.
■ Nuclear pleomorphism is mild.
■ This variant is reminiscent of intestinal villous adenomas and adenocarcinomas.

Grade II

■ Papillary and tubular growth, with more of a tubular pattern as compared with grade I.
■ The cells lining the irregularly shaped glands are cuboidal to columnar, with variation in the nuclear appearance that ranges from uniform and moderately hyperchromatic to markedly pleomorphic with coarse chromatin and prominent nucleoli.
■ This variant is reminiscent of the typical intestinal colonic adenocarcinoma.

Alveolar-Mucoid or Alveolar-Goblet and Signet Ring

■ Arises from the seromucous glands and is confined to the lamina propria.
■ Characterized by abundant mucus production (mucus pools), within which goblet cells, signet-ring cells, or epithelial glands or strands are seen.
■ This variant is reminiscent of intestinal colloid carcinoma.

Differential Diagnosis

■ Adenoma of minor salivary glands.
■ Metastatic adenocarcinoma from the gastrointestinal tract, lungs, and breast.

Treatment and Prognosis

■ The treatment for all the histologic variants of sinonasal tract adenocarcinomas is complete surgical excision, generally via a lateral rhinotomy; depending on the extent and histology of the neoplasm, the surgery varies from local excision to more radical procedures (maxillectomy, ethmoidectomy, and additional exenterations).
■ Radiotherapy may be used for extensive disease or for higher grade neoplasms.
■ Low-grade neoplasms have an excellent prognosis.
■ High-grade neoplasms have a dismal prognosis, with approximately 20% 3-year survival rates.
■ All the intestinal-type adenocarcinomas are considered high-grade neoplasms; however, papillary-tubular grade I appears to behave more indolently than the other variants; nevertheless, it may still be lethal.

■ Death results from uncontrollable locoregional disease with extension and invasion of vital structures (orbit and anterior cranial cavity) or metastatic disease (nodal or systemic).

References

Barnes L: Intestinal-type adenocarcinoma of the nasal cavity and paranasal sinuses. Am J Surg Pathol 10:192–202, 1986.

Franquemont DW, Fechner RE, Mills SE: Histologic classification of sinonasal intestinal-type adenocarcinoma. Am J Surg Pathol 15:368–375, 1991.

Heffner DK, Hyams VJ, Hauck KW, Lingeman C: Low-grade adenocarcinoma of the nasal cavity and paranasal sinuses. Cancer 50:312–322, 1982.

Hyams VJ, Batsakis JG, Michaels L: Adenocarcinoma of the sinonasal tract. *In*: Hyams VJ, Batsakis JG, Michaels L, eds. Tumors of the upper respiratory tract and ear. Fascicle 25, second series. Washington, DC: Armed Forces Institute of Pathology, 1988; pp 95–100.

Kleinsasser O, Schroeder HG: Adenocarcinoma of the inner nose after exposure to wood dust: morphological findings and relationships between histopathology and clinical behavior in 79 cases. Arch Otorhinolaryngol 245:1–15, 1988.

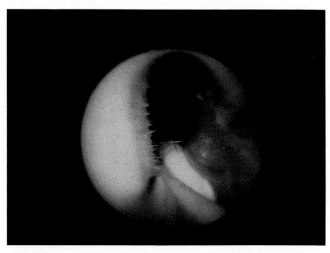

Figure 4–60. Nasal cavity adenocarcinoma, appearing as a raised, oval mucosal-covered mass along the lateral wall of the nasal cavity.

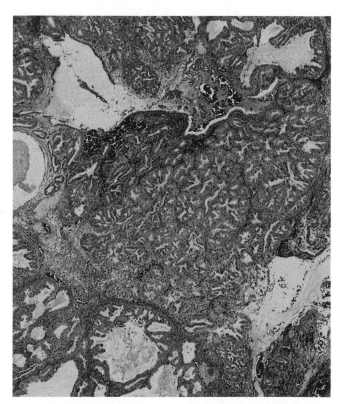

Figure 4–61. Well-differentiated sinonasal adenocarcinoma with a glandular and papillary growth; large, irregular cystic spaces can be seen.

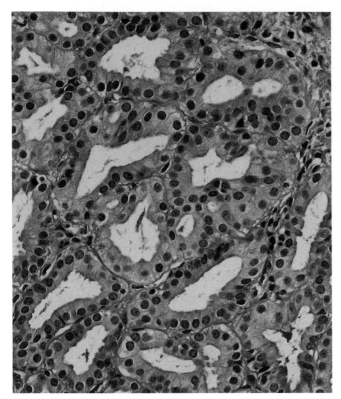

Figure 4–62. Complex glandular growth with back-to-back glands and cribriform pattern is identified without an intervening stromal component; glands are lined by a single layer of nonciliated, cuboidal to columnar cells with uniform, round nuclei, often oriented along the basal aspect of the cell or demonstrating stratification with loss of nuclear polarity, and an eosinophilic cytoplasm.

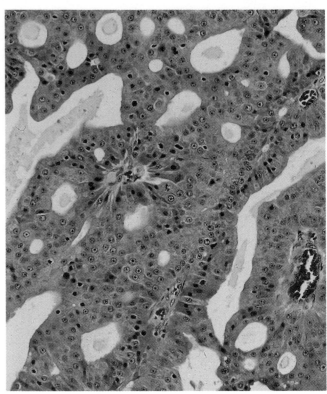

Figure 4–63. Well-differentiated sinonasal oncocytic adenocarcinoma characterized by cells with abundant eosinophilic granular cytoplasm (oncocytes); histologic features of adenocarcinoma include complex glandular growth with back-to-back glands lined by a single layer of cells and increased mitotic activity.

Figure 4–64. Well-differentiated sinonasal adenocarcinoma, characterized by a complex glandular growth with back-to-back glands, absence of an intervening stromal component, glands lined by a single layer of cells, and prominent clear-cell cytoplasmic features; necrotic material can be seen within glandular lumens.

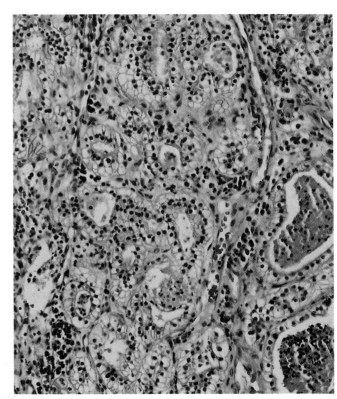

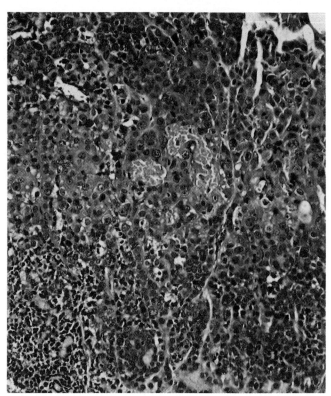

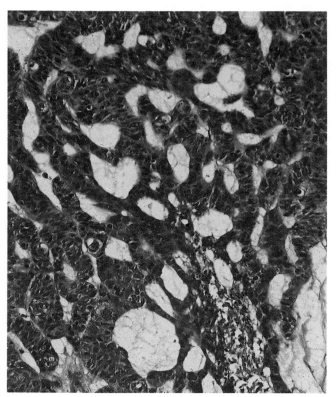

Figure 4–65. Poorly differentiated sinonasal adenocarcinoma, demonstrating a complex glandular growth pattern with moderate to marked cellular pleomorphism, loss of nuclear polarity, and increased mitotic activity.

Figure 4–66. Poorly differentiated sinonasal adenocarcinoma, demonstrating a predominantly solid growth pattern with occasional glandular differentiation. Marked cellular pleomorphism, enlarged nuclei with prominent nucleoli, and increased mitotic activity are seen.

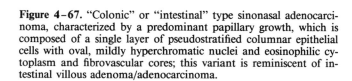

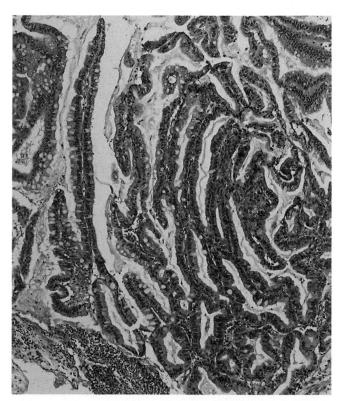

Figure 4–67. "Colonic" or "intestinal" type sinonasal adenocarcinoma, characterized by a predominant papillary growth, which is composed of a single layer of pseudostratified columnar epithelial cells with oval, mildly hyperchromatic nuclei and eosinophilic cytoplasm and fibrovascular cores; this variant is reminiscent of intestinal villous adenoma/adenocarcinoma.

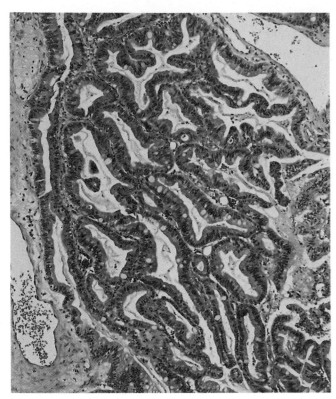

Figure 4–68. "Colonic" or "intestinal" type sinonasal adenocarcinoma, characterized by a papillary and tubular growth, with more of a tubular pattern; this variant is reminiscent of intestinal colonic adenocarcinoma.

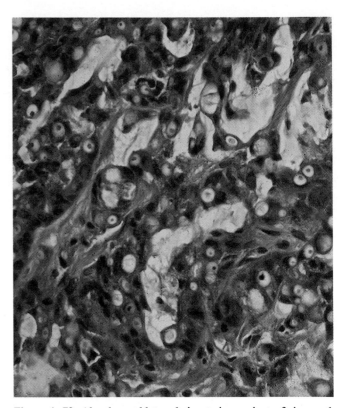

Figure 4–70. Alveolar–goblet and signet ring variant of sinonasal "intestinal" type adenocarcinoma, characterized by the presence of goblet cells and signet ring cells with marked cellular pleomorphism.

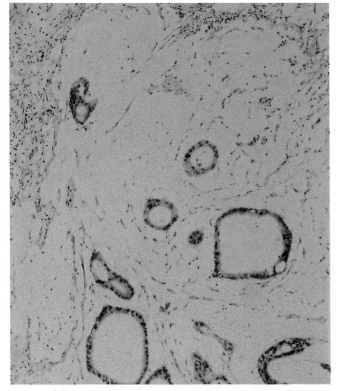

Figure 4–69. Alveolar–mucoid variant of sinonasal "intestinal" type adenocarcinoma, characterized by abundant production of mucus (mucus pools), within which malignant glandular components are seen. This variant is reminiscent of intestinal colloid carcinoma.

3. Mucosal Malignant Melanoma

Definition: Malignant neural crest–derived neoplasm originating from melanocytes that have migrated to the mucosa of the upper respiratory tract.

Clinical

- Primary (noncutaneous) upper respiratory tract malignant melanoma accounts for <2% of all malignant melanomas.
- Affects men more than women; wide age range, but most frequently occurs in the sixth to eighth decades of life.
- Can be identified in all upper respiratory tract sites, but is most commonly seen in the nasal cavity and paranasal sinuses; less common sites of involvement include nasopharynx, pharynx, larynx, and middle ear.
- Symptoms vary according to the site of occurrence and include nasal obstruction, epistaxis, painful mass, hoarseness, and dysphagia.
- Nasal cavity malignant melanomas occur more frequently than those arising in the paranasal sinuses; however, concurrent nasal cavity and paranasal sinus melanomas frequently occur, either as a result of direct extension or as multicentric tumors.
  - Primary sites of involvement in the nasal cavity are septum > lateral wall > middle and inferior turbinates; the left side is affected more often than the right.
  - Primary sites of involvement in the paranasal sinuses are maxillary (antrum) > ethmoid; other sinuses are rarely involved as primary sites.

Pathology

Gross

- A variety of appearances can be seen, including polypoid or sessile with or without ulceration; brown, black, pink, or white; friable to rubbery; and measuring from 1.0 cm to large tumors occluding the nasal cavity or paranasal sinus.

Histology

- In general, surface ulceration is a common finding.
- In tumors with intact surface epithelium, continuity of the tumor with the surface epithelium (junctional or pagetoid changes) can usually be identified.
- Cytomorphologic features include epithelioid or spindled cells; tumors with mixed epithelioid and spindle cells can be seen.
- Epithelioid cell features:
  Growth pattern varies and includes solid, organoid, nested, trabecular, alveolar, and any combination of these patterns.
  Round to oval, markedly pleomorphic cells with increased nuclear–cytoplasmic ratio, vesicular to hyperchromatic nuclei, prominent eosino-philic nucleoli, nuclear grooving, nuclear pseudoinclusions, eosinophilic to clear cytoplasm; plasmacytoid features may be prominent, but a paranuclear clear zone is not seen.
- Spindle cell features:
  Growth pattern varies, including storiform or fascicular, which may be associated with a myxoid stroma.
  Oblong to cigar-shaped, markedly pleomorphic cells with large vesicular to hyperchromatic nuclei, absent to prominent nucleoli, and scant eosinophilic cytoplasm.
- For both cytomorphologic types:
  Necrosis and increased mitoses with atypical mitotic figures are common findings.
  Rarely, glandular differentiation may be seen.
  Neoplastic giant cells can be found.
- Melanin may be heavily deposited, with easy identification, or may be limited or absent.
- Histochemistry: tumor cells are argentaffin and argyrophilic positive; PAS-positivity may be seen.
- Immunohistochemistry: diffuse S-100 protein and HMB-45 positive in both epithelioid and spindle cells.
- Electronmicroscopic: melanosomes and premelanosomes.

Differential Diagnosis

- Paraganglioma (Chapter 9A, #4).
- Squamous cell carcinoma and spindle-cell carcinoma (Chapter 14B, #1,2).
- Malignant schwannoma (Chapter 9B, #6).
- Neuroendocrine carcinoma (Chapter 14B, #6).
- Olfactory neuroblastoma (Chapter 4B, #5).
- Malignant fibrous histiocytoma (Chapter 4B, #6).
- Fibrosarcoma (Chapter 4B, #7).
- Rhabdomyosarcoma (Chapter 9B, #5).
- Alveolar soft part sarcoma (Chapter 9A, #4).
- Melanotic neuroectodermal tumor of infancy (see below).
- Metastatic malignant melanoma.

Treatment and Prognosis

- Irrespective of the site of origin, aggressive radical surgical excision is indicated.
- Adjuvant radiotherapy may be used.
- In general, prognosis is poor, with 5-year survival rates in the range of 6% to 17%.
- No correlation between size, location, or histologic appearance of the tumor and survival.
- Up to 2/3 of patients with sinonasal melanoma have recurrent disease in the first postoperative year; treatment for recurrent tumor includes surgery, radiotherapy, and chemotherapy.
- In contrast to squamous carcinoma, sinonasal melanomas metastasize less frequently to regional lymph nodes (<20%); metastatic disease occurs most frequently to the lungs, lymph nodes, and brain.

Additional Facts

■ Nasal cavity melanomas may have a better prognosis than paranasal sinus melanomas.

■ Oral cavity melanomas tend to metastasize more frequently to regional lymph nodes than those melanomas originating in the sinonasal tract.

■ Despite the overall poor prognosis, patients may experience long quiescent periods, even with recurrent or metastatic disease.

■ The possibility of metastasis to a mucosal site from a cutaneous melanoma should always be considered.

■ Laryngeal malignant melanomas are most frequently identified in supraglottic sites.

■ *Melanotic neuroectodermal tumor of infancy (MNTI):*

Rare, primitive neuroectodermal tumor, occurring most often in infants in the first year of life and primarily arising in head and neck sites (anterior maxilla ≫ other craniofacial sites); rarely, MNTI may occur in non–head and neck sites.

Presents as a rapidly growing soft-tissue mass in the area of the upper jaw (canine teeth), with or without bone destruction.

Histopathology characterized by an alveolar or pseudoglandular growth, composed of a biphasic cell population consisting of (1) small, round, lymphocytic-like cells with hyperchromatic nuclei and scant cytoplasm (neuroblastic cells); and (2) epithelioid cells with vesicular nuclei, prominent nucleoli, and eosinophilic cytoplasm; the latter cell population is noteworthy for the presence of melanin.

Immunohistochemistry: polyphenotypic expression of neural, epithelial, and melanocytic cell markers.

Majority of MNTI are benign; however, a small percentage behave in a malignant manner (metastatic disease); treatment is surgical, and conservative procedures can be used as long as these procedures completely eradicate the tumor.

References

Berthelsen A, Andersen AP, Jensen TS, Hansen HS: Melanomas of the mucosa in the oral cavity and upper respiratory passages. Cancer 54:907–912, 1984.

Blatchford SJ, Koopmann CF, Coulthard SW: Mucosal melanoma of the head and neck. Laryngoscope 96:929–934, 1986.

Conley J: Melanomas of the mucous membranes of the head and neck. Laryngoscope 99:1248–1253, 1989.

Cove H: Melanosis, melanocytic hyperplasia, and primary malignant melanoma of the nasal cavity. Cancer 44:1424–1433, 1979.

Panje WR, Moran WJ: Melanoma of the upper aerodigestive tract: a review of 21 cases. Head Neck Surg 8:309–312, 1986.

Pettinato G, Manivel JC, d'Amore ESG, Jaszcz W, Gorlin RJ: Melanotic neuroectodermal tumor of infancy: a reexamination of a histogenetic problem based on immunohistochemical, flow cytometric, and ultrastructural study of 10 cases. Am J Surg Pathol 15:233–245, 1991.

Wick MR, Swanson PE, Rocamora A: Recognition of malignant melanoma by monoclonal antibody HMB-45: an immunohistochemical study of 200 paraffin-embedded cutaneous tumors. J Cutan Pathol 15:201–207, 1988.

Figure 4-71. Sinonasal malignant melanoma, characterized by focal surface ulceration and a diffuse invasive cellular infiltrate of epithelioid-appearing pleomorphic cells.

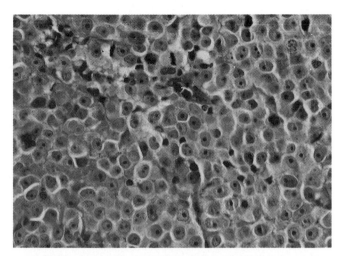

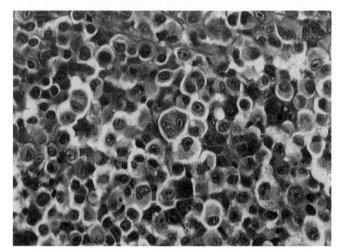

Figure 4-73. (*Top*) More often than not the cellular infiltrate of sinonasal epithelioid malignant melanoma demonstrates absence of melanin production. (*Bottom*) Occasionally, melanin production appearing as cytoplasmic brown granular pigment may be heavily deposited within the neoplastic cellular infiltrate, aiding in diagnosis.

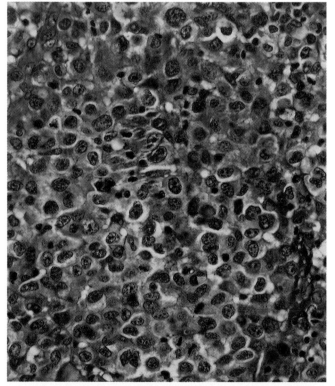

Figure 4-72. Sinonasal epithelioid malignant melanoma with a solid cellular growth pattern composed of round to oval, markedly pleomorphic cells with increased nuclear–cytoplasmic ratio, vesicular to hyperchromatic nuclei, prominent eosinophilic nucleoli, numerous mitotic figures, and eosinophilic to clear cytoplasm.

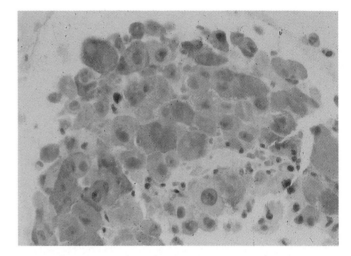

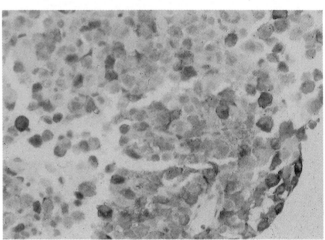

Figure 4–74. Diagnosis of malignant melanoma is greatly facilitated by immunohistochemical evaluation, as seen by the presence of both S-100 protein (*top*) and HMB-45 (*bottom*).

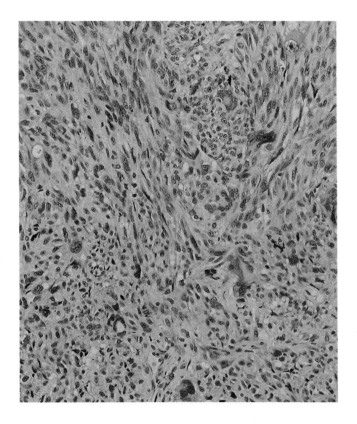

Figure 4–75. Sinonasal spindle cell malignant melanoma, demonstrating a storiform or fascicular growth pattern with oblong to cigar-shaped, markedly pleomorphic cells with large vesicular to hyperchromatic nuclei, absent to prominent nucleoli, and scant eosinophilic cytoplasm. The growth pattern and cytomorphologic features are indistinguishable from other spindle cell neoplasms (carcinoma and sarcoma).

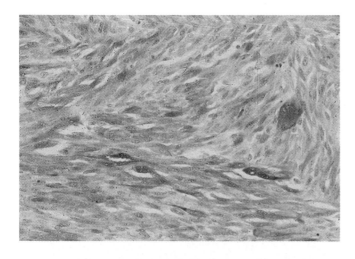

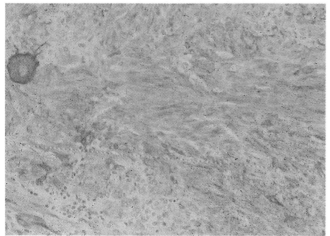

Figure 4–76. Similar to epithelioid malignant melanoma, the diagnosis of spindle cell malignant melanoma is greatly facilitated by the presence of immunoreactivity with both S-100 protein (*top*) and HMB-45 (*bottom*).

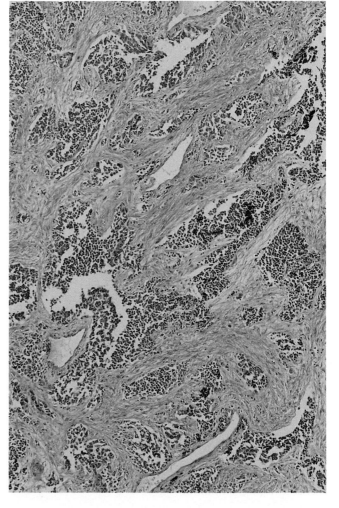

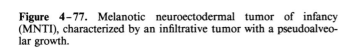

Figure 4–77. Melanotic neuroectodermal tumor of infancy (MNTI), characterized by an infiltrative tumor with a pseudoalveolar growth.

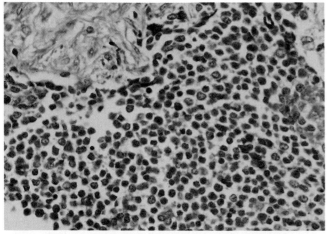

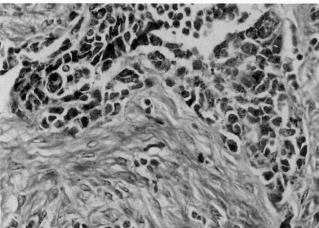

Figure 4–78. MNTI, showing the dual cell population including (*top*) small, round, lymphocytic-like cells with hyperchromatic nuclei and scant cytoplasm (neuroblastic cells) and (*bottom*) larger epithelioid cells with vesicular nuclei, eosinophilic cytoplasm, and melanin.

4. Midline Malignant Reticulosis

Definition: Upper respiratory tract neoplastic, lymphoproliferative disorder, characterized by either a polymorphous (with atypical lymphoid cells) or monomorphous cellular infiltrate that has ulcerative and destructive properties, angiocentricity, and a predominantly but not exclusively T-cell phenotype.

Synonyms: Lethal midline granuloma; Stewart's granuloma; polymorphic reticulosis; peripheral, angiocentric T-cell malignant lymphoma; angiocentric lymphoproliferative lesion.

Clinical (Table 4–3)

■ Affects males more than females; occurs over a wide age range, including in childhood, but is most common in the fifth to sixth decades of life.
■ Most commonly affects the nasal cavity or the paranasal sinuses (maxillary antrum in particular); nasal lesions are often bilateral.
■ Involvement of the oral cavity (destructive lesion of the hard palate) and nasopharynx, as well as extension of disease to the base of skull and orbit, may occur; laryngeal and tracheal involvement occur but are uncommon.

■ Symptoms include nasal obstruction, unilateral facial swelling, mucosal ulceration or a mass, purulent nasal discharge, constitutional symptoms (fever, weight loss), and, less frequently, proptosis, pain, epistaxis, and paresthesias; with progression, destruction of soft tissue, cartilage (septal perforation), and bone may occur.
■ May be associated with systemic manifestations, including malaise, fatigue, night sweats, and fever; involvement of the lower respiratory tract, gastrointestinal tract, genitourinary system (necrotizing glomerulonephritis is absent), adrenal glands, skin, and central nervous system may occur.

Radiology

■ Radiographic findings are essentially similar and indistinguishable from carcinomas or sarcomas.
■ Involvement of the lungs results in radiographic findings similar to those of Wegener's granulomatosis.

Pathology

Gross

■ Polypoid, soft to rubbery mass with a homogeneous appearance and a pink to tan-white color.

Table 4–3.

CLINICOPATHOLOGIC COMPARISON BETWEEN WEGENER'S GRANULOMATOSIS, MIDLINE MALIGNANT RETICULOSIS, AND SINONASAL LYMPHOMA

	Wegener's Granulomatosis	Midline Malignant Reticulosis	Sinonasal Malignant Lymphoma (A) Western (B) Asian
Sex/age	♂ > ♀; 4th–5th decades	♂ > ♀; 5th–6th decades	(A) ♂ = ♀; 6th decade (B) ♂ > ♀; 7th decade
Location	Sinonasal region is most common; may involve oral cavity, nasopharynx, larynx, trachea, ear, salivary glands	Similar to Wegener's granulomatosis	Generally limited to the sinonasal region; extrasinonasal disease occurs and represents a higher stage tumor
Symptoms	Nasal obstruction, epistaxis, pain, anosmia, purulent rhinorrhea; dyspnea, hoarseness; hearing loss	Nasal obstruction, unilateral facial swelling, constitutional symptoms (fever, weight loss), purulent nasal discharge, a mass, otitis media	Similar to polymorphic type
Systemic involvement	Lungs, kidney, skin, orbit	Lower respiratory tract, genitourinary system, adrenal glands, skin and central nervous system	Similar to midline malignant reticulosis; lymph nodes, spleen and bone marrow may be involved also
Serology	ANCA (antineotrophil cytoplasmic antibodies) increased in both primary disease and recurrent disease	No specific serologic marker	No specific serologic marker
Histology	1. Polymorphous benign cellular infiltrate 2. Vasculitis 3. Ischemic-type necrosis 4. Giant cells invariably identified 5. Negative cultures and stains for organisms	1. Polymorphous atypical cellular infiltrate 2. Angiocentric and angioinvasive 3. Necrosis 4. Negative cultures and stains for organisms	1. Monomorphous overtly malignant cellular infiltrate of various types 2. Necrosis, angiocentricity, angioinvasion seen in Asian and usually not in Western patients 3. Negative cultures and stains for organisms
Immunohistochemistry	Polymorphous and polyclonal	"Atypical" cells, predominantly of T-cell phenotype	Malignant cells, predominantly of: (A) B-cell phenotype (B) T-cell phenotype
Treatment	Corticosteroids; cyclophosphamide	Radiotherapy; chemotherapy in higher stages	Radiotherapy; chemotherapy in higher stages
Prognosis	Limited disease associated with a good to excellent prognosis and occasional spontaneous remissions	Dependent on stage and, if localized, prognosis is generally good, with >50% 5-year survival; higher stage disease usually is rapidly lethal	(A) Dependent on stage but generally good with >50% 5-year survival (B) Often rapidly fatal

■ Locally destructive ulcerated and crusted lesion; with advanced disease, extension of this process may involve adjacent structures, leading to a communicating orifice between normally separated anatomic structures (i.e., septal perforation).

Histology

■ Subepithelial polymorphous cellular infiltrate growing in a diffuse pattern, composed of mononuclear cells that include mature and atypical lymphocytes, immunoblasts, histiocytes, and plasma cells; infrequently, eosinophils and polymorphonuclear leukocytes can be seen in association with the surface ulceration.

■ Atypical cells do not form sheets but are interspersed among the other cells; some cases may have a predominance of atypical cells (>70% in one or more high-power fields) that may have clear cytoplasmic changes.

■ The cellular infiltrate typically is angiocentrically located, with angioinvasive properties; compromise of the vascular lumens results in ischemic (coagulative-type) necrosis, which may be focal or confluent, forming large necrotic zones; a proliferation of medium-sized, nonarborizing capillaries may be prominent.

■ The associated acute and chronic inflammatory cell infiltrate is seen and may obscure the atypical lymphocytic infiltrate.

■ Giant cells may be seen but are uncommon, and granulomas are typically absent.

■ Special stains for microorganisms are negative.

■ Immunohistochemistry: monoclonality associated

with the atypical lymphocytic infiltrate is predominantly of T-cell lineage; there is polyclonality for immune globulins.

Differential Diagnosis

- Infectious diseases.
- Wegener's granulomatosis (Chapter 3, #8).
- Histiocytosis X (Chapter 24B, #4).
- Non-Hodgkin's malignant lymphoma (see below; Chapter 9B, #4).
- Extramedullary plasmacytoma (Chapter 9B, #4).
- Carcinoma (squamous cell; undifferentiated) (Chapter 4B, #1; Chapter 9B, #2).
- Neuroendocrine carcinoma (Chapter 14B, #6).
- Olfactory neuroblastoma (Chapter 4B, #5).
- Malignant melanoma (Chapter 4B, #3).
- Ewing's sarcoma.

Treatment and Prognosis

- Following the diagnosis, patients must be clinically staged (staging is similar to Waldeyer ring malignant lymphomas, see chapter 9B, #4), with therapy based on the stage of disease:
  For localized disease, radiotherapy in curative doses (at least 4000 rads) is the treatment of choice.
  In patients with multifocal or disseminated (higher stage) disease, radiotherapy and chemotherapy are used.
- Prognosis is dependent on stage: if localized (lower grade) prognosis is considered good, with >50% 5-year survival; higher stage disease usually is rapidly lethal.
- In 10% to 50% of patients, a "transformation" into a conventional non-Hodgkin's malignant lymphoma occurs, usually accompanied with dissemination; this overtly malignant lymphoma is often of the large cell or immunoblastic cell type, but may also be of small cell or mixed small and large cell types.

Additional Facts

- The polymorphic variant is notoriously difficult to diagnose, resulting in delays in identification and in the establishment of treatment protocols.
- Relapse of tumor is generally accompanied by relapse in other extranodal sites.
- Bacterial superinfection of the diseased mucosa, particularly *Staphylococcus aureus,* may complicate the clinical picture.
- *Sinonasal non-Hodgkin's malignant lymphoma* (classified according to the Working Formulation) is an uncommon neoplasm in Western countries, being much more prevalent in Asia; differences between Western and Asian populations include:
  Predilection for males in Asian countries; no sex predilection in Western populations.
  Cellular infiltrates are essentially similar, composed of a monomorphic population of overtly malignant-appearing lymphocytes, predominantly growing in a diffuse pattern with varied cytologic appearance, but most often infiltrates are large cell or immunoblastic, mixed small and large cells, and small cleaved-cell type.
  Overwhelming majority of lymphomas of Asian populations are of a T-cell phenotype; a much higher percentage of cases in Western populations are of a B-cell phenotype.
  The histologic findings of angioinvasion, ischemic-type necrosis, and epitheliotropism are most often seen in association with lymphomas of T-cell phenotype and are, therefore, more common in association with lymphomas in Asian populations; in Western populations, with a majority of B-cell lymphomas, prominent necrosis, angiocentric location, and angioinvasion are seen only in a minority of cases.
  Prognosis for Asian patients as compared with Western patients is much worse, often resulting in rapidly fatal disease; this probably relates to the angioinvasive and destructive properties associated with T-cell lymphomas, which are more commonly seen in Asian patients; in Western patients, a good response to radiotherapy is seen in localized neoplasms.
- Factors adversely affecting prognosis include:
  Higher stage disease at presentation.
  A large primary tumor.
  Unfavorable histology (immunoblastic and diffuse large cell).
- In general, sinonasal malignant lymphomas are primary neoplasms that occasionally may be associated with systemic disease.
- Prognosis and therapy depend on the clinical stage of disease.

References

Batsakis JG, Luna MA: Midfacial necrotizing lesions. Semin Diagn Pathol 4:90–116, 1987.

Chan JKC, Ng CS, Lau WH, Lo STH: Most nasal/nasopharyngal lymphomas are peripheral T-cell neoplasia. Am J Surg Pathol 11:418–429, 1987.

Frierson HF JR, Innes DJ, Mills SE, Wick MR: Immunophenotypic analysis of sinonasal non-Hodgkin's lymphomas. Hum Pathol 20:636–642, 1989.

Ho FCS, Choy D, Loke SL, et al: Polymorphic reticulosis and conventional lymphomas of the nose and upper aerodigestive tract: a clinicopatholgoic study of 70 cases, and immunophenotypic studies of 16 cases. Hum Pathol 21:1041–1050, 1990.

Ferry JA, Sklar J, Zukerberg LR, Harris NL: Nasal lymphoma: a clinicopathologic study with immunophenotypic and genotypic analysis. Am J Surg Pathol 15:268–279, 1991.

Jaffe ES: Post-thymic lymphoid neoplasia. *In*: Jaffe ES, ed. Surgical pathology of the lymph nodes and related organs, vol. 16. Philadelphia: W.B. Saunders Co., 1985; pp 218–248.

Lipford EH, Margolick JB, Longo DL: Angiocentric immunoproliferative lesions: a clinico-pathologic spectrum of post-thymic proliferations. Blood 72:1674–1681, 1988.

Ratech H, Burke JS, Blayney DW, Sheibani K, Rappaport H: A clinicopathologic study of malignant lymphomas of the nose, paranasal sinuses, and hard palate, including cases of lethal midline granuloma. Cancer 64:2525–2531, 1989.

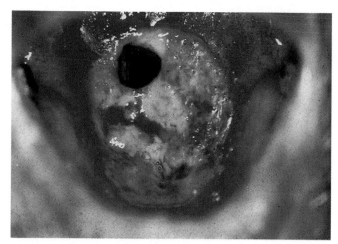

Figure 4–79. Midline malignant reticulosis with a locally destructive, ulcerated lesion of the floor of the maxillary sinus with perforation of the palate; the lesion has an associated purulent exudate.

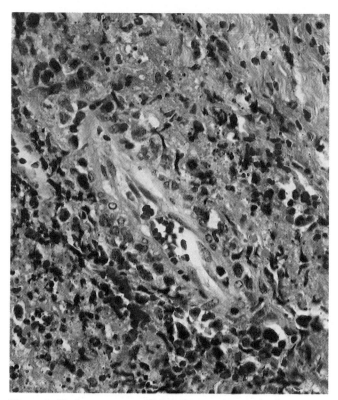

Figure 4–81. In contrast to Wegener's granulomatosis, the cellular infiltrate seen in midline malignant reticulosis includes atypical lymphocytic cells interspersed among the other cells; in this field, the atypical cells are seen invading a blood vessel.

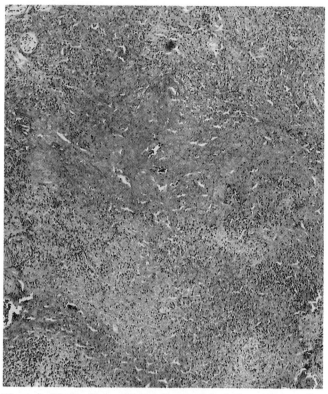

Figure 4–80. Similar to Wegener's granulomatosis, midline malignant reticulosis has a polymorphic cellular infiltrate with angiocentric and angioinvasive properties involving small- and medium-sized vessels, and resulting in an "ischemic" or "geographic" type of necrosis with a basophilic, smudgy appearance.

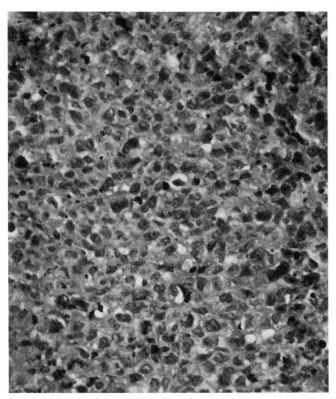

Figure 4–82. Sinonasal non-Hodgkin's malignant lymphoma, T-cell phenotype, is characterized by a diffuse infiltrate of a pleomorphic overtly malignant-appearing cell infiltrate with hyperchromatic, irregularly shaped large nuclei and clear-appearing cytoplasm.

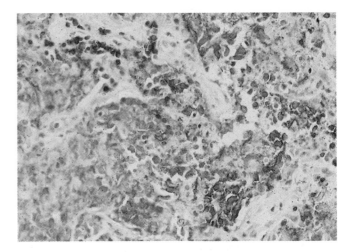

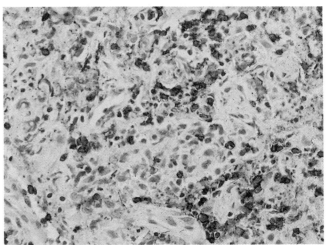

Figure 4–84. Sinonasal non-Hodgkin's malignant lymphoma. (*Top*) The cellular infiltrate is of lymphoid cell origin, as seen by the presence of immunoreactivity with leukocyte common antigen (LCA). (*Bottom*) This non-Hodgkin's malignant lymphoma demonstrates a T-cell phenotype, as seen by the presence of immunoreactivity with UCHL, a T-cell marker (L-26, a B-cell marker, was nonreactive in the malignant cellular infiltrate).

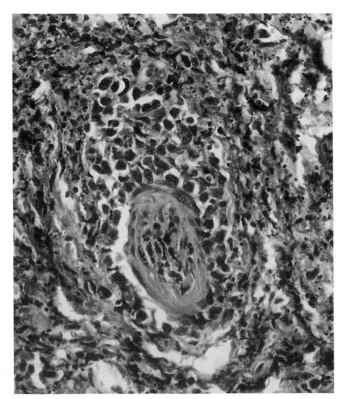

Figure 4–83. Sinonasal non-Hodgkin's malignant lymphoma, T-cell phenotype, demonstrates angiocentric and angioinvasive properties.

5. Olfactory Neuroblastoma

Definition: Malignant neoplasm arising from the olfactory membrane of the sinonasal tract.

Clinical

- Uncommon malignant neoplasm.
- Slight female predominance; ages at onset range from 3 years to the ninth decade, with a bimodal peak in the second and sixth decades of life.
- Appears to take origin from the olfactory membrane located in the upper nasal cavity, which is the most common site of presentation.
- Main presenting symptoms are unilateral nasal obstruction and epistaxis; less common manifestations include anosmia, headache, pain, excessive lacrimation, and ocular disturbances.
- No known etiologic agent; cytogenetic abnormalities (translocations) have been seen in association with olfactory neuroblastomas.

Radiology

- Sinus opacification with or without bone erosion.
- Angiographic studies disclose a hypervascular neoplasm.
- Speckled pattern of calcification may be seen.

Pathology

Gross

- Glistening, mucosal-covered, soft, polypoid mass, varying from a small nodule less than 1 cm to a mass filling the nasal cavity, with possible extension into adjacent paranasal sinuses and nasopharynx.

Histology

- Four grades (I–IV) (Table 4–4):

Grade I (the most differentiated)

- Lobular architecture with intercommunication of the neoplasm between lobules.
- Neoplastic cells are well differentiated, with uniform round to vesicular nuclei with or without nucleoli.
- Cells do not have distinct borders; rather, the nuclei are surrounded by a neurofibrillary material, suggesting cytoplasmic extension.
- Pseudorosette pattern (Homer Wright rosettes) are frequently seen.
- Varying amounts of calcification may be noted.
- Interlobular fibrous stroma is often extremely vascular.
- No mitotic activity; necrosis is absent.

Grade II

- Exhibit many of the histologic features described for Grade I lesions, but the neurofibrillary element

Table 4–4.
HYAMS' HISTOLOGIC GRADING SYSTEM FOR OLFACTORY NEUROBLASTOMA

Microscopic Feature	Grade I	Grade II	Grade III	Grade IV
Architecture	Lobular	Lobular	±Lobular	±Lobular
Pleomorphism	Absent to slight	Present	Prominent	Marked
NF matrix	Prominent	Present	May be present	Absent
Rosettes	Present*	Present*	May be present†	May be present†
Mitoses	Absent	Present	Prominent	Marked
Necrosis	Absent	Absent	Present	Prominent
Glands	May be present	May be present	May be present	May be present
Calcification	Variable	Variable	Absent	Absent

* Homer Wright rosettes (pseudorosettes).
† Flexner-Wintersteiner rosettes (true neural rosettes).
NF, neurofibrillary.

is less well defined, and the neoplastic nuclei show increased pleomorphism.
- Scattered mitoses can be seen.

Grade III

- Although the micromorphology suggests a lobular architecture with an interstitial vascular stroma, there is a hypercellularity of the neoplastic cell proliferation.
- Individual cells are more anaplastic and hyperchromatic, and have increased mitotic activity compared with those of either grade I or II.
- The neurofibrillary component is less conspicuous.
- Identification of true neural rosettes (Flexner-Wintersteiner).
- Calcification is absent, but necrosis is seen.

Grade IV

- Overall lobular architecture may be retained, and the neoplastic element is the most undifferentiated and anaplastic of all the grades.
- Nuclei are hyperchromatic and anaplastic.
- Cytoplasm is indistinct and difficult to associate with neural origin.
- True rosettes may be seen.
- Increased mitotic activity.
- Necrosis is commonly seen; calcifications are uncommon.

Special Studies

- Histochemistry: positive staining with Bodian and Grimelius; periodic acid-Schiff may be positive.
- Immunohistochemistry: consistent positive staining with neuron-specific enolase (NSE); variably positive reactivity with S-100 protein (usually seen at the periphery of the neoplastic lobules), cytokera-

tin, glial fibrillary acidic protein (GFAP), neurofibrillary protein (NFP), β-tubulin, microtubule-associated protein, chromogranin, synaptophysin, Ber-EP4, and Leu-7.

■ Electronmicroscopy: identification of neuronal processes and dense core neurosecretory granules.

Differential Diagnosis

■ Vascular neoplasms (hemangiopericytoma) (Chapter 4, #3).
■ Paraganglioma (Chapter 9A, #4).
■ Extracranial meningioma (Chapter 25B, #4).
■ Undifferentiated or anaplastic carcinoma (see below; Chapter 9B, #2).
■ Neuroendocrine carcinoma (Chapter 14B, #6).
■ Respiratory carcinoma (Chapter 4B, #1).
■ Malignant melanoma (Chapter 4B, #3).
■ Malignant lymphoproliferative disorder (lymphoma, plasmacytoma) (Chapter 4B, #4; Chapter 9B, #4).
■ Ewing's sarcoma.
■ Chordoma (Chapter 9B, #7).

Treatment and Prognosis

■ Radical surgery is the treatment of choice, followed by full-course radiotherapy.
■ Limited success using chemotherapeutic modalities has been achieved for disseminated disease.
■ Survival figures vary, depending on the clinical stage (Kadish staging): stage A, tumor confined to the nasal cavity, 3-year survival of better than 90%; stage B, tumor involves the nasal cavity plus one or more paranasal sinuses, >80% 3-year survival; and stage C, extension of tumor beyond the sinonasal cavities, <50% 3-year survival.
■ The majority of tumors behave as locally aggressive lesions, mainly involving adjacent structures (orbit and cranial cavity).
■ From 20% to 40% metastasize to regional lymph nodes, lungs, and bone.

Additional Facts

■ All histologic grades may metastasize locally or distantly.
■ Included in the areas of proposed origin are Jacobson's organ (vomeronasal organ), sphenopalatine (pterygoid palatine) ganglion, olfactory placode, and the ganglion of Loci (nervus terminalis).
■ Light microscopic and ultrastructural studies support the bipolar neurons of the olfactory membrane as the cell of origin.

■ "Ectopic" origin within one of the paranasal sinuses may occur.
■ Sinonasal undifferentiated (anaplastic) carcinoma:
Highly aggressive and invasive tumor typically affecting adults and identified in the nasal cavity and/or multiple paranasal sinuses.
Absence of any histologic differentiating features (squamous, glandular, neurofibrillary material or rosettes); possibly arises from schneiderian epithelium, but histogenesis remains speculative.
Pleomorphic cellular infiltrate with trabecular, nested, or sheet-like growth composed of medium-sized cells with pleomorphic round to oval nuclei, variable cytoplasm and prominent nucleoli; increased mitotic activity and associated necrosis are commonly seen.
Immunohistochemistry: reactive for epithelial markers (cytokeratin and epithelial membrane antigen); also, often reactive for neuron-specific enolase.
May be difficult to differentiate from higher-grade olfactory neuroblastoma (see above).
Poor prognosis despite all attempts at therapeutic intervention.

References

Frierson HF JR, Mills SE, Fechner RE, Taxy JB, Levine PA: Sinonasal undifferentiated carcinoma: an aggressive neoplasm derived from schneiderian epithelium and distinct from olfactory neuroblastoma. Am J Surg Pathol 10:771–779, 1986.

Frierson HF JR, Ross GW, Mills SE, Frankfurter A: Olfactory neuroblastoma: additional immunohistochemical characterization. Am J Clin Pathol 94:547–553, 1990.

Hyams VJ, Batsakis JG, Michaels L: Olfactory neuroblastoma. In: Hyams VJ, Batsakis JG, Michaels L, eds. Tumors of the upper respiratory tract and ear. Fascicle 25, second series. Washington, DC: Armed Forces Institute of Pathology, 1988; pp 240–248.

Kadish S, Goodman M, Wine CC: Olfactory neuroblastoma: a clinical analysis of 17 cases. Cancer 37:1571–1576, 1976.

Sandberg AA, Turc-Carel C: The cytogenetics of solid tumors: relation to diagnosis, classification and pathology. Cancer 59:387–395, 1987.

Silva EG, Butler JJ, Mackay B, Goepfert H: Neuroblastomas and neuroendocrine carcinomas of the nasal cavity: a proposed new classification. Cancer 50:2388–2405, 1982.

Schmidt JL, Zarbo RJ, Clark JL: Olfactory neuroblastoma: clinicopathologic and immunohistochemical characterization of four representative cases. Laryngoscope 100:1052–1058, 1990.

Taxy JB, Bharani NK, Mills SE, Frierson HF JR, Gould VE: The spectrum of olfactory neural tumors: a light-microscopic, immunohistochemical and electron microscopic analysis. Am J Surg Pathol 10:687–695, 1986.

Whang-Peng J, Freier RE, Knutsen T, Nanfro JJ, Gazdar A: Translocation t(11;22) in esthesioneuroblastoma. Cancer Genet Cytogenet 29:155–157, 1987.

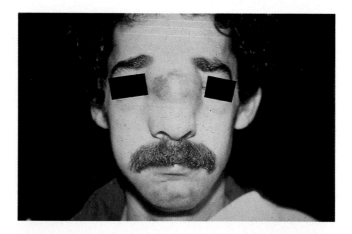

Figure 4–85. Patient with an enormous olfactory neuroblastoma destroying much of the soft tissue and bony structures in the upper nasal cavity; its appearance along the bridge of the nose results in marked facial deformity.

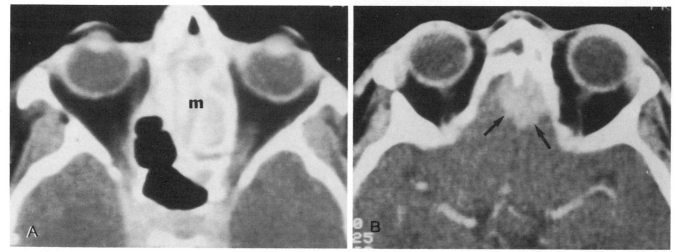

Figure 4–86. (*A*) Axial CT, contrast-enhanced olfactory neuroblastoma of the ethmoid sinus with an enhancing soft tissue mass (m) opacifying the ethmoid sinus and destroying the bony septa and walls. (*B*) Axial CT, contrast-enhanced, showing the lesion extending through the cribriform plate, and presenting as a contrast-enhanced frontal lobe mass (*arrows*) (Courtesy of Franz J. Wippold II, M.D., Mallinckrodt Institute of Radiology, St. Louis, MO.)

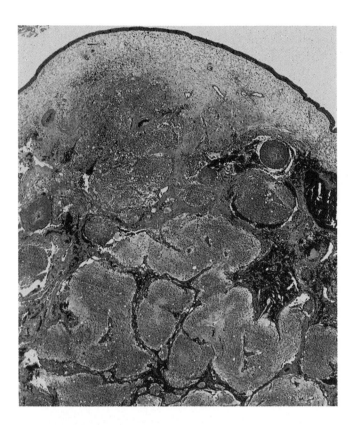

Figure 4–87. Olfactory neuroblastoma (ONB), grade I: common to all grades of ONB is the lobular growth pattern; in higher grade neoplasms, the lobular growth is maintained but may be only focally present.

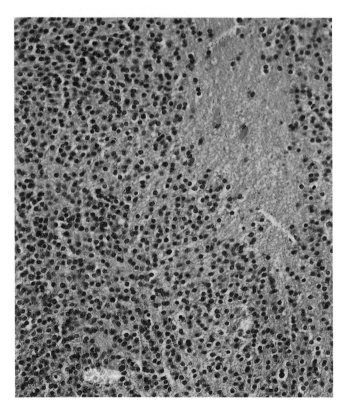

Figure 4–88. ONB, grade I: neoplastic cells are well differentiated, with uniform round to vesicular nuclei surrounded by abundant neurofibrillary material, suggesting cytoplasmic extensions; mitotic figures are rarely seen.

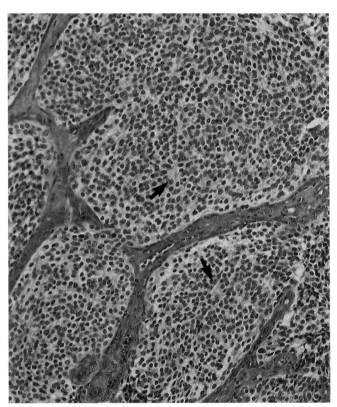

Figure 4–89. ONB, grade II: lobules of neoplastic cells surrounded by a neurofibrillary matrix, which is less well defined as compared with grade I ONB; in addition, the cellular component of grade II demonstrates greater pleomorphism with scattered mitoses, in contrast to the features seen in grade I ONB. Homer Wright rosettes can be seen (*arrowheads*).

Figure 4–90. ONB, grade III: hypercellular neoplastic cell proliferation demonstrating greater pleomorphism and a less conspicuous neurofibrillary component as compared with grades I or II ONB.

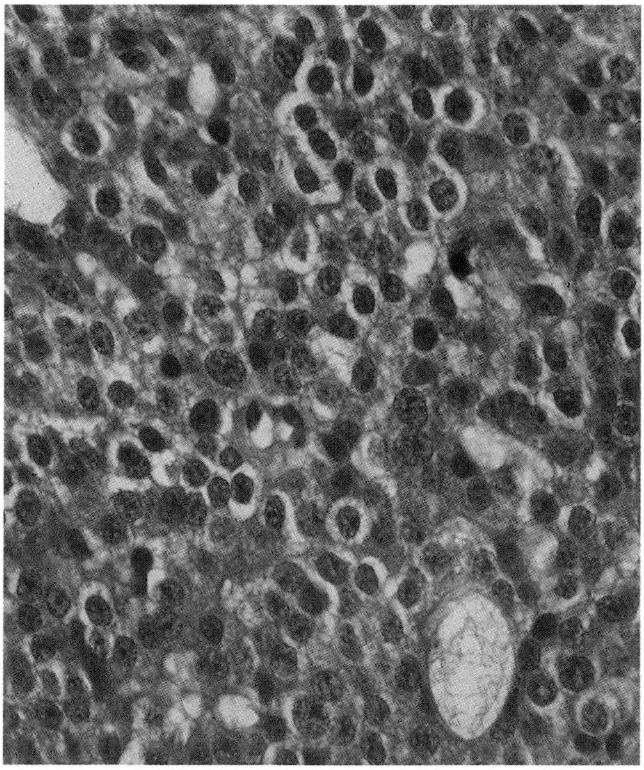

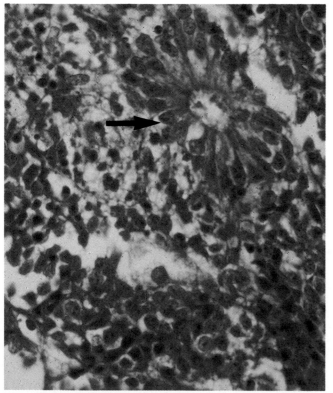

Figure 4–91. ONB, grade III: anaplastic, hyperchromatic nuclei are seen, as well as the presence of a true neural rosette (*arrow;* Flexner-Wintersteiner rosette).

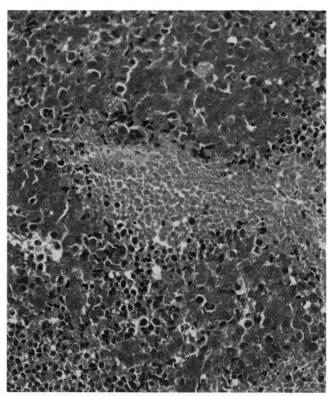

Figure 4–92. ONB, grade IV: most undifferentiated and anaplastic of all the grades, characterized by hyperchromatic nuclei, indistinct cytoplasm, increased mitotic activity, and necrosis. The neurofibrillary component is minimal to absent, making identification of this neoplasm as an ONB difficult, with the diagnosis often hinging on location of the tumor, presence of a lobular growth pattern, and the immunohistochemical antigenic profile.

6. Malignant Fibrous Histiocytoma (MFH)

Definition: Malignant neoplasm, composed of an admixture of fibroblastic and histiocytic cells.

Clinical

- Most common soft tissue sarcoma of late adult life, primarily affecting the soft tissues of the lower extremity.
- Uncommon neoplasm in the head and neck.
- Affects males more than females; occurs over a wide age range, but is most commonly seen in adults.
- Most common noncutaneous locations in the head and neck are the sinonasal cavity and the neck.
- Symptoms vary and include a mass with or without associated pain, nasal obstruction, epistaxis, facial asymmetry, and proptosis.

Pathology

Gross

- Nodular appearing tan-white to gray lesion of varying size.
- May have a translucent, gelatinous, or hemorrhagic appearance.

Histology

- Most common histologic variant is the storiform-pleomorphic type, composed of fascicular and pleomorphic growth patterns.
- Cellular neoplasm, consisting of spindle-shaped cells admixed with histiocytic cells and marked by prominent pleomorphism and increased mitotic activity (typical and atypical forms).
- Many giant cells with multiple hyperchromatic nuclei and necrosis are commonly seen.
- Variable amounts of chronic inflammatory cells (lymphocytes, plasma cells, xanthoma cells), fibrosis, hyalinization, myxoid change, and stromal vascularity are seen.
- Special stains are of little assistance in the diagnosis.
- Other histologic variants include:
  Myxoid (second most common type).
  Giant cell.
  Inflammatory.
  Angiomatoid.

Differential Diagnosis

- Nodular fasciitis (Chapter 8, #5).
- Dermatofibrosarcoma protuberans (Chapter 4A, #4).
- Pleomorphic or anaplastic carcinoma (Chapter 14B, #2).
- Rhabdomyosarcoma (Chapter 9B, #5).
- Liposarcoma (Chapter 9B, #8).

Treatment and Prognosis

- Complete surgical excision is the treatment of choice.
- Radiotherapy is of questionable efficacy.
- Lymph node metastases occur in approximately 15% of cases and, unless clinically suspect, neck dissection is of limited value.
- Recurrence rates vary according to histologic type, ranging from 44% (storiform-pleomorphic) to 66% (myxoid).
- Metastatic rates vary according to histologic type, ranging from as few as 23% (myxoid) to 42% (storiform-pleomorphic).
- Metastases occur to the lung > lymph nodes > liver and bone.
- Prognosis is dependent on the depth and size of tumor.

Additional Facts

- Majority of malignant fibrous histiocytomas occur *de novo*; however, evidence supports that some of these tumors are radiation induced.
- Histologic features are of limited prognostic importance, except for the myxoid variant, which is associated with a better prognosis as compared with the storiform-pleomorphic type of MFH.

References

Barnes L, Kanbour A: Malignant fibrous histiocytoma of the head and neck. Arch Otolaryngol Head Neck Surg 114:1149–1156, 1988.

Blitzer A, Lawson W, Biller HF: Malignant fibrous histiocytoma of the head and neck. Laryngoscope 87:1479–1499, 1977.

Enzinger FW, Weiss SW: Malignant fibrohistiocytic tumors. *In*: Enzinger FW, Weiss SW, eds. Soft tissue tumors; 2nd ed. St. Louis: C. V. Mosby, 1988; pp 269–300.

Perzin KH, Fu YS: Non-epithelial tumors of the nasal cavity, paranasal sinuses, and nasopharynx: a clinicopathologic study. XI: fibrous histiocytomas. Cancer 45:2616–2626, 1980.

Merrick RE, Rhone DP, Chilis TJ: Malignant fibrous histiocytoma of the maxillary sinus: case report and literature review. Arch Otolaryngol Head Neck Surg 106:365–367, 1980.

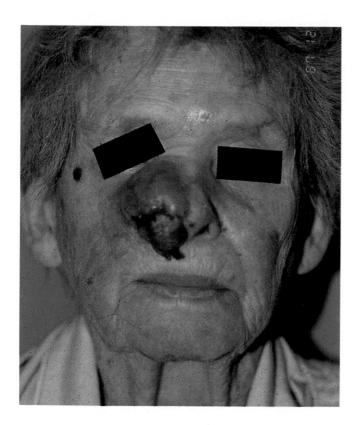

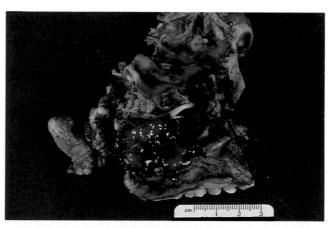

Figure 4–93. Nasal cavity–based malignant fibrous histiocytoma (MFH) protruding from the left nasal vestibule and invading into the subcutaneous compartment, resulting in facial deformity.

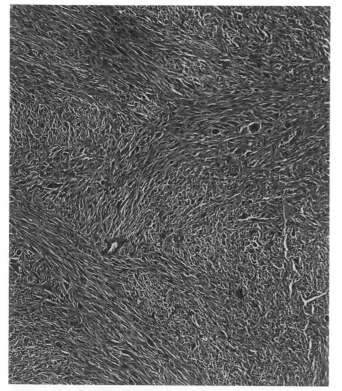

Figure 4–95. Recurrent maxillary sinus myxoid variant of MFH with a gelatinous/mucoid appearance, necessitating a radical surgical removal procedure, including orbital exenteration.

Figure 4–94. Histologic appearance of the storiform-pleomorphic type of MFH, composed of fascicular and pleomorphic growth pattern with a spindle-shaped cellular infiltrate admixed with histiocytic cells and many giant cells, and marked by prominent pleomorphism and increased mitotic activity (typical and atypical forms).

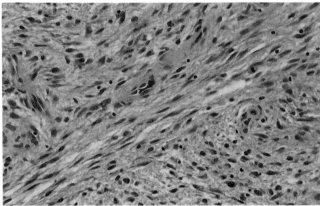

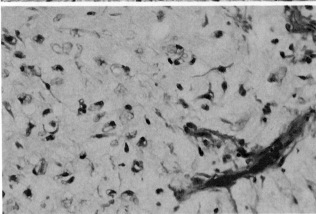

Figure 4-96. Myxoid MFH. The diagnosis of myxoid MFH is facilitated by the presence of more recognizable histomorphologic pattern of MFH (*top*) characterized by a cellular area with a storiform pattern and (*bottom*) myxoid areas characterized by the presence of spindle- to stellate-shaped cells in a myxoid matrix with an associated network of narrow curvilinear vascular spaces; the storiform pattern is absent in the myxoid areas.

7. Fibrosarcoma

Definition: Malignant tumor of fibroblasts, lacking evidence of other types of cellular differentiation.

Clinical

- Found predominantly in the soft tissues of the lower extremities.
- Approximately 10% to 15% occur in the head and neck region.
- No sex predilection; may affect all age groups, with the majority of cases occurring in the fourth to sixth decades of life.
- Common head and neck sites are nasal cavity and paranasal sinuses > larynx > neck.
- Symptoms vary according to site and include nasal obstruction, epistaxis, pain, dysphagia, or as a solitary mass with or without associated pain.
- Generally arise *de novo*, but may be linked with prior radiation treatment.

Pathology

Gross

- Unencapsulated, polypoid or sessile, tan-white, firm tumor, usually measuring less than 10 cm in diameter.
- Sinonasal fibrosarcomas are often associated with bone erosion or destruction.

Histology

- Fasciculated growth pattern, composed of spindle-shaped cells with scanty cytoplasm and indistinct cell borders.
- Histologic grade based on cellularity, cellular maturity, and the amount of collagen production:
  1. Low-grade fibrosarcoma:
     Cellular neoplasm with uniform spindle cells, absence of nuclear hyperchromasia, scattered mitoses, and variable amount of collagen.
     Fasciculated growth pattern is distinct.
  2. High-grade fibrosarcoma:
     Hypercellular neoplasm with pleomorphism, hyperchromatic, rounded to oval nuclei, increased mitotic activity, necrosis, and less collagen production.
     Loss or indistinct fasciculated growth.
- Both low- and high-grade neoplasms lack the marked pleomorphism or multinucleated giant cells more typically seen in malignant fibrous histiocytoma.
- Heterologous metaplastic elements (bone and cartilage) may be seen, particularly in the low-grade types.
- Myxoid stromal changes may be seen and may be prominent.
- Special stains of limited assistance in the diagnosis.

Differential Diagnosis

- Nodular fasciitis (Chapter 8, #5).
- Fibromatosis (Chapter 4A, #5).
- Malignant fibrous histiocytoma (Chapter 4B, #6).
- Spindle cell carcinoma (Chapter 14B, #2).
- Spindle cell melanoma (Chapter 4B, #3).
- Malignant schwannoma (Chapter 9B, #6).
- Synovial sarcoma, monophasic type (Chapter 14B, #8).

Treatment and Prognosis

- Radical surgical excision is the treatment of choice.
- Adjunctive radiotherapy may be of assistance, but there is no definitive proof as to its efficacy in treating fibrosarcomas.
- Prognosis is primarily related to the adequacy of surgical excision.
- Overall survival statistics vary considerably.
- Recurrent tumor is usually noted within the first postoperative year, but may be latent and occur many years after resection.
- Metastatic disease primarily occurs to the lungs and bone; lymph node metastasis is rare, and therefore radical neck dissections are not warranted.

Additional Facts

- Histologic grading schema has been proposed based on tumor differentiation (grades I and II, well differentiated; grades III and IV, poorly differentiated).
- Five-year survival statistics vary according to grade (approximate percentages): grade I, 80%; grade II, 55% to 75%; grade III, 35% to 40%; grade IV, 25%.
- Additional factors of importance in prognosis include size of tumor, location of the tumor, and number of mitoses.

References

Enzinger FW, Weiss SW: Malignant fibrohistiocytic tumors. *In*: Enzinger FW, Weiss SW, eds. Soft tissue tumors; 2nd ed. St. Louis; C. V. Mosby, 1988; pp 201–222.

Fu YS, Perzin KH: Non-epithelial tumors of the nasal cavity, paranasal sinuses, and nasopharynx: a clinicopathologic study. VI: fibrous tissue tumors (fibroma, fibromatosis, and fibrosarcoma). Cancer 37:2912–2928, 1976.

Heffner DK, Gnepp DR: Sinonasal fibrosarcoma, malignant schwannomas, and "Triton" tumors. Cancer 70:1089–1101, 1992.

Mark RJ, Tran L, Sercarz JA, Selch M, Calcaterra TC: Fibrosarcoma of the head and neck: the UCLA experience. Arch Otolaryngol Head Neck Surg 117:396–401, 1991.

Swain RE, Sessions DG, Ogura JH: Fibrosarcoma of the head and neck: a clinical analysis of forty cases. Ann Otol Rhinol Laryngol 83:439–444, 1974.

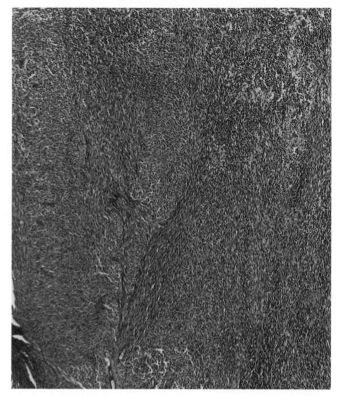

Figure 4–97. Sinonasal fibrosarcoma, characterized by a fasciculated growth pattern with long, sweeping fascicles and a dense, spindle-shaped cellular infiltrate.

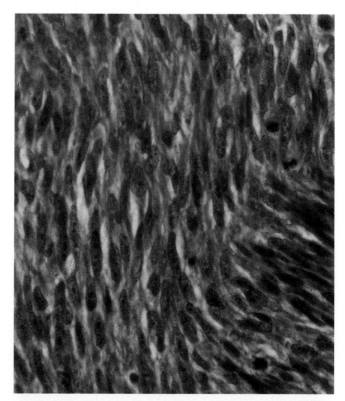

Figure 4–98. Fibrosarcoma, composed of a dense, pleomorphic cellular infiltrate of spindle-shaped cells with scanty cytoplasm, indistinct cell borders, and multiple mitotic figures.

8. Leiomyosarcoma

Definition: Malignant tumor of smooth muscle.

Clinical

■ Up to 10% of all leiomyosarcomas arise in the head and neck.

■ No sex predilection; occurs in a wide age range but is most common in the sixth decade of life.

■ In the head and neck, the most common sites of occurrence are nasal cavity and paranasal sinuses > skin > oral cavity (buccal mucosa, gingiva, tongue, floor of mouth) > larynx; other sites of occurrence include trachea, neck, hypopharynx, external auditory canal.

■ Most common symptoms are nasal obstruction, pain, and epistaxis.

■ Given the relative lack of smooth muscle in the head and neck region, the histogenesis of these neoplasms appears to arise from vascular structures.

Radiology

■ Soft tissue density.

■ Sinus opacification.

■ Bone erosion or invasion.

Pathology

Gross

■ Circumscribed but not encapsulated, tan-white to pink-red, polypoid or sessile lesion, usually measuring > 5 cm in diameter.

■ Ulceration, hemorrhage, necrosis, and invasion of adjacent structures are often identified.

Histology

■ Cellular neoplasm, composed of interlacing bundles of spindle-shaped cells with elongated, centrally located, blunt-ended, cigar-shaped nuclei and eosinophilic cytoplasm.

■ Infiltrative growth, cellular anaplasia/pleomorphism, nuclear hyperchromasia, and increased mitotic activity are hallmarks of this tumor and represent the features for the diagnosis of malignancy.

■ Multinucleated giant cells are common.

■ Nuclear palisading may be prominent.

■ A perinuclear vacuole or clear halo may be seen, giving the nucleus an indented or concave contour.

■ Stroma tends to be richly vascular, with close apposition of the tumor with the vascular structures.

■ Epithelioid cells and myxomatous change may be seen and occasionally may predominate, giving rise to so-called epithelioid leiomyosarcoma and myxoid leiomyosarcoma, respectively.

■ Histochemistry: cytoplasmic myofibrils can be seen in better differentiated tumors as deep red, longitudinal lines by Masson trichrome stain and purple by phosphotungstic acid-hematoxylin (PTAH) stain; glycogen is demonstrable as diastase-sensitive, PAS-positive material.

■ Immunohistochemistry: actin (smooth muscle and muscle-specific) positive; desmin generally is negative.

■ Electronmicroscopy: deeply indented nuclei, well-oriented myofilaments, pinocytotic vesicles, intercellular connections, and a basal lamina enveloping the entire cell membrane.

Differential Diagnosis

■ Leiomyoma (Chapter 4A, #6).

■ Spindle cell carcinoma (Chapter 14B, #2).

■ Malignant peripheral nerve sheath tumors (Chapter 9B, #6).

■ Fibrosarcoma (Chapter 4B, #7).

■ Rhabdomyosarcoma (Chapter 9B, #5).

Treatment and Prognosis

■ Radical surgical excision is the treatment of choice.

■ Radio- and chemotherapy are of questionable utility.

■ Prognosis is dependent on the site and extent of tumor and is not contingent on the histology:

Tumors limited to the nasal cavity are associated with a good prognosis and are cured after complete removal.

Tumors involving both the nasal cavity and paranasal sinuses result in an aggressive neoplasm, which is associated with increased recurrence, morbidity, and mortality rates.

■ Local recurrence occurs frequently and is usually associated with extensive uncontrollable local infiltration.

■ Metastases (hematogenous) occur infrequently, usually involving the lung; lymph node metastases are seen late in the disease course.

Additional Facts

■ Vascular derivation of the sinonasal tract leiomyosarcomas is supported by:

Close association of the neoplastic cells with vessel walls.

Relative lack of desmin immunoreactivity in these neoplasms (in general, desmin is seen in tumors of smooth muscle derivation; however, vascular smooth muscle has little, if any, desmin).

References

Fu YS, Perzin KH: Non-epithelial tumors of the nasal cavity, paranasal sinuses, and nasopharynx: a clinicopathologic study. IV: smooth muscle tumors (leiomyoma, leiomyosarcoma). Cancer 35:1300–1308, 1975.

Gabbiani G, Schmid E, Winter S, et al: Vascular smooth muscle cells differ from other smooth muscle cells: predominance of vimentin filaments and a specific alpha-type actin. Proc Natl Acad Sci USA 78:298–302, 1981.

Kuruvilla A, Wenig BM, Humphrey DM, Heffner DK: Leiomyosarcoma of the sinonasal tract: a clinicopathologic study of nine cases. Arch Otolaryngol Head Neck Surg 116:1278–1286, 1990.

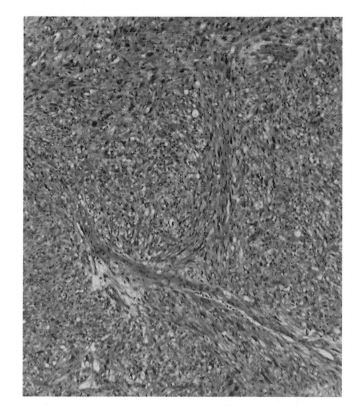

Figure 4–99. Leiomyosarcoma of the nasal cavity: cellular neoplasm composed of interlacing bundles of spindle-shaped cells and numerous hyperchromatic and enlarged nuclei are seen.

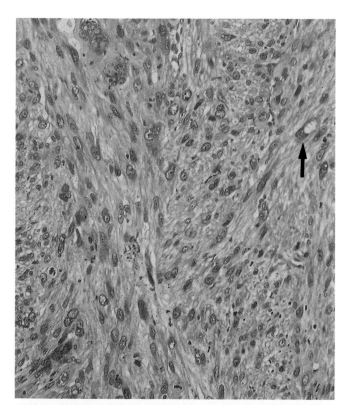

Figure 4–100. Cellular components of leiomyosarcoma include elongated, centrally located, blunt-ended, cigar-shaped nuclei with eosinophilic cytoplasm; cellular anaplasia and pleomorphism, nuclear hyperchromasia, and increased mitotic activity are seen; the presence of perinuclear vacuole or clear halo gives the nucleus an indented or concave contour (*arrow*).

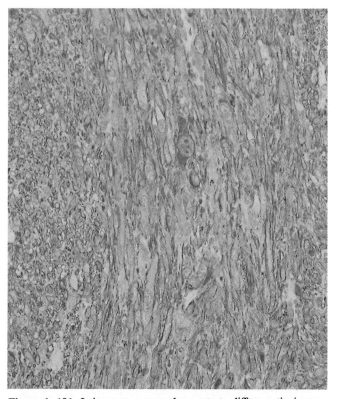

Figure 4–101. Leiomyosarcomas demonstrate diffuse actin immunoreactivity.

9. Angiosarcoma

Definition: Malignant tumor of endothelial cell origin.

Clinical

- In general, a rare neoplasm, accounting for <1% of all sarcomas.
- In contrast to other sarcomas, angiosarcomas have a predilection for cutaneous and superficial soft tissue sites.
- In the head and neck, the most common site of occurrence is in the skin and subcutaneous tissue, particularly the scalp.
- Cutaneous angiosarcomas affect males more than females; most often seen in the seventh and eighth decades of life.
- Noncutaneous angiosarcomas:
  No sex predilection; occur in a younger age population as compared with their cutaneous counterparts, with the average age of occurrence in the fifth decade of life.
  Are seen in the nasal cavity and paranasal sinuses > oral cavity (gingiva, buccal mucosa, palate, tongue, tonsil) > nasopharynx and larynx.
  Symptoms vary according to the site of occurrence and include a mass lesion, epistaxis, nasal obstruction, and headaches.

Pathology

Gross

- Nodular or ulcerative, ill-defined lesion with a bluish color, sometimes surrounded by an erythematous ring.
- Bleeding is common.
- Clinically, the extent of the tumor is often difficult to determine.
- May be unifocal or multifocal.

Histology

- Proliferation of ramifying and anastomosing vascular channels that "dissect" through surrounding structures.
- Endothelial cells lining the vascular spaces are plump; increased in number; pleomorphic; pile up along the lumen, creating papillations; and demonstrate mitotic activity.
- Depending on the cellularity, pleomorphism and mitotic activity tumors are graded as either low or high grade.
- Necrosis is a prominent finding.
- Endothelial cells may appear spindled, epithelioid, or polygonal.
- Histochemistry: reticulin stains delineate the vascular lumina, with the endothelial cells identified on the luminal side of the reticulin framework (this contrasts with the reticulin staining seen in hemangiopericytomas).
- Immunohistochemistry: factor VIII-related antigen, *Ulex europaeus,* and CD34 positive.

- Electronmicroscopy: partial envelopment of basal lamina along the antiluminal border, pinocytotic bodies, tight junctions between cells, and occasional identification of rod-shaped microtubulated bodies (Weibel-Palade bodies).

Differential Diagnosis

- Angiolymphoid hyperplasia with eosinophilia (Chapter 24A, #4).
- Hemangioma and lobular capillary hemangioma (Chapter 4A, #2; Chapter 19A, #4).
- Epithelioid hemangioendothelioma.
- Kaposi's sarcoma (Chapter 9B, #9).
- Malignant melanoma (Chapter 4B, #3).
- Poorly differentiated carcinoma (Chapter 4B, #1).
- Fibrosarcoma (Chapter 4B, #7).

Treatment and Prognosis

- Complete surgical excision is the treatment of choice, especially with well-delineated and solitary tumors.
- Surgery and radiotherapy may be of benefit in multifocal, ill-defined tumors.
- Prognosis is generally poor, with 10% to 15% 5-year survival rates.
- Recurrences and metastases occur within 2 years of diagnosis; the common sites for metastases are lymph nodes and lung.
- The most important factor in prognosis is tumor size, with tumors <5 cm in diameter having a better prognosis than larger tumors.

Additional Facts

- Angiosarcomas often extend beyond their apparent macroscopic limits, which must be accounted for in therapeutic management of these tumors.
- Upper respiratory tract angiosarcomas may have a better prognosis than their cutaneous counterparts, which may be related to earlier symptomatology and diagnosis and to a younger age at initial presentation.

References

Barnes L: Angiosarcoma. *In*: Barnes L, ed. Surgical pathology of the head and neck. New York: Marcel Dekker, 1985; pp 826–831.

Enzinger FW, Weiss SW: Malignant vascular tumors. *In*: Enzinger FW, Weiss SW, eds. Soft tissue tumors; 2nd ed. St. Louis: C. V. Mosby, 1988; pp 545–561.

Fu YS, Perzin KH: Non-epithelial tumors of the nasal cavity, paranasal sinuses, and nasopharynx: a clinicopathologic study. I: general features and vascular tumors. Cancer 33:1275–1288, 1974.

Holden CA, Spittle MF, Wilson Jones E: Angiosarcoma of the face and scalp, prognosis and treatment. Cancer 59:1046–1057, 1987.

Traweek ST, Kandalaft PL, Mehta P, Battifora H: The human hematopoietic progenitor cell antigen (CD34) in vascular neoplasia. Am J Clin Pathol 96:25–31, 1991.

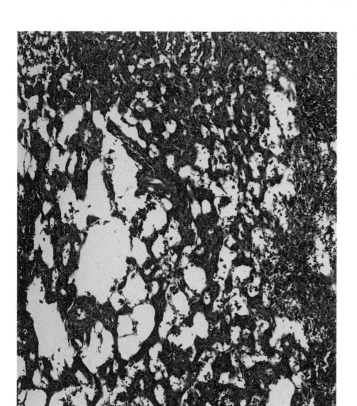

Figure 4–102. Nasal cavity angiosarcoma, characterized by proliferation of ramifying and anastomosing vascular channels with piling up of the endothelial cells along the lumen, thereby creating papillations or endothelial tufts.

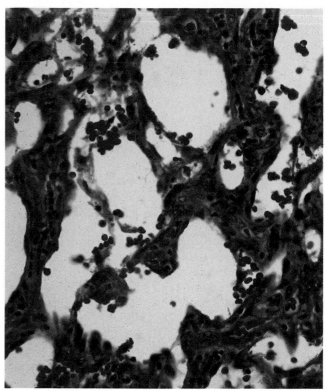

Figure 4–103. Angiosarcoma, with ramifying and interconnecting vascular spaces lined by plump, hyperchromatic and pleomorphic endothelial cells with increased mitotic activity.

10. Osteosarcoma

Definition: Malignant (osteoid-producing) neoplasm arising from bone.
Synonym: Osteogenic sarcoma.

Clinical

■ Second to multiple myeloma, osteosarcoma is the most common malignant bone tumor and commonly arises in the metaphyseal area of long bones, occurring primarily in the second decade of life.

■ Head and neck osteosarcomas are rare, representing approximately 6% of all osteogenic sarcomas.

■ Osteosarcomas of the head and neck (excluding those arising in the setting of Paget's disease) have no sex predilection and occur in a slightly older age group as compared with osteosarcomas of long bones, affecting individuals in the third to fourth decades of life.

■ The most common site of involvement in the head and neck is the mandible (body > symphysis > angle > ramus); other sites of involvement include the maxilla, paranasal sinuses (maxillary and ethmoid), and skull.

■ Symptoms vary according to the site of occurrence and include painful swelling of the face, dentition problems, nasal obstruction, epistaxis.

■ Most osteosarcomas arise *de novo*; however, some are related to prior radiotherapy, Paget's disease, fibrous dysplasia, and thorotrast injection.

■ Elevated serum alkaline phosphatase represents the sole laboratory value of clinical import in osteosarcoma; an abrupt elevation in patients with preexisting benign bone lesions may be indicative of malignant transformation.

Radiology

■ Destructive, poorly delineated osteolytic, osteosclerotic, or mixed lesion.

■ Periosteal reactions include cupping out of subperiosteal cortical bone; thin, bulging, opaque, noncontinuous line of new bone formation beneath the periosteum in the adjacent soft tissue; irregular, sclerotic mass of subperiosteal new bone with multiple laminations; Codman's triangle (where tumor strips the periosteum from the bone and new bone is laid down, creating a "sunburst" pattern that represents radiating spicules within the tumor itself; this pattern can be seen in a small percentage of cases and is not pathognomonic for osteosarcoma).

■ Involvement of the alveolar bone between teeth may result in projection of sclerotic material beyond the height of the crestal bone into adjacent soft tissue; this is highly suggestive of osteosarcoma.

■ Widening of the periodontal membrane space along one side of one or more roots is a highly characteristic feature of malignant neoplasms.

Pathology

Gross

■ Gross appearance is dependent on the extent of mineralization versus the extent of the stromal component, such that the tumor may vary from firm, hard, and gritty to fleshy and fibrous.

■ Gnathic osteosarcomas generally do not exceed 5.0 cm in greatest diameter.

Histology

■ Sarcomatous stroma intimately admixed and giving rise to osteoid.

■ Osteoid, the calcified precursor of bone, appears by hematoxylin and eosin stain as eosinophilic, hyalin-like material with irregular contours and surrounded by a rim of osteoblasts.

■ Stromal cells display variable anaplasia and are spindled to polygonal, composed of hyperchromatic nuclei with or without nucleoli.

■ Tumor giant cells are often seen; benign, osteoclast-like multinucleated giant cells are identified in approximately 25% of cases.

■ Necrosis, invasive growth, and mitotic activity (normal and bizarre mitoses) are commonly seen.

■ Vascularity varies from relatively inconspicuous to dominant.

■ Tumor cells demonstrate strong alkaline phosphatase activity.

■ Osteoblasts are multipotential cells capable of producing chondroblastic and fibroblastic foci; depending on which component predominates, osteosarcomas are divided into osteoblastic, chondroblastic, and fibroblastic types; however, prognosis does not appear to be altered based on this subdivision.

■ Telangiectatic variant is rarely identified in head and neck osteosarcomas and is composed of prominent, blood-filled cystic spaces separated by septa containing the malignant stroma; osteoid tends to be fine and lacelike in this variant.

Differential Diagnosis

As a result of the histomorphologic variability of osteosarcoma, the differential diagnosis may include:

■ Benign lesions: fracture callus, myositis ossificans, fibrous dysplasia (Chapter 4A, #7a), aneurysmal bone cyst.

■ Benign tumors: osteoblastoma, giant-cell tumor, juvenile active ossifying fibroma (Chapter 4A, #7c).

■ Malignant tumors: chondrosarcoma (Chapter 14B, #7), fibrosarcoma (Chapter 4B, #7).

Treatment and Prognosis

■ Complete surgical excision, generally encompassing radical procedures including mandibulectomy or maxillectomy.

■ Radiation and chemotherapy are used as adjuncts to surgery.

■ Gnathic osteosarcomas have a tendency to recur, with maxillary osteosarcomas recurring in a higher percentage of cases as compared with mandibular tumors; recurrence appears within the first postoperative year.

■ Metastases occur late in the course of disease, usually disseminate to the lungs and brain, and are associated with a mean survival of 6 months.

■ Prognostic factors include:
Stage of disease.
Site of origin of the tumor: in general, gnathic osteosarcomas have a better prognosis as compared with those of their long bone counterparts; however, skull-based and maxillary antral osteosarcomas have a worse prognosis compared with mandibular osteosarcomas.
Multifocality: considered uniformly fatal.
Serum alkaline phosphatase level: elevations of this enzyme are associated with a worse prognosis and may be indicative of residual viable tumor or metastatic disease.
Osteosarcomas arising in Paget's disease: highly malignant, with negligible 5-year survival.

Additional Facts

■ Juxtacortical (paraosteal) osteosarcoma is an infrequently occurring variant of conventional osteosarcoma and is associated with a better prognosis; this variant rarely occurs within the head and neck.

■ Osteosarcomas may occur in extraosseous sites such as soft tissue and viscera but are decidedly uncommon, and in the head and neck they are rare.

References

Barnes L: Osteosarcoma. *In*: Barnes L, ed. Surgical pathology of the head and neck. New York: Marcel Dekker, 1985; pp 985–999.

Caron AS, Hajdu SI, Strong EL: Osteogenic sarcoma of the facial and cranial bones. Am J Surg 122:719–725, 1971.

Chan CW, Kung TM, Ma L: Telangiectatic osteosarcoma of the mandible. Cancer 58:2110–2115, 1986.

Clark JC, Unni KK, Dahlin DC, Devine KD: Osteosarcoma of the jaw. Cancer 52:2311–2316, 1983.

Garrington GE, Scofield HH, Cornyn J, Hooker SP: Osteosarcoma of the jaws: analysis of 56 cases. Cancer 20:377–391, 1967.

Gupta D, Vishwakarma SK: Osteogenic sarcoma of the frontal sinus. Ann Otol Rhinol Laryngol 99:489–490, 1990.

Langlais RP: Osteosarcoma (osteogenic sarcoma). *In*: Delbalso AM, ed. Maxillofacial imaging. Philadelphia: W. B. Saunders Co., 1990; pp 359–261.

Roca AN, Smith JL, Jing BS: Osteosarcoma and paraosteal osteogenic sarcoma of the maxilla and mandible: study of 20 cases. Am J Clin Pathol 54:625–636, 1970.

Rufus RJ, Sercarz JA, Tran L, Dodd LG, Selch M, Calcaterra TC: Osteosarcoma of the head and neck; the UCLA experience. Arch Otolaryngol Head Neck Surg 117:761–766, 1991.

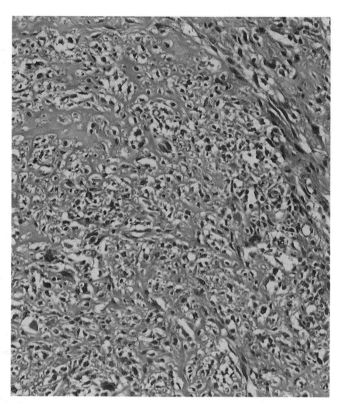

Figure 4–105. Histologic appearance of osteosarcoma composed of a sarcomatous stroma intimately admixed with osteoid, which appears as eosinophilic, hyalin-like material with irregular contours; the stromal cells are anaplastic and vary from spindled to polygonal in shape, with scattered tumor giant cells.

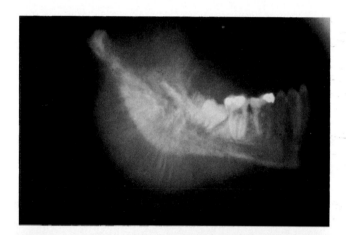

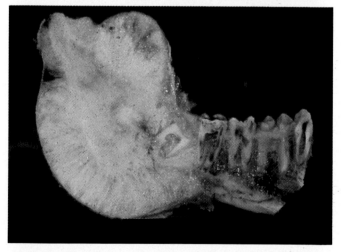

Figure 4–104. Osteosarcoma of the mandible. (*Top*) Radiograph of resected specimen showing a large mass at the angle of the mandible. Multiple radial densities representing new bone formation beneath an elevated periosteum and termed "sun-burst" pattern can be seen. Although not pathognomonic, this pattern is typically associated with osteogenic sarcoma. (*Bottom*) The corresponding gross specimen showing destruction of the mandible and extension into adjacent soft tissue by a tan-white mass with spiculations at its peripheral portion. Both osseous and chondroid differentiation can be appreciated.

11. Teratocarcinosarcoma

Definition: Malignant sinonasal tract neoplasm with combined histologic features of carcinosarcoma and teratoma.

Clinical

- Affects males more than females; occurs over a wide age range, with a median age of 60 years.
- Rapidly growing neoplasm whose symptoms primarily include nasal obstruction and epistaxis.
- The most common site of involvement is the nasal cavity; other sites of involvement include the ethmoid and maxillary sinuses.

Radiology

- Nasal cavity mass or clouding of a sinus.
- Associated bone destruction may be seen.

Pathology

Gross

- Friable to firm, red-brown mass.

Histology

- All neoplasms are characterized by a combination of epithelial and mesenchymal tissue components with heterogeneic or variegated architectural growth patterns.
- Epithelial components include:
  Glandular or ductal structures lined by benign-appearing, partly ciliated columnar epithelium with transitional areas to nonkeratinizing clear-cell squamous epithelium and to squamous epithelium without clear cells.
  Areas of squamous carcinoma and adenocarcinoma.
  Poorly differentiated malignant epithelial elements.
- Mesenchymal components include:
  Benign- and malignant-appearing fibroblasts or myofibroblasts.
  Rhabdomyosarcoma.
  Benign cartilage with an immature or "fetal" appearance and chondrosarcoma.
  Osteoid.
- Teratoid components include:
  "Fetal-appearing" clear-cell squamous epithelium.
  Organoid structures.
  Neural tissue component in the form of poorly differentiated neuroepithelial tissue occasionally associated with neural rosettes and neurofibrillary matrix.
- No areas of seminoma, germinoma, choriocarcinoma, or embryonal carcinoma are seen.
- Histochemistry: abundant glycogen as demonstrated by diastase-sensitive, PAS-positive material seen in clear cells; mucin and PAS-positive material seen within the lumen or cytoplasm of the glandular component.

- Immunohistochemistry: dependent on the cytologic components and includes reactivity with cytokeratin, epithelial membrane antigen, S-100 protein, chromogranin, Ber-EP4, Leu-7, neuron-specific enolase, desmin, vimentin, glial fibrillary acidic protein (GFAP).

Differential Diagnosis

- Squamous carcinoma and adenocarcinoma (Chapter 4B, #1,2).
- Olfactory neuroblastoma (Chapter 4B, #5).
- Mixed tumor (Chapter 19A, #1) and malignant mixed tumor (Chapter 19B, #4).
- Malignant teratoma (Chapter 8, #3).
- Rhabdomyosarcoma (Chapter 9B, #5).
- Craniopharyngioma.

Treatment and Prognosis

- Aggressive therapy, including radical surgical extirpation and irradiation.
- Highly malignant neoplasm, with an average survival of <2 years.
- Recurrence of tumor is common, with extensive local invasion.
- Metastatic disease primarily to cervical lymph nodes.

Additional Facts

- Teratocarcinosarcoma represents a unique clinicopathologic entity.
- "Fetal-appearing" clear-cell squamous epithelium represents:
  A characteristic histologic finding for diagnosis.
  Supportive evidence of the teratoid nature of this neoplasm, given its description in teratomas of other organ systems.

Reference

Heffner DK: Teratocarcinosarcoma (malignant teratoma?) of the nasal cavity and paranasal sinuses: a clinicopathologic study of 20 cases. Cancer 53:2140–2154, 1984.

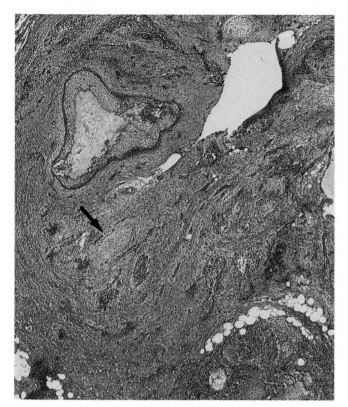

Figure 4-106. Sinonasal teratocarcinosarcoma (STCS) showing squamous epithelial nests, neurofibrillary matrix (*arrow*), and a variably cellular stroma composed of a spindle-shaped to small round cell infiltrate.

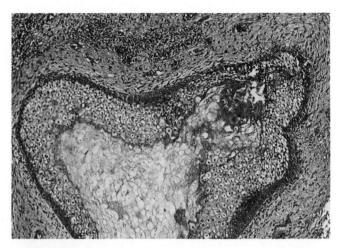

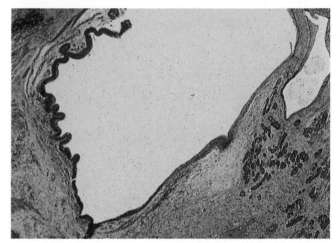

Figure 4-107. STCS. (*Top*) Nonkeratinizing clear cell squamous epithelium. (*Bottom*) Dilated glandular space lined by an epithelium demonstrating a transition from a bland-appearing cuboidal and columnar epithelium (benign) to a cellular columnar epithelium with hyperchromatic, stratified nuclei (malignant).

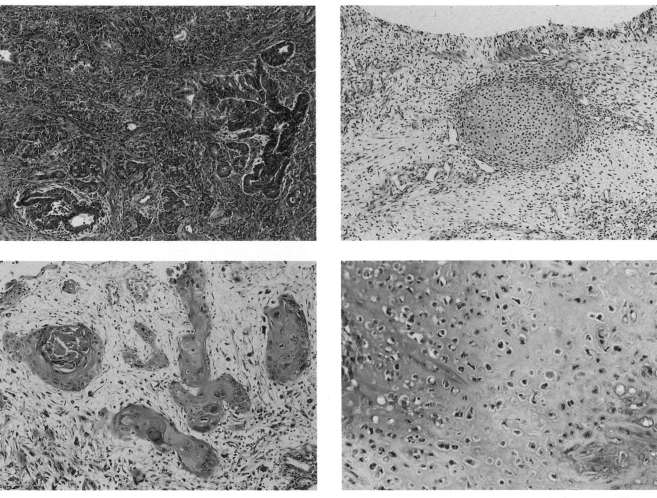

Figure 4-108. STCS. (*Top*) Adenocarcinoma associated with a malignant fibroblastic stromal component. (*Bottom*) Squamous cell carcinoma admixed with a malignant pleomorphic mesenchymal component.

Figure 4-109. STCS. (*Top*) Immature cartilaginous nest. (*Bottom*) Focus of chondrosarcoma.

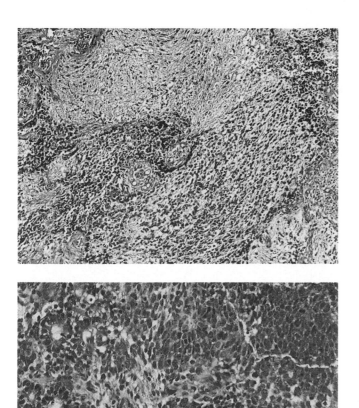

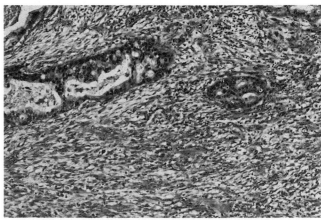

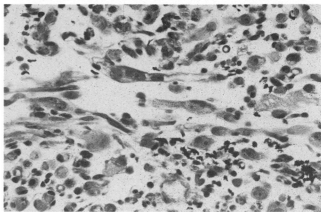

Figure 4-111. STCS. (*Top*) Adenocarcinomatous foci associated with a fibrosarcomatous stromal component. (*Bottom*) Rhabdomyosarcomatous foci with strap cells, one of which has identifiable cross striations (*center*).

Figure 4-110. STCS. (*Top*) Neurofibrillary matrix associated with an immature and undifferentiated small round cell infiltrate. (*Bottom*) Neural rosettes associated with a neurosarcomatous cellular infiltrate.

CHAPTER 5

Tumor, Nodes, and Metastases (TNM) Classification of Maxillary Sinus Neoplasms

ANATOMIC SITE
Maxillary Sinus

CLASSIFICATION
CLINICAL STAGE

ANATOMIC SITE

Maxillary Sinus

Ohngren's line: the plane that passes through the inner canthus and the mandibular angle, dividing the upper jaw into the superoposterior (suprastructure) and inferoanterior (infrastructure) structures.

CLASSIFICATION

1. T = extent of the primary tumor.
   - Includes both the clinical (T) and pathologic (pT) categories.
   - T designation varies according to the anatomic site involved:
     TX—primary tumor cannot be assessed.
     T0—no evidence of primary tumor.
     Tis—carcinoma in situ.
     T1—tumor limited to the antral mucosa, with no erosion or destruction of bone.
     T2—tumor with erosion or destruction of the infrastructure, including the hard palate or middle nasal meatus.
     T3—tumor invades the skin of cheek, posterior wall of the maxillary sinus, floor or medial wall of orbit, or anterior ethmoid sinus.
     T4—tumor invades the orbital contents or the cribriform plate, posterior ethmoid or sphenoid sinuses, nasopharynx, soft palate, pterygomaxillary or temporal fossae, base of skull.
2. N = absence/presence and extent of regional lymph node metastasis; includes both the clinical (N) and pathologic (pN) categories.
   NX—regional lymph nodes cannot be assessed.
   N0—no regional lymph node metastasis.

N1—metastasis in a single ipsilateral lymph node, 3 cm or less in greatest dimension.
N2—metastasis in a single ipsilateral lymph node, >3 cm but not >6 cm in greatest dimension *or* metastasis in multiple ipsilateral lymph nodes, none >6 cm in greatest dimension, *or* metastasis in bilateral or contralateral lymph nodes, none >6 cm in greatest dimension.
N2a—metastasis in a single ipsilateral lymph node, >3 cm but not >6 cm in greatest dimension.
N2b—metastasis in multiple ipsilateral lymph nodes, none >6 cm in greatest dimension.
N2c—metastasis in bilateral or contralateral lymph nodes, none >6 cm in greatest dimension.
N3—metastasis in a lymph node >6 cm in greatest dimension.

3. M = absence or presence of distant metastasis; includes both the clinical (M) and pathologic (pM) categories.
   MX—not assessed.
   M0—no distant metastasis.
   M1—distant metastasis present.

CLINICAL STAGE

Stage I—T1N0M0.
Stage II—T2N0M0.
Stage III—T3N0M0 or T1–T3N1M0.
Stage IV—T4, or N2, N3, or M1.

Reference

Spiessl B, Beahrs OH, Hermanek P, Hutter RVP, Scheibe O, Sobin LH, Wagner G (eds): TNM atlas: illustrated guide to the TNM/PTNM-classification of malignant tumours, 3rd ed. Berlin, Springer-Verlag; 1989.

SECTION ■2

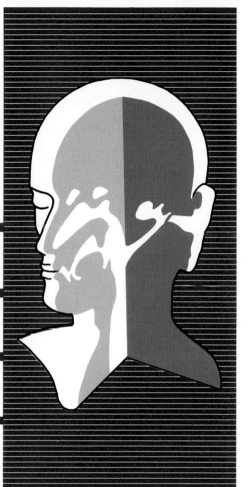

ORAL CAVITY, NASOPHARYNX, AND NECK

CHAPTER 6

Anatomy and Histology of the Oral Cavity, Nasopharynx, and Neck

ORAL CAVITY
Contents
Anatomic Borders
Histology

NASOPHARYNX AND OROPHARYNX
Contents
Anatomic Borders
Histology
NECK
Anatomy

ORAL CAVITY

Contents

■ The structures within the anatomic confines of the oral cavity include lips, buccal mucosa (includes all membrane lining of the interior surface of the cheeks and lips), alveolar ridges (upper and lower), retromolar trigone, floor of mouth, anterior two thirds of the tongue, the hard palate, gingivae (gums), and teeth.

Anatomic Borders

■ Anterior—vermilion border of the lips.
■ Posterior—line drawn from the junction of the hard and soft palate to the circumvallate papillae of the tongue.
■ Superior—hard palate until its junction with the soft palate.
■ Inferior—anterior two thirds of the tongue to the line of the circumvallate papillae.
■ Lateral—buccal mucosa of the cheeks.

Histology

■ The epithelial surface of the oral cavity is covered by a stratified squamous epithelium, and, unlike the skin, keratinization is not seen under normal conditions.
■ Minor salivary glands are seen throughout the oral cavity submucosa.
■ Tongue: The epithelial lining is a stratified squamous epithelium; a submucous layer is present only on the ventral surface; underneath the mu-

cosa, the tongue is characterized by the presence of interlacing bundles of striated muscle.
■ The dorsal aspect of the tongue, in particular the anterior portion, is characterized by the presence of numerous mucosal projections forming papillae; these papillae are absent on the ventral surface.
■ Taste buds are seen as pale, oval bodies within the papillae epithelium along the dorsal and lateral aspects of the tongue.
■ Minor salivary glands are identified within the muscular tissue.

NASOPHARYNX AND OROPHARYNX

Contents

1. **Nasopharynx:** the nasopharyngeal tonsils (adenoids) lie along the posterior and lateral wall of the nasopharynx.
2. **Oropharynx:** soft palate, tonsillar pillars, palatine tonsils, posterior tonsillar pillars, uvula, and base of tongue, including the lingual tonsils.
3. **Waldeyer's ring** is formed by a ring or group of lymphoid tissues about the upper end of the pharynx and consists of the palatine tonsils, pharyngeal tonsils (adenoids), the lingual tonsils, and the adjacent submucosal lymphatics.

Anatomic Borders

1. **Nasopharynx:** lies behind the nasal cavity and above the soft palate.
   ■ Anterior—continuous with the nasal cavities through the choanae.

101

■ Posterior—continuous with the roof and is further supported by the first cervical vertebra (anterior arch of the atlas).
■ Superior (roof)—base of skull (occipital bone) and posterior part of the body of the sphenoid bone.
■ Inferior (floor)—continuous with the oropharynx; during swallowing, the palate and uvula provide a functional floor.
■ Lateral—each side contains the pharyngeal orifice of the eustacian tube, which, in the posterior portion, has a submucosal cartilaginous elevation called the torus tubarius; behind this is a shallow depression called the fossa of Rosenmüller.

2. **Oropharynx:**
■ Anterior—continuous with the mouth through the oropharyngeal isthmus.
■ Posterior—on a level with the second and third cervical vertebrae.
■ Superior—horizontal plane of the palate.
■ Inferior—horizontal plane of the hyoid bone (upper border of the epiglottis).
■ Lateral—palatopharyngeal arch.

Histology

1. **Nasopharynx:**
■ The epithelium varies from stratified squamous to ciliated pseudostratified (respiratory) to a transitional type; although these types of epithelia may be associated with a specific part of the nasopharyngeal region, this is not constant, so that any site may be covered by any type of epithelium.
■ The submucosa contains minor salivary glands as well as a prominent lymphoid component; the basement membrane of the epithelium is inconspicuous, and the lymphoid component may normally be present in the epithelium (lymphoepithelium).
■ Adenoids: lymphoid tissue contains germinal centers but does not have a capsule or sinusoids, nor are there epithelial crypts; the lymphoid component is normally present in the epithelial layer.

2. **Oropharynx:**
■ The epithelium throughout is a stratified squamous epithelium, which normally does not have a keratin layer.
■ The submucosa contains minor salivary glands as well as a scattered lymphoid component.
■ Tonsils: like the adenoids, the tonsils contain a prominent lymphoid component, including germinal centers, but do not have a capsule or sinusoids; unlike the adenoids, the tonsils have crypts lined by stratified squamous epithelium.
■ The lymphoid component is normally seen in the surface and crypt epithelium.
■ Minor salivary glands are seen embedded in the underlying muscle.

NECK

Anatomy

■ The prominent landmarks in the neck are the hyoid bone, the thyroid cartilage, the trachea, and the sternocleidomastoid muscles.
■ The neck is divided into the anterior and posterior triangles by the sternocleidomastoid muscles.
■ Anterior triangle:
Lateral limit—anterior border of the sternocleidomastoid muscle.
Medial limit—anatomic midline of the neck.
Above—lower border of the mandible.
■ Subdivisions of the anterior triangle include:
Carotid triangle.
Submandibular (submaxillary) triangle.
Inferior carotid (muscular) triangle.
Submental or suprahyoid triangle.
■ The contents of the anterior triangle include the common carotid artery with its internal and external branches, cranial nerves IX to XII, the internal jugular vein, and the superficial and deep cervical lymph nodes.
■ Posterior triangle:
Anteromedial—posterior border of the sternocleidomastoid muscle.
Posterolateral—anterior border of the trapezius muscle.
Below—the clavicle.
■ The contents of the posterior triangle include subclavian artery, external jugular vein, branches of the cervical plexus, cranial nerve XI (accessory), and numerous lymph nodes, including the posterior cervical and supraclavicular lymph nodes.

References

Embryology, Anatomy, and Histology

Fawcett DW: Oral cavity and associated glands. *In*: Fawcett DW, ed. Bloom and Fawcett's A textbook of histology, 11th ed. Philadelphia: W.B. Saunders Co., 1986; pp 579–601.
Hollinshead WH: The jaws, palate and tongue. *In*: Hollinshead WH, ed. Anatomy for surgeons, vol. 1, 3rd ed. Philadelphia: Harper & Row, 1982; pp 325–387.
Hollinshead WH: The pharynx and larynx. *In*: Hollinshead WH, ed. Anatomy for surgeons, vol. 1, 3rd ed. Philadelphia: Harper & Row, 1982; pp 389–441.
Hollinshead WH: The neck. *In*: Hollinshead WH, ed. Anatomy for surgeons, vol. 1, 3rd ed. Philadelphia: Harper & Row, 1982; pp 443–531.
Moore KL: The branchial apparatus and the head and neck. *In*: Moore ML, ed. The developing human: clinically oriented embryology, 4th ed. Philadelphia: W.B. Saunders Co., 1988; pp 170–206.
Moore KL: The respiratory system. *In*: Moore ML, ed. The developing human: clinically oriented embryology, 4th ed. Philadelphia: W.B. Saunders Co., 1988; pp 207–216.
Warwick R, Williams PL: The oral cavity. *In*: Warwick R, Williams PL, eds. Gray's anatomy, 35th British ed. Philadelphia: W.B. Saunders Co., 1973; pp 1205–1209.
Warwick R, Williams PL: The pharynx. *In*: Warwick R, Williams PL, eds. Gray's anatomy, 35th British ed. Philadelphia: W.B. Saunders Co., 1973; pp 1243–1250.

CHAPTER 7

Classification of Non-neoplastic Lesions and Neoplasms of the Oral Cavity, Nasopharynx, Tonsils, and Neck

NON-NEOPLASTIC LESIONS

Table 7–1
CLASSIFICATION OF NON-NEOPLASTIC LESIONS OF THE ORAL CAVITY, NASOPHARYNX, TONSILS, AND NECK

Developmental anomalies: branchial cleft anomalies; others
Heterotopias; hamartomas; teratomas
Cysts: mucocele, ranula
Necrotizing sialometaplasia
Nodular fasciitis
Tangier disease
Reactive and infectious lymphadenopathies:
  Epstein-Barr virus (infectious mononucleosis)
  Mycobacterial *(M. tuberculosis)*
  Sarcoidosis
  Actinomycosis
  Cat scratch disease
  Human immunodeficiency virus (HIV) and acquired immune deficiency syndrome–related infections of the head and neck and lymphadenopathies
  Others

Table 7–2
CLASSIFICATION OF NEOPLASMS OF THE ORAL CAVITY, NASOPHARYNX, TONSILS, AND NECK

I . Benign
  A. Epithelial
    Squamous papilloma
    Minor salivary gland tumors
  B. Mesenchymal/neuroectodermal
    Angiofibroma
    Granular cell tumor
    Lymphangioma/cystic hygroma
    Hemangioma
    Neurilemmoma/Neurofibroma

NEOPLASMS

Table 7–2
Continued

    Lipoma
    Paraganglioma
    Fibrous histiocytoma
    Leiomyoma
    Rhabdomyoma
    Others
II. Malignant
  A. Epithelial
    Squamous cell carcinoma including:
      "Conventional-type"
      Spindle cell or sarcomatoid
      Exophytic/papillary
    Verrucous carcinoma
    Nasopharyngeal carcinoma (keratinizing, nonkeratinizing, undifferentiated)
    Low-grade papillary adenocarcinoma
    Adenosquamous carcinoma
    Minor salivary gland tumors:
      Adenoid cystic carcinoma
      Mucoepidermoid carcinoma
      Acinic cell adenocarcinoma
      Polymorphous low-grade adenocarcinoma
      Others
  B. Mesenchymal/neuroectodermal
    Malignant melanoma
    Lymphomas (non-Hodgkin's and Hodgkin's)
    Rhabdomyosarcoma
    Malignant fibrous histiocytoma/fibrosarcoma
    Malignant schwannoma
    Chordoma
    Angiosarcoma
    Kaposi's sarcoma
    Liposarcoma
    Synovial sarcoma
    Leiomyosarcoma
    Others
  C. Metastatic neoplasms to the neck

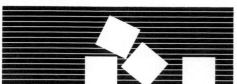

CHAPTER 8

Non-neoplastic Lesions of the Oral Cavity, Nasopharynx, Tonsils, and Neck

1. BRANCHIAL CLEFT ANOMALIES

Definition: Cysts, sinuses, or fistulas related to developmental alterations of the branchial apparatus.

Clinical

- No sex preference; seen at any age but most commonly become evident in young adults.
- Predominantly occur in the lateral neck along the anterior portion of the sternocleidomastoid muscle; also seen in the area around the external ear, in the external auditory canal, and in the parotid gland.
- Generally occur as an isolated phenomenon but may be familial or rarely may be associated with other congenital defects (malformed auricles, hearing abnormalities, patent ductus arteriosus, tear duct atresia).
- Cysts present as nontender, fluctuant masses in appropriate locations; cysts may become inflamed and abscesses may develop, potentially associated with dysphagia, dyspnea, or stridor.
- Sinuses and fistulas are associated with discharge of mucoid or purulent secretions from the tract opening.

- Up to 10% of cases may be bilateral.
- Branchial cleft anomalies are divided according to the branchial apparatus involved.

First Branchial Cleft Anomalies

- Rare as compared with anomalies of the second branchial cleft; represent from 1% to 8% of all branchial apparatus defects.
- Identified in a variety of locations, including pre-, post-, or infra-auricular; at the angle of the jaw; associated with the ear lobe; and in the external auditory canal.
- May involve the parotid gland, resulting in a mass or inflammation.
- Involvement of the external auditory canal may result in otalgia or otorrhea.

Pathology

Gross

- May occur as a cyst (68%), sinus (16%), or fistula (16%).
- Fistulous tract connects the skin and the external auditory canal.

Histology

Divided by Work into two types.

- Type I contains only ectodermal elements, as represented by the presence of a keratinized squamous epithelium.
- Type II contains both ectodermal and mesodermal elements, including keratinized squamous epithelium, cutaneous adnexa, and cartilage.

Differential Diagnosis

- Epidermoid cyst.
- Dermoids.
- Cystic sebaceous lymphadenoma.

Treatment and Prognosis

- Complete surgical excision is the treatment of choice.
- Incision and drainage are indicated in cases where abscesses have developed; complete surgical excision must wait until resolution of the infection.
- Inadequate excision results in recurrence and increased risk of infection.
- Work type II anomalies are often intimately associated with the parotid gland and may require a superficial parotidectomy to ensure complete excision.
- Although there is no consistent relationship of the tract with the facial nerve as it courses through the parotid gland, exposure and dissection of the nerve and its branches are required in Work type II anomalies.

Second Branchial Cleft Anomalies

- Account for the majority of the branchial apparatus anomalies representing from 92% to 99% of all cases.
- Cysts:
  Are much more common than fistulas.
  Affect both sexes equally; typically occur in the third to fifth decades of life and are uncommon in patients older than 50 years of age.
  Occur along the anterior border of the sternocleidomastoid muscle, most commonly at the level of the angle of the mandible.
  Present as a painless, fluctuant neck mass that may increase in size in conjunction with an upper respiratory tract infection, at which time they may become painful.
- Sinuses and fistulas:
  Are most often identified at birth or in early childhood.
  Present as a small opening above the clavicle through which mucoid secretions may be expressed.
  Are divided into three types:
  1. Incomplete external, having an external (cutaneous) but no internal (pharyngeal) opening.

2. Incomplete internal, having a pharyngeal but no cutaneous opening.
3. Complete, having both pharyngeal and cutaneous openings: the cutaneous opening is seen anywhere along the anterior border of the sternocleidomastoid muscle from the hyoid bone to the sternum with the epithelial tract coursing cephalad, between the internal and external carotid arteries, over cranial nerves IX and XII, deep to the posterior belly of the digastric muscle and terminating close to the middle constrictor muscle or with an internal opening in the pharyngeal wall or tonsillar region.

Radiology

- Cyst: well-defined, low-density lesion surrounded by a thin, uniform wall.
- Non-inflamed cysts have no or minimal computed tomography (CT) mural enhancement; infected cysts have increased CT density of the central fluid with rim enhancement and poorly defined cyst wall.
- Fistula or sinus tract: may extend either toward the skin surface, supratonsillar fossa, or between the internal and external carotid arteries.

Pathology

Gross

- Thin-walled, cystic structures filled with cheesy material or serous, mucoid, or purulent fluid.
- Nodular excrescences may be seen lining the cyst wall.

Histology

- Lining epithelium is predominantly a stratified squamous epithelium, seen in approximately 90% of cases; less frequently, a purely columnar epithelial lining or a mixed lining may be seen.
- Cyst wall typically contains a nodular or diffuse lymphoid infiltrate, often with germinal centers.
- Fibrosis and granulation tissue may be prominent and even replace the surface epithelium in cases associated with repeated infections.
- Fistulas often are composed of a stratified squamous epithelium associated with the external segments and a columnar epithelium with the internal segments.
- No evidence of thymic (thymic cyst) or thyroid tissue (thyroglossal duct cyst).

Differential Diagnosis

- Thymic cyst.
- Thyroglossal duct cyst (see below).
- Metastatic cystic squamous cell carcinoma of Waldeyer's tonsillar tissue (Chapter 9B, #10).
- Metastatic papillary carcinoma of thyroid gland origin.

Treatment and Prognosis

- Complete surgical excision is the treatment of choice.
- Depending on the extent of the fistula tract, a tonsillectomy may be needed.

Third Branchial Cleft Anomalies

- Rare.
- Cysts occur in the region of the laryngeal ventricle.
- Fistulas open externally anterior to the lower third of the sternocleidomastoid muscle; if complete, the internal opening is in the pyriform sinus, following the passage of the tract along the carotid sheath that penetrates the thyrohyoid membrane.

Fourth or Sixth Branchial Cleft Anomalies

- Extremely rare.
- Thought to arise within the mediastinum.

Additional Facts

- Histogenesis of branchial cleft cysts is controversial; among the structures proposed as the origins for these anomalies are:
  Branchial apparatus (considered to represent the origin for these abnormalities).
  Salivary gland inclusions.
  Thymic duct.
- Branchial cleft cysts occur in the oral cavity and are referred to as *lymphoepithelial cysts:*
  Affect men more than women; occur primarily in the fourth to fifth decades of life.

Submucosal cystic lesions are most commonly identified along the floor of the mouth.
Histologic similarity to those occurring in the neck.
Cured by conservative surgical excision.
Thought to occur as a result of cystic transformation of the glandular epithelium included within the oral lymphoid tissue during embryogenesis.

- *Thyroglossal duct cysts:*
  No sex predilection; occur over a wide age range, but a large percentage of cases occur before the fourth decade of life.
  Majority occur in the midline of the neck below the level of the hyoid bone; some occur lateral to midline.
  Cysts are lined by a respiratory or squamous epithelium; presence of thyroid tissue varies and may be dependent on the extent of specimen sampling.
  Surgery is the treatment of choice and may include all or part of the hyoid bone; recurrence rates are low, and development of a carcinoma (majority of those reported are papillary carcinomas) is rare.

References

Barnes L: Branchial cleft cysts, fistulas, and sinuses. *In:* Barnes L, ed. Surgical pathology of the head and neck. New York: Marcel Dekker, 1985; pp 1285–1292.

Bhaskar SN, Bernier JL: Histogenesis of branchial cysts: a report of 468 cases. Am J Pathol 35:407–423, 1959.

Little JW, Rickles RH: The histogenesis of the branchial cyst. Am J Pathol 50:533–547,1967.

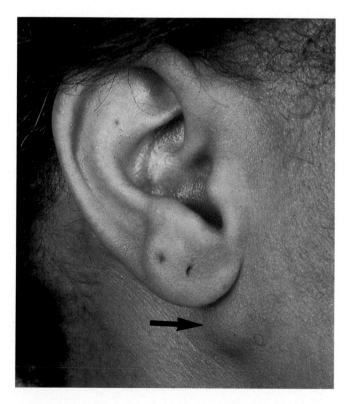

Figure 8-1. First branchial cleft cyst identified as an infra-auricular, freely movable and fluctuant mass *(arrow).*

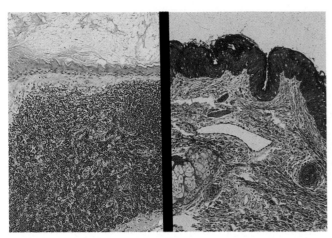

Figure 8–2. *(Left)* First branchial cleft cyst (type I), composed of a cyst with a keratinized squamous epithelial lining devoid of adnexa or mesodermal structures; a dense lymphoid infiltrate is seen in the cyst wall. *(Right)* First branchial cleft cyst (type II), composed of a cyst with a keratinized squamous epithelial lining with associated adnexal structures (sebaceous glands and hair follicle).

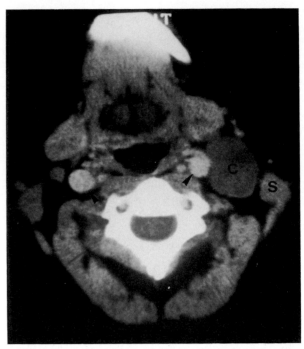

Figure 8–4. Branchial cleft cyst—axial CT, enhanced: fluid-filled cyst (c) anterior to the left sternocleidomastoid muscle (s). The thin-walled cyst does not enhance after administration of intravenous contrast. Jugular veins *(arrowheads)*. (Courtesy of Franz J. Wippold II, M.D., Mallinckrodt Institute of Radiology, St. Louis, MO.)

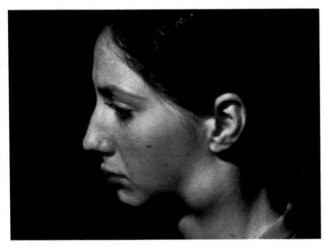

Figure 8–3. Second branchial cleft cyst occurring along the anterior border of the sternocleidomastoid muscle as a painless, fluctuant neck mass.

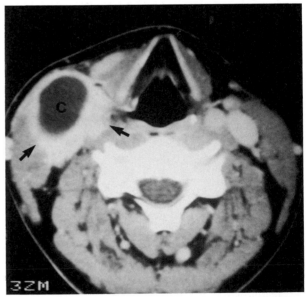

Figure 8–5. Infected branchial cleft cyst—axial CT, contrast enhanced: after administration of intravenous contrast material, the thick walls *(arrows)* of the cyst (c) densely contrast enhance, a typical finding in infected cysts. (Courtesy of Franz J. Wippold II, M.D., Mallinckrodt Institute of Radiology, St. Louis, MO.)

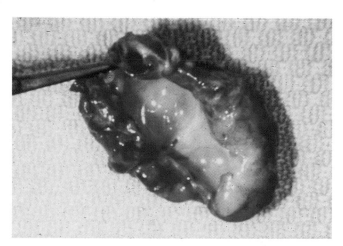

Figure 8–6. Resected, smooth-walled second branchial cleft cyst.

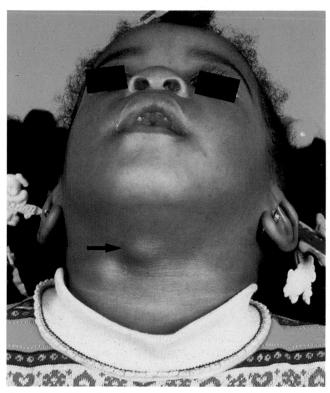

Figure 8–8. Thyroglossal duct cyst, presenting in this young girl as a midline neck mass at the level of the hyoid bone *(arrow)*.

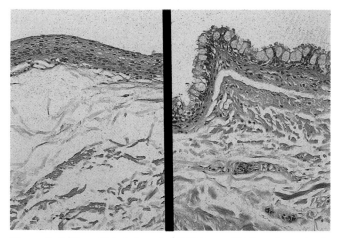

Figure 8–7. Branchial cleft cyst wall lining epithelium is predominantly a stratified squamous epithelium *(left)*, and less frequently a purely ciliated columnar epithelium *(right)*; although not depicted here, the cyst wall typically contains a nodular or diffuse lymphoid infiltrate, often with germinal centers.

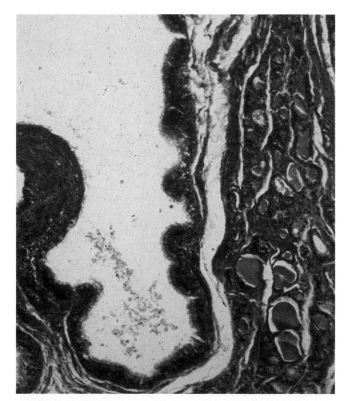

Figure 8–9. Histologic appearance of a thyroglossal duct cyst, composed of a ciliated columnar epithelial-lined cyst that contains thyroid follicles in the cyst wall.

2. HETEROTOPIAS, HAMARTOMAS, AND TERATOMAS

Definitions

Heterotopia—the presence of otherwise normal-appearing tissue in an abnormal location.

Synonyms: aberrant rests; ectopia; choristoma.

Hamartoma—benign, tumor-like proliferation or overgrowth of tissue indigenous to a specific anatomic location.

Teratoma—true neoplasm, composed of a variety of tissue types representing all three germ layers (ecto-, endo-, and mesoderm), occurring in areas in which these tissues are not natively identified.

a. Fordyce's Granules

Definition: Heterotopic collections of sebaceous glands at various sites in the oral cavity.

Synonyms: Fordyce's disease or condition.

Clinical

- No sex predilection; occurs primarily in adults and is only rarely identified in children.
- Present in approximately 80% of the normal adult population.
- Most commonly seen in a bilateral symmetrical distribution on the buccal mucosa opposite the molar teeth; also seen on the inner surfaces of the lips, retromolar area, tongue, gingiva, and palate.
- Generally are asymptomatic.

Pathology

Gross

- Small, yellow raised spots that may be discretely separated or coalesce to form large plaques.

Histology

- Sebaceous glands are identical to those found in the skin, but are not associated with hair follicles.
- Glands are generally seen in superficial locations and vary in the composition of lobules from one to many.

Treatment and Prognosis

- No treatment is required.
- Very rarely a sebaceous adenoma may develop from these structures.

Additional Facts

- Paucity in children is probably related to the fact that sebaceous glands and hair follicles do not attain maximal development until puberty.
- Other than the oral cavity, head and neck sebaceous gland ectopia may be seen in the parotid gland, larynx, middle ear, and sinonasal region.

b. Ectopic Thyroid Tissue

Definition: Presence of thyroid tissue in abnormal locations.

Clinical

- Excluding and in comparison to thyroid tissue seen in association with thyroglossal duct cysts, the presence of ectopic thyroid tissue is rare and is almost exclusively seen in suprahyoid locations.
- The most common ectopic focus for thyroid tissue is the base of the tongue, referred to as lingual thyroid; however, ectopic thyroid may be seen in any location from the tongue to the suprasternal notch.

Lingual Thyroid

- Affects females more than males; occurs from birth to the seventh decade of life.
- Most frequently seen along the midline of the base of the tongue between the foramen cecum and the epiglottis; in rare instances, the body of the tongue is affected.
- Most common symptom is dysphagia, which varies in severity; other symptoms include voice changes, dyspnea, orthopnea, bleeding, and a foreign body sensation.
- The majority of patients with symptomatic lingual thyroid have hypothyroid function; about 10% suffer from clinical manifestations of hypothyroidism.
- In >70% of patients, cervical thyroid tissue is absent and the lingual thyroid represents the sole thyroid tissue present; if completely removed, hypothyroidism results; therefore, scintigraphy with technetium or radioiodine studies are mandatory preoperatively in order to:
  Determine the presence or absence of normally placed or other ectopic foci of thyroid tissue.
  Determine the functional activity of the lingual thyroid tissue.

Pathology

Gross

- Red, soft to firm, smooth or lobulated, nodular mass ranging in size from 2 to 3 cm.
- Overlying mucosa may be intact or ulcerated.

Histology

- Unencapsulated embryonic or mature thyroid tissue.
- Thyroid tissue may extend into skeletal muscle.

Treatment and Prognosis

- Treatment modalities include:
  Shrinking the mass by using thyroid hormones.
  Radioactive iodine-131 to kill the lingual thyroid; however, this modality also destroys other thyroid tissue and, in addition, may cause sloughing of the gland and hemorrhage.
  Surgical excision (intraorally or pharyngotomy); indications for surgery are for symptomatic patients (dysphagia, dysphonia, dyspnea, uncontrollable hyperthyroidism, hemorrhage); in

those individuals with absent cervical thyroid tissue or other ectopic thyroid sites, autotransplantation of thyroid tissue into the neck muscles can be done.

■ Prognosis is good; malignant transformation is uncommon; rarely, metastasis to cervical lymph nodes and to the lungs has been reported (limited to men who were older than 35 years of age).

Additional Facts

■ Incisional biopsies must be performed with caution because this may cause sloughing of the gland, infection, necrosis, or hemorrhage.
■ Overwhelming majority of patients who are symptomatic are women, and contributing factors are thought to be related to puberty, pregnancy, and menopause.

c. Benign Teratoma

Clinical

■ Teratomas in the head and neck are rare neoplasms, accounting for less than 2% of all teratomas.
■ No sex predilection; may be seen in the adult population, but the majority occur in newborns or infants and are rarely seen over the age of 1 year (cervical teratoma) and 2 years (nasopharyngeal teratoma).
■ The most common locations for teratomas seen within the head and neck are the neck and nasopharynx; other less commonly involved sites include the oral cavity (tonsil, tongue, palate), sinonasal cavity, external and middle ear including the temporal bone, mandible, and maxilla.
■ Presenting symptoms include cervical teratoma—neck mass that may compress the trachea, resulting in airway obstruction (stridor, apnea); nasopharyngeal teratoma—a mass protruding into the oral cavity or pharynx, causing associated dysphagia or airway obstruction.
■ Teratomas may be associated with maternal hydramnios and stillbirth.

Pathology

Gross

■ Encapsulated cystic, solid, or multiloculated mass measuring from 5 to 17 cm in diameter.

Histology

■ Composition of teratomas includes the identification of tissue arising from all three germ layers, including epithelia (keratinizing squamous, columnar, ciliated respiratory, or gastrointestinal-type epithelium), cutaneous adnexae, minor salivary glands, neuroectodermal and central nervous system tissue, cartilage, bone, fat, and smooth muscle.
■ Epithelial-lined cystic spaces are prominent.

■ Immature or embryonal tissue components can be identified throughout the tumor.
■ Necrosis and hemorrhage may be seen.

Differential Diagnosis

■ Teratoid lesions (dermoid cysts, nasopharyngeal "hairy polyp").
■ Heterotopic central nervous system tissue or encephalocele (Chapter 3, #4).
■ Cystic hygroma (Chapter 9A, #3).

Treatment and Prognosis

■ Complete surgical excision is the treatment of choice.
■ Morbidity may be high due to the size and location of the tumors; mortality rates are low if surgical intervention is initiated early; however, death may ensue if not adequately treated and is usually caused by complications of respiratory obstruction.
■ Nasopharyngeal teratomas may extend intracranially.
■ Lymph node metastases may be seen, but may reflect "benign" metastases rather than an indication of malignancy.
■ In the pediatric age group, malignant transformation or behavior of a head and neck teratoma has not been reported.

Additional Facts

■ The finding of immature or embryonic tissue components is not of any prognostic significance.
■ Particularly in nasopharyngeal teratomas, neuroectodermal and neural tissue components predominate.
■ In contrast to teratomas occurring in the pediatric population, teratomas of the head and neck in adults occur much less frequently; however, a much larger percentage of these tumors demonstrate malignancy, and some advocate considering these malignant teratomas until proven otherwise. Clinicopathologic features of *malignant teratomas* include:
 Equal sex predilection; occur over a wide age range, from the third through the eighth decades of life.
 Histologic evaluation demonstrates a prominent neural component associated with poorly differentiated carcinoma or sarcoma.
 In the adult setting, increased cellular immaturity has prognostic significance as demonstrated by a greater malignant potential; additionally, teratomas with benign histology may recur or metastasize.
 Metastases commonly occur via both lymphatic and vascular routes.
 Aggressive therapy is indicated.
 Prognosis is poor.

References

Fordyce's Granules

Shafer WG, Hine MK, Levy BM: Fordyce's granules. *In:* Shafer WG, Hine MK, Levy BM, eds. A textbook of oral pathology, 4th ed. Philadelphia: W.B. Saunders Co., 1983; pp 20–22.

Ectopic Thyroid Tissue

Aguirre A, de la Piedra M, Ruiz R, Portilla J: Ectopic thyroid tissue in the submandibular gland. Oral Surg Oral Med Oral Pathol 71:73–76, 1991.

Barnes L: Ectopic thyroid tissue. *In:* Barnes L, ed. Surgical pathology of the head and neck. New York: Marcel Dekker, 1985; pp 230–231.

LiVolsi V: Lingual thyroid. *In:* LiVolsi V, ed. Surgical pathology of the thyroid. Philadelphia: W. B. Saunders Co., 1991; pp. 352–353.

Teratoma

Gnepp DR: Teratomas. *In:* Barnes L, ed. Surgical pathology of the head and neck. New York: Marcel Dekker, 1985; pp 1416–1433.

Hyams VJ, Batsakis JG, Michaels L: Teratomas. *In:* Hyams VJ, Batsakis JG, Michaels L, eds. Tumors of the upper respiratory tract and ear. Fascicle 25, second series. Washington, D.C.: Armed Forces Institute of Pathology, 1988; pp 204–206.

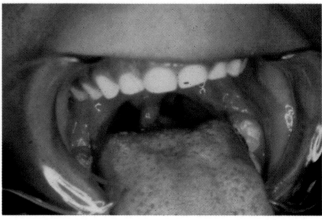

Figure 8–11. Lingual thyroid, seen as a raised, red, lobulated mass behind the uvula.

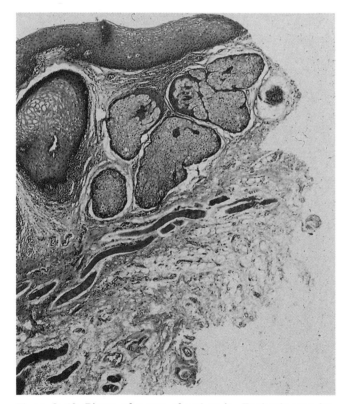

Figure 8–10. Biopsy of a case of oral cavity Fordyce's granules, showing sebaceous gland lobules immediately subjacent to the oral cavity stratified squamous epithelium.

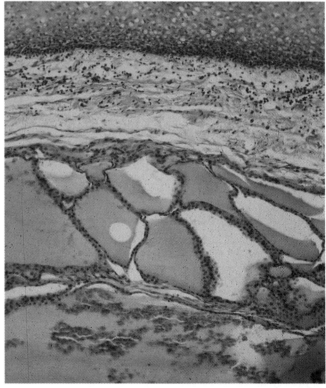

Figure 8–12. Biopsy specimen of the tongue mass, showing intact stratified squamous epithelium with unencapsulated mature thyroid tissue within the submucosal compartment.

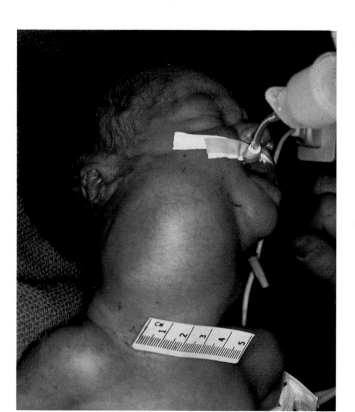

Figure 8–13. Large, benign teratoma of the lateral neck; the mass compressed the trachea, resulting in airway obstruction.

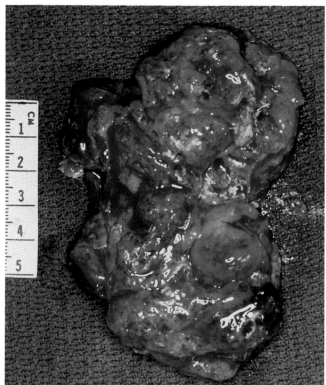

Figure 8–14. Section from the teratoma, showing an encapsulated solid and focally cystic tissue with a tan-brown to fleshy appearance.

Figure 8–15. Histologic composition of teratomas includes elements from all germ cell layers, including epithelial tissue (squamous and columnar), mesenchymal structures (cartilage), and central nervous system tissue (along the left upper third of the illustration).

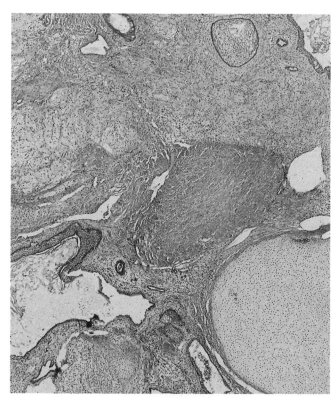

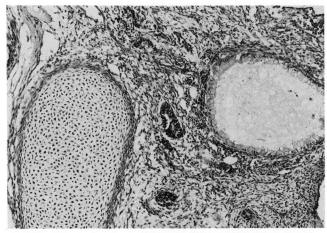

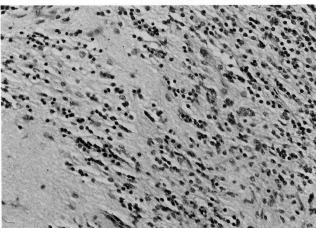

Figure 8-16. Benign teratoma. *(Top)* Ciliated respiratory epithelium and immature cartilage. *(Bottom)* Central nervous system tissue.

3. MUCOUS CYSTS

a. Mucocele

Definition: Dilatation of minor salivary glands with accumulated mucus secretion, often associated with mucus extravasation into the connective tissue without an associated epithelial lining.

Synonyms: Mucous retention cyst; mucus escape phenomenon; ranula.

Clinical

- Relatively common lesion.
- No sex predilection; occurs in all age groups, but is most common in the second to third decades of life.
- Most common site of occurrence is the lower lip; other sites affected include the buccal mucosa, floor of mouth, palate, tongue, retromolar fossa, tonsillar region, and upper lip.
- Usually asymptomatic, but may be associated with pain or a burning sensation.

- Initially considered to arise as a result of obstruction of an excretory duct of a minor salivary gland; however, etiology is thought to be traumatic in nature, resulting in rupture of a duct with mucus extravasation into surrounding tissue.

Pathology

Gross

- Superficial lesions are movable, smooth, soft to firm, raised vesicles with a blue or green appearance that measure in size from a few millimeters to several centimeters.
- Deeper seated lesions are movable, firm, nodular, and covered by normal-appearing mucosa.

Histology

Two patterns may be seen:

1. Well-circumscribed cavity lined by granulation tissue and filled with eosinophilic material that con-

tains an admixture of polymorphonuclear leukocytes, eosinophils, and histiocytes (represents the more common histologic pattern).
2. Extravasation of mucus into adjacent tissue, intermixed with granulation tissue and inflammatory cells.
■ Overlying epithelium is thinned.
■ Associated minor salivary glands show variable degrees of atrophy, ductal dilatation, fibrosis, and a chronic inflammatory cell infiltrate.
■ Associated epithelial-lined cyst is seldom identified.

Differential Diagnosis

■ Mucoepidermoid carcinoma (Chapter 19B, #1).

Treatment and Prognosis

■ Surgical excision of the mucocele as well as the associated salivary gland acini.
■ Except in cases treated by inadequate surgery (incision), recurrences rarely occur.

b. Ranula

Definition: Specific form of mucocele or mucous retention phenomenon occurring in the floor of the mouth in association with the ducts of the sublingual or submaxillary gland.

Clinical

■ Rare as compared with the usual mucocele.
■ No sex predilection; may affect any age group.
■ Most commonly a unilateral lesion, but may be bilateral.
■ Etiology considered similar to the usual mucocele.
■ Divided into two types: simple and plunging.

Simple Ranula

■ Occurs in the lateral aspect of the floor of the mouth.
■ Presenting symptoms include loud snoring and a painless mass; if large, deviation of the tongue may occur.

Pathology

Gross

■ Fluctuant mass, measuring up to several centimeters.
■ Superficial lesions may impart a bluish color; more commonly, the lesions are deep-seated, with the color of the overlying intact mucosa.

Histology

■ Unilocular or multilocular cystic lesion often associated with an epithelial lining (squamous, cuboidal, columnar).
■ Cysts contain amorphous eosinophilic material.

Differential Diagnosis

■ Mucocele (Chapter 8, #3a).
■ Dermoid cyst .
■ Benign mixed tumor (Chapter 19A, #1).
■ Lipoma (Chapter 9A, #5).

Treatment and Prognosis

■ Adequate excision, including removal of the entire associated salivary gland; some prefer to simply unroof the lesion (marsupialization of the cyst wall), rather than performing total excision.
■ Occasionally, the lesion recurs.

Plunging Ranula

■ Ranula that extends beyond the mucous membranes and has herniated through the mylohyoid muscle into the neck, resulting from mucus extravasation.
■ Clinical presentation is that of a painless neck mass in the submental or submandibular triangle, with or without an associated lesion in the floor of the mouth.

Pathology

Histology

■ Pools of mucus surrounded by fibrous tissue, chronic inflammatory cells including histiocytes; an associated epithelial lining is not seen.

Differential Diagnosis

■ Dermoid cyst.
■ Cystic hygroma (Chapter 9A, #3).
■ Thyroglossal duct cyst (Chapter 8; #1).

Treatment and Prognosis

■ Meticulous excision of the lesion, including excision of the associated salivary gland of origin, is the treatment of choice.
■ Failure to include resection of the salivary gland results in recurrence.

Additional Facts

■ Simple ranulas are considered true cysts based on the presence of an epithelial lining.
■ Plunging ranulas are considered pseudocysts based on the absence of an associated epithelial lining.

References

Koudelka BM: Mucus escape reaction. *In:* Ellis GL, Auclair PL, Gnepp DR, eds. Surgical pathology of salivary glands. Philadelphia: W.B. Saunders Co., 1991; pp 26–31.
Verbin RS: Mucocele and ranula. *In:* Barnes L, ed. Surgical pathology of the head and neck. New York: Marcel Dekker, 1985; pp 1295–1300.

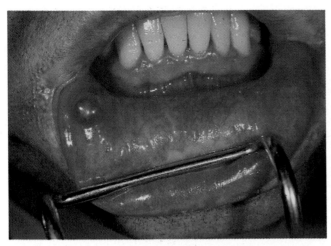

Figure 8–17. Mucocele (mucous retention cyst) of the lip appears as a superficial raised vesicle with a bluish appearance.

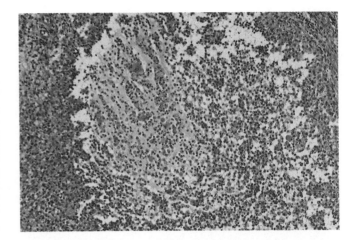

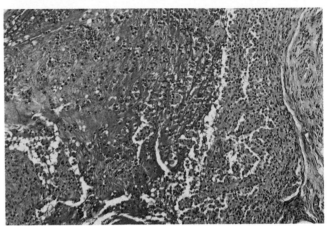

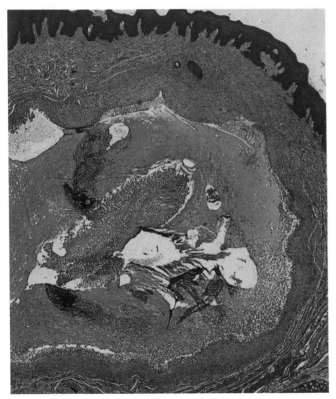

Figure 8–18. Histologic appearance of a mucocele composed of a well-circumscribed submucosal cavity lined with granulation tissue.

Figure 8–19. Mucocele (mucous retention cyst). *(Top)* Portion of the cyst lined by granulation tissue and an absent epithelium, with the cyst cavity filled with eosinophilic material containing an admixture of polymorphonuclear leukocytes, eosinophils, and histiocytes. *(Bottom)* Mucin stains depict the presence of mucinous material admixed with the inflammatory infiltrate.

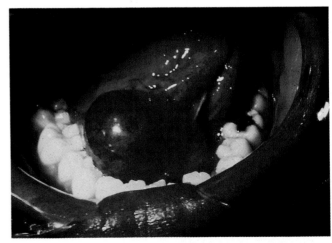

Figure 8–20. Simple ranula, identified as a large, fluid-filled mass in the lateral aspect of the floor of the mouth.

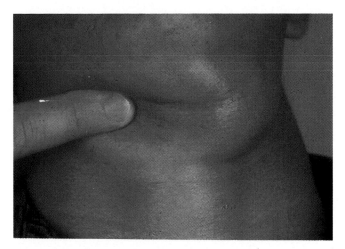

Figure 8–21. Plunging ranula that has extended from the floor of the mouth, herniated through the mylohyoid muscle, and presented as a painless neck mass.

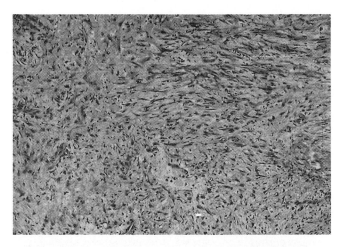

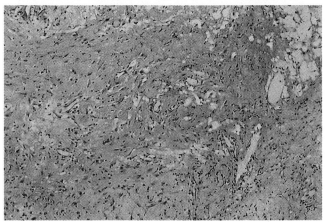

Figure 8–22. *(Top)* Histologically, plunging ranulas appear as mucinous material surrounded by fibrous tissue and chronic inflammatory cells including histiocytes, without an associated epithelial lining. *(Bottom)* The presence of mucin within the fibroinflammatory tissue can be identified with mucin stains.

4. NECROTIZING SIALOMETAPLASIA

Definition: Benign, self-healing (reactive) inflammatory process of salivary gland tissue that clinically and histologically mimics a malignant neoplasm.

Clinical

■ Affects men more than women; occurs over a wide age range, with the average age of occurrence in the fifth to sixth decades of life.
■ Most commonly involves the minor salivary glands of the palate, but other intraoral sites as well as the minor salivary glands of virtually every site in the upper aerodigestive tract can be affected; major salivary gland involvement occurs as well.
■ The most common presenting problem is that of a painless ulcerated lesion or a nodular swelling, which is usually unilateral but may be bilateral; in general, the lesions are asymptomatic, but may be associated with pain, numbness, or a burning sensation.
■ Palatal-based lesions occur spontaneously and are of unknown causes; the majority of cases involving extrapalatal minor salivary glands and major salivary glands are iatrogenically induced following operative procedures, trauma, or radiotherapy, with a mean duration of 18 days from the insult to the development of the lesion.
■ The pathogenesis for the iatrogenically induced lesions is primarily but not exclusively thought to be ischemic; a similar pathogenesis is implicated for the palate lesions, but this remains unproved.

Pathology

Gross

■ The typical appearance is that of deep, crater-like ulcerative lesions measuring from 1 to 3 cm; however, the lesion may appear as a submucosal nodular swelling that may slough, leaving a crater-like ulcer.

Histology

■ Lobular necrosis of the salivary glands with preservation of the lobular architecture and squamous metaplasia of residual acinar and ductal elements are the histologic hallmarks.

■ Necrotic lobules consist of acinus-sized pools of mucin that may extend into adjacent tissue, eliciting a granulation tissue reaction with associated acute and chronic inflammation (neutrophils and foamy histiocytes).

■ The squamous metaplasia is bland in appearance, composed of squamous cells with uniform nuclei and abundant eosinophilic cytoplasm, with occasional preservation of ductal lumina or scattered mucous cells; the lobular architecture is maintained and the metaplastic lobules vary slightly to moderately in size and shape and have smooth edges surrounded by granulation tissue and an intense mixed acute and chronic inflammatory reaction.

■ With regeneration, mitoses, individual cell necrosis, enlarged nuclei, and prominent nucleoli can be seen; occasionally, the metaplastic cells have a predominantly basaloid appearance with hyperchromatic nuclei.

■ Associated findings include ulcerated mucosa and pseudo-epitheliomatous hyperplasia; the latter, resulting when the metaplastic lobules present in excretory ducts and merge with surface epithelium, may be so striking that it presents a diagnostic nightmare in separating it from an infiltrating squamous cell carcinoma.

Differential Diagnosis

■ Squamous cell carcinoma (Chapter 9B, #1).
■ Mucoepidermoid carcinoma (Chapter 19B, #1).

Treatment and Prognosis

■ These lesions are self-limiting and heal by secondary intention; depending on the size of the lesion, the healing process in most cases occurs in 3 to 12 weeks.

■ Debridement and saline rinses may aid in the healing process.

■ Recurrences do not usually occur.

Additional Facts

■ Small biopsy specimens of the lesion may cause diagnostic difficulties and may necessitate additional biopsy material for diagnosis.

■ Pitfalls in diagnosis may be avoided, given the distinctive clinical and pathologic features.

References

Abrams AM, Melrose RJ, Howell FV: Necrotizing sialometaplasia: a disease simulating malignancy. Cancer 32:13–135,1973.

Batsakis JG, Manning JT: Necrotizing sialometaplasia of major salivary glands. J Laryngol Otol 101:962-966,1987.

Brannon RB, Fowler CB, Hartman KS: Necrotizing sialometaplasia: a clinicopathologic study of sixty-nine cases and review of the literature. Oral Surg Oral Med Oral Pathol 71:317–325,1991.

Jensen JL: Necrotizing sialometaplasia. In: Ellis GL, Auclair PL, Gnepp DR, eds. Surgical pathology of salivary glands. Philadelphia: W.B. Saunders Co., 1991; pp 60–66.

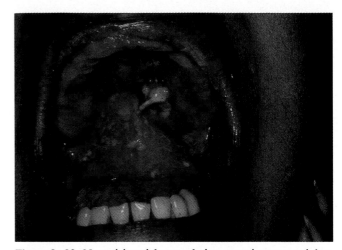

Figure 8-23. Necrotizing sialometaplasia presenting as a painless, deep, crater-like ulcerative lesion on the palate.

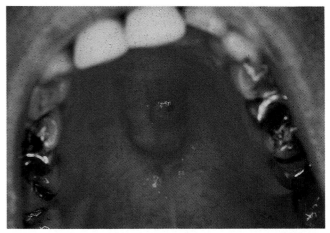

Figure 8-24. Necrotizing sialometaplasia may also clinically present as palatal-based nodular swelling.

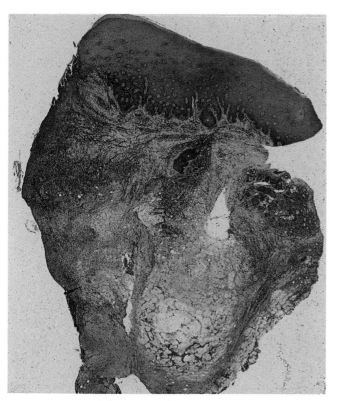

Figure 8–25. Necrotizing sialometaplasia, histologically appearing as lobular necrosis of the salivary glands and consisting of acinus-sized pools of mucin with preservation of the lobular architecture and squamous metaplasia of residual acinar and ductal elements.

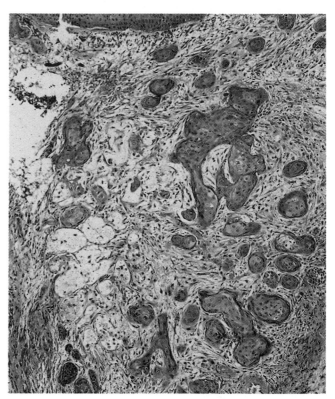

Figure 8–26. The squamous metaplasia is bland in appearance, composed of squamous cells with uniform nuclei, abundant eosinophilic cytoplasm with occasional preservation of ductal lumina or scattered mucous cells. The lobular architecture is maintained and the metaplastic lobules vary slightly to moderately in size and shape and have smooth edges surrounded by granulation tissue and a mixed acute and chronic inflammatory reaction.

5. NODULAR FASCIITIS

Definition: Non-neoplastic (reactive) proliferation of fibroblasts.
Synonyms: Pseudosarcomatous fasciitis, pseudosarcomatous fibromatosis, infiltrative fasciitis.

Clinical

- One of the more common soft tissue lesions.
- Most commonly occurs in the upper extremities, but is seen involving head and neck sites in up to 20% of cases.
- In the head and neck, the most common site of involvement is the neck.
- No sex predilection; predominantly occurs in the third to fifth decades of life.
- Although nodular fasciitis is considered to occur primarily in adults and infrequently affects infants and children, head and neck involvement is common in infants and children and rare in adults.

- Nodular fasciitis characteristically arises from the superficial fascia, accounting for its predominant occurrence in subcutaneous areas.
- Most common symptom is that of a painless mass noted for its rapid growth which occurs over a 1 to 2-week period.
- Lesions are solitary and rarely, if ever, multiple.
- Etiology is unknown; however, trauma is considered a likely initiating factor.

Pathology

Gross

- Firm, nodular, tan-white, nonencapsulated but well-delineated mass, usually measuring less than 3 to 4 cm in size.
- On cut section, the lesion may be smooth or whorled, varying from firm and tan-white to soft and gelatinous or myxoid.
- Cystic areas may be seen.

Histology

- Circumscribed but unencapsulated lesion composed of a proliferation of plump-appearing fibroblasts arranged in short, irregular fascicles and bundles or in a whorled appearance.
- The fibroblasts have little variation in size and shape; nuclei are pale-staining with an oval, plump, or spindle shape and have prominent nucleoli.
- Cellularity varies and may demonstrate hyper- and hypocellular areas, even within the same lesion.
- Mitoses are a prominent feature; however, atypical mitoses are not seen.
- The stroma is rich in mucopolysaccharides, and this abundance of ground substance imparts a loose or "feathery" growth pattern characteristic of nodular fasciitides.
- Lymphocytes and extravasated erythrocytes are commonly seen admixed with the fibroblasts.
- Less commonly identified features include the presence of multinucleated giant cells and lipid-laden macrophages in the central portions of the lesion, with plasma cells and histiocytes at the periphery of the lesion.
- Nonendothelial-lined slits or clefts are seen throughout the lesion.
- Collagen fibers may be seen, but are thin and delicate, rather than arranged in thick bundles.
- With time, fibrosis and microcysts are seen; microcysts may coalesce to form large cystic spaces.
- Immunohistochemistry: actin (muscle-specific and smooth muscle), vimentin, and KP-1 immunoreactivity; absence of reactivity with S-100 protein or desmin.

Differential Diagnosis

- Benign fibrous histiocytoma (Chapter 4A, #4) and fibromatosis (Chapter 4A, #5).
- Malignant fibrous histiocytoma (Chapter 5B, #6).
- Fibrosarcoma (Chapter 5B, #7).
- Benign and malignant peripheral nerve sheath tumors (Chapter 9A, #6; Chapter 9B, #6).

Treatment and Prognosis

- Local excision is the treatment of choice.
- Local recurrence may occur in approximately 2% of all cases; usually occurs shortly after surgery; however, this is not necessarily an indication for additional surgery.
- Benign, self-limiting process.
- Spontaneous regression can be seen.

Additional Facts

- The most important aspect of the pathologic diagnosis of nodular fasciitis is not to mistake it for a sarcoma.
- Nodular fasciitis can also arise within muscle (intramuscular fasciitis), deep fascia (fascial fasciitis), blood vessels (intravascular fasciitis), soft tissues of the scalp or skull (cranial fasciitis), and in areas lacking fascia, including the trachea, oral mucosa, and esophagus.
- Immunohistochemical profile suggests dual myofibroblastic and histiocytic differentiation.

References

Barnes L: Nodular fasciitis. *In:* Barnes L, ed. Surgical pathology of the head and neck. New York: Marcel Dekker, 1985; pp 758–762.

Dahl I, Jarlstedt J: Nodular fasciitis of the head and neck: a clinicopathological study of 18 cases. Acta Otolaryngol (Stockh) 90:152–159, 1980.

DiNardo LJ, Wetmore RF, Potsic WP: Nodular fasciitis of the head and neck in children: a deceptive lesion. Arch Otolaryngol Head Neck Surg 117:1001–1002, 1991.

Konwaler BE, Keasbey L, Kaplan L: Subcutaneous pseudosarcomatous fibromatosis (fasciitis). Am J Clin Pathol 25:241–252, 1955.

Montgomery EA, Meis JM: Nodular fasciitis: its morphologic spectrum and immunohistochemical profile. Am J Surg Pathol 15:942–948, 1991.

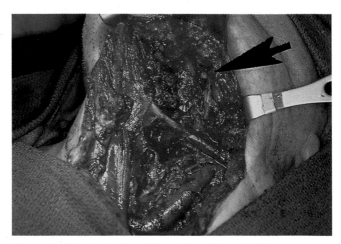

Figure 8–27. Surgical excision of nodular fasciitis, seen as a roughly rectangular soft tissue mass *(arrow)* just above and to the right of the tendon identified in the center of the illustration.

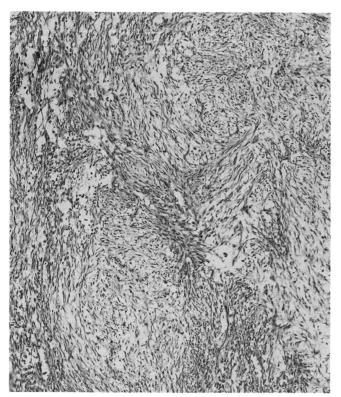

Figure 8–28. Nodular fasciitis appears as a proliferation of fibroblasts arranged in short, irregular fascicles or bundles or in a whorled appearance set within a stroma with an abundance of ground substance, imparting a loose or "feathery" growth pattern.

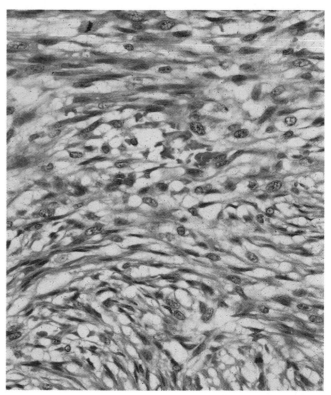

Figure 8–29. The fibroblasts have pale-staining, oval, plump or spindle-shaped nuclei, occasional prominent nucleoli, prominent mitotic activity, and extravasated erythrocytes admixed with the fibroblasts.

6. TANGIER DISEASE

Definition: Autosomal recessive disorder of lipoprotein metabolism that results in deposition of xanthomatous cells in the tonsils, liver, spleen, lymph nodes, and palate.

Clinical

- Initially observed on Tangier Island in the Chesapeake Bay area of the United States.
- Deficiency of high-density lipoproteins and low levels of apoproteins, low to normal low-density lipoprotein levels, and high plasma triglyceride levels.
- No sex predilection; occurs in all age groups.
- Clinical manifestations relate to deposition of cholesterol esters in various tissue sites, including the tonsils, spleen, liver, lymph nodes, and peripheral nerves and the cornea.
- Tonsillar involvement results in symptoms of pharyngotonsillitis.

Pathology

Gross

- Tonsils are enlarged and yellow in appearance.

Histology

- Multifocal deposition of clear (xanthomatous) cells throughout the involved tissue.

Differential Diagnosis

- Lipid storage diseases.
- Nonspecific tonsillitis.

Treatment and Prognosis

- Management is essentially symptomatic.
- Prognosis is good; however, coronary artery disease is common in patients over 40 years of age.

References

Schoenberg BS, Schoenberg DG: Tangerine tonsils in Tangier: high density lipoprotein deficiency. South Med J 71:453–454, 1978.

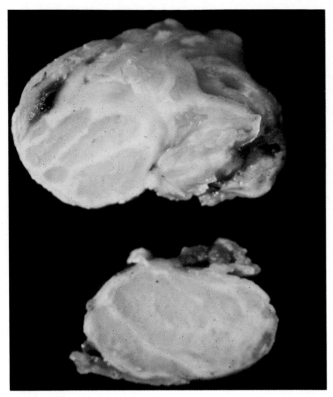

Figure 8–30. Tonsils removed from a patient with Tangier disease are enlarged and yellow in appearance.

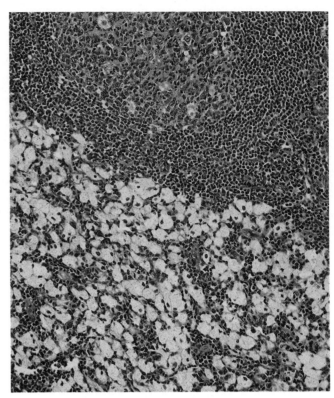

Figure 8–31. The histologic appearance of Tangier disease consists of (multifocal) deposition of clear (xanthomatous) cells throughout the tonsillar parenchyma.

7. INFECTIOUS DISEASES

a. Infectious Mononucleosis

Definition: Systemic, benign, self-limiting infectious lymphoproliferative disease, primarily caused by but not limited to the Epstein-Barr virus (EBV).

Clinical

■ No sex predilection; may occur in all age groups, but primarily affects adolescents and young adults.

■ EBV is estimated to cause from 80% to 95% of the cases of infectious mononucleosis; other microorganisms associated with mononucleosis-like syndromes include cytomegalovirus (CMV), *Toxoplasma gondii,* rubella, hepatitis A virus, and adenoviruses.

■ Clinical presentation of EBV-associated infectious mononucleosis includes acute pharyngotonsillitis, with patients experiencing sore throat, fever, and malaise; in addition, lymphadenopathy and hepatosplenomegaly with chemical evidence of hepatitis may represent the systemic manifestations of the disease.

■ Pharyngotonsillitis is often severe and may be exudative; lymphadenopathy commonly affects posterior cervical lymph nodes, but both anterior and posterior nodes may be involved.

■ A prodromal period of from 2 to 5 days consists of malaise and fatigue and frequently occurs prior to the onset of the full syndrome.

■ The diagnosis of infectious mononucleosis is established in a patient with typical clinical presentations and appropriate laboratory findings; tissue confirmation of the diagnosis is usually not required.

■ Laboratory findings include:

Absolute lymphocytosis with more than 50% lymphocytes in a total leukocyte population of over 5000/mm³.

Prominent atypical lymphocytes, which are often over 10% of the total leukocyte count.

Mild to moderate elevations of liver enzymes, including aspartate and alanine aminotransferase.

Diagnosis can be confirmed by the demonstration of serum antibodies to horse red cells (positive Mono-Spot test) or sheep erythrocytes (positive Paul-Bunnell heterophile antibody test).

- With patients who consistently prove to be heterophile antibody or Mono-Spot negative, serodiagnosis is invaluable and includes:

  An appreciable serum response to EBV viral capsid antigen (VCA) with both IgM and IgG antibodies at the time of clinical presentation.

  At presentation or shortly thereafter, many infected patients develop antibodies to early antigen complex (EA).

  During the early phase of primary infection, antibodies to EBV nuclear antigens (EBNA) are usually not demonstrable.

  IgM antibodies to VCA disappear within 2 to 3 months after infection; antibodies to EA disappear within 2 to 6 months following infection; IgG antibodies to VCA and anti-EBNA antibodies persist for life and are indicative of a chronic carrier state.

Pathology

Gross

- Pharynx (tonsils): moderate to severe pharyngitis, with marked swollen and enlarged tonsils covered by a dirty gray exudate.
- Lymph nodes: tender lymphadenopathy, particularly of the posterior cervical lymph nodes.

Histology

- Distorted or partially effaced nodal/tonsillar architecture with the following findings:

  Reactive follicular hyperplasia with enlarged and irregularly shaped germinal centers.

  Expansion of the interfollicular areas with proliferation of immunoblasts, plasma cells, Reed–Sternberg-like cells, and lymphocytes.

  Cellular proliferation (lymphocytes and immunoblasts) often displays marked cytologic atypia with one or more prominent nucleoli, increased mitotic activity, and phagocytosis.

  Necrosis may be seen and is usually focal, but occasionally may be extensive.

Differential Diagnosis

- Nonspecific reactive tonsillitis/lymphadenopathy.

- Non-Hodgkin's malignant lymphomas (Chapter 9B, #4).
- Hodgkin's disease (Chapter 9B, #4).

Treatment and Prognosis

- Favorable clinical course, with resolution of symptoms over a period of several months.
- Therapy is supportive, including rest and fluids.
- Rarely, serious and potentially fatal complications may develop and include airway obstruction and splenic rupture.

Additional Facts

- The atypical lymphocytes in the peripheral blood are thought to represent mostly activated T-lymphocyte populations in response to B-cell infection.
- In patients with infectious mononucleosis who exhibit the typical clinical presentation and hematologic findings but who are heterophile antibody-negative, the most likely agents are EBV and CMV; the non-EBV infectious agents that cause infectious mononucleosis are not associated with a positive heterophile antibody test or Mono-Spot test.
- It is in the atypical case where the patient presents with adenotonsillar or lymph node enlargement without fever, sore throat, or splenomegaly that a biopsy specimen may be needed in order to establish a diagnosis and rule out a malignant process.
- Advances in molecular biologic techniques permit the generation of proteins that contain EBV-encoded polypeptide sequences and represent a more reliable and sensitive means for detecting the presence of virus than serodiagnosis.

References

Brown NA: The Epstein-Barr virus (infectious mononucleosis, B-lymphoproliferative disorders). *In:* Feigin RD, Cherry JD, eds. Textbook of pediatric infectious diseases. Philadelphia: W.B. Saunders Co., 1987, pp 1566–1577.

Childs CC, Purham DM, Berard CW: Infectious mononucleosis: the spectrum of morphologic changes simulating lymphoma in lymph nodes and tonsils. Am J Surg Pathol 11:122–132, 1987.

Salvador AH, Harrison EG, Kyle RA: Lymphadenopathy due to infectious mononucleosis: its confusion with malignant lymphoma. Cancer 27:1029–1040, 1971.

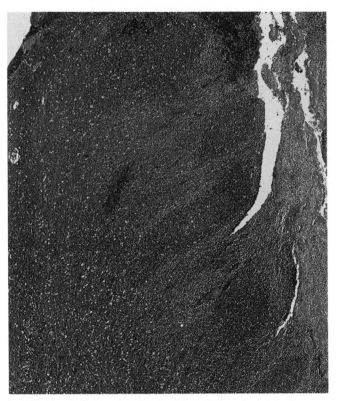

Figure 8-32. Tonsil removed in a case of infectious mononucleosis shows distortion and partial effacement of tonsillar architecture, with preservation of germinal centers, which are enlarged and irregularly shaped.

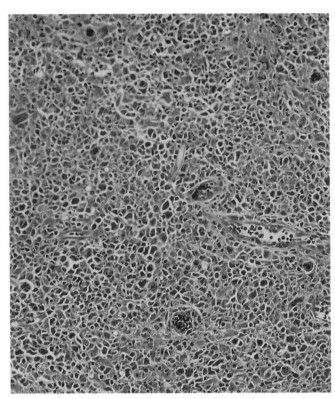

Figure 8-33. Interfollicular area with proliferation of immunoblasts, plasma cells, Reed-Sternberg-like cells, and lymphocytes.

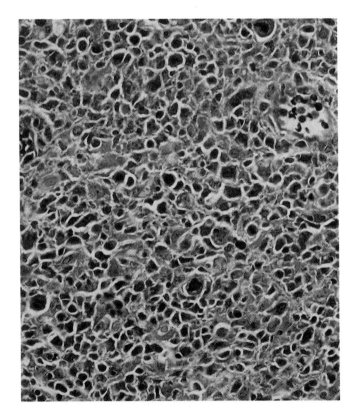

Figure 8-34. Infectious mononucleosis displays marked cytologic atypia, with cells having one or more prominent nucleoli and increased mitotic activity with atypical forms. Without analyzing the overall clinical-pathologic features, this morphologic appearance is easily mistaken for a malignant lymphoma.

b. Mycobacterial Infection

Definition: Infectious disease caused by *Mycobacterium,* a microorganism classified in the order Actinomycetales and the family Mycobacteriaceae.

Clinical

- Involvement of the head and neck is relatively uncommon.
- Overall incidence of *Mycobacterium tuberculosis* has decreased over the last five decades; however, with the advent of acquired immunodeficiency syndrome (AIDS), increased incidence of infection by mycobacteria, especially caused by the nontuberculous ("atypical") mycobacteria, has been noted in select patient populations.
- In the head and neck, all sites may be involved, but infection involves lymph nodes, tonsils, pharynx, oral cavity, sinonasal region, larynx, salivary glands, middle ear, and temporal bone.
- Head and neck involvement may result as a complication of pulmonary involvement (via expectoration of infected sputum) or as an isolated occurrence.
- Symptoms vary according to the site infected and include a neck mass (cervical adenopathy), sore throat, nasal obstruction, hoarseness, dysphagia.
- Clinical work-up includes chest radiograph, tuberculin skin test, and microbiologic cultures.

Scrofula

- Cervical lymph node involvement is referred to as scrofula, and although the causative organism may include *M. tuberculosis,* scrofula is most commonly caused by nontuberculous mycobacteria *(M. scrofulaceum, M. avium-intracellulare, M. kansasii).*
- Affects women more than men; primarily affects children.
- Most commonly involves high cervical lymph nodes in the region of the submandibular gland; periparotid and periauricular lymph nodes may also be involved.
- Usually presents as a unilateral neck mass when caused by nontuberculous mycobacteria; bilateral involvement generally is related to systemic involvement caused by dissemination of *M. tuberculosis.*

Pathology

Gross

- Enlarged, firm lymph nodes.
- Granular inflammation or ulceration of the mucosae.

Histology

- Caseating granulomas, characterized by central necrosis surrounded by histiocytes and giant cells.
- Organisms are often extremely difficult to identify and may defy detection despite an extensive and diligent effort.
- Microorganism identification requires special stains and is based on the capability of forming stable mycolate complexes with certain aryl methane dyes, referred to as "acid-fastness"; depending on the stain, the organisms, when identified, appear beaded, showing a red or purple color.

Differential Diagnosis

- Sarcoidosis (Chapter 8, #7c).
- Cat scratch disease (Chapter 8, #7e).
- Wegener's granulomatosis (Chapter 3, #8).

Treatment and Prognosis

- For infection caused by *M. tuberculosis,* treatment consists of antituberculous chemotherapy.
- For scrofula caused by nontuberculous mycobacteria, surgical excision is considered curative.

Additional Facts

- Irrespective of the causative organism, the histologic picture of mycobacterial infection is the same.
- Up to 25% of cases of nontuberculous mycobacterial infections will not produce a caseating granulomatous tissue response.

References

Harrison NK, Knight RK: Tuberculosis of the nasopharynx misdiagnosed as Wegener's granulomatosis. Thorax 41:219–220, 1986.

MacKeller A: Diagnosis and management of atypical mycobacterial lymphadenitis in children. J Pediatr Surg 11:85–89, 1976.

Myerowitz RL, Barnes L: Tuberculosis and nontuberculous mycobacterial cervical lymphadenitis. *In:* Barnes L, ed. Surgical pathology of the head and neck. New York: Marcel Dekker, 1985; pp 1780–1783.

Rohwedder JJ: Upper respiratory tract tuberculosis: sixteen cases in a general hospital. Ann Intern Med 80:708–713, 1974.

Waldman RH: Tuberculosis and the atypical mycobacteria. Otolaryngol Clin North Am 15:581–596, 1982.

Wolinsky E: Nontuberculous mycobacteria and associated diseases. Am Rev Respir Dis 119:107–159, 1979.

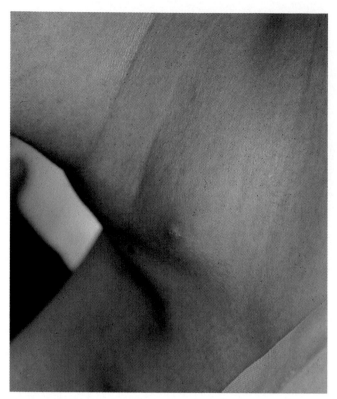

Figure 8–35. Mycobacterial involvement of cervical lymph nodes (scrofula) presenting as a unilateral, firm, red neck mass with focal ulceration of the skin.

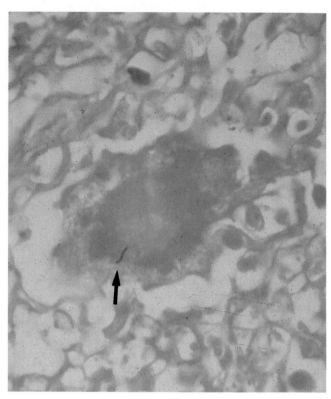

Figure 8–37. Acid-fast bacilli (AFB) stain aids in the identification of the *M. tuberculosis* organism, which appears as a slender, beaded, red/purple rod within the giant cell (*arrow*).

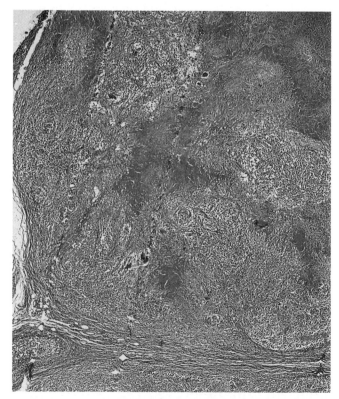

Figure 8–36. Characteristic histologic appearance of mycobacterial infection, consisting of replacement of the lymph node architecture by caseating granulomas, which are characterized by central necrosis surrounded by histiocytes and giant cells.

c. Sarcoidosis

Definition: Multisystem chronic granulomatous disease of unknown etiology.

Clinical

■ Affects virtually every organ system.
■ No sex predilection; occurs in all age groups, but most commonly is seen in young adults.
■ Any organ system may be involved, but typically pulmonary and cutaneous involvements are identified; most common clinical presentation is with fever, weight loss, and hilar adenopathy.
■ Isolated extranodal head and neck involvement only occurs in a small percentage of cases and includes the pharynx and tonsils, ear and temporal bones, sinonasal region, salivary glands, and larynx; site-specific involvement may occur as an isolated phenomenon or may coexist with systemic disease.
■ Otolaryngic symptoms vary according to site and include cervical adenopathy, pharyngotonsillitis with tonsillar enlargement, airway obstruction, nasal discharge, epistaxis.
■ Salivary gland involvement may clinically simulate Sjögren's syndrome, with salivary gland enlargement, xerostomia, and xerophthalmia; involvement of the parotid gland and uveal tract, referred to as *uveoparotid fever or Heerfordt's syndrome,* may present with facial nerve paralysis.
■ There are no laboratory findings specific for or diagnostic of sarcoidosis; cutaneous anergy to skin test antigens may be seen.
■ The diagnosis of sarcoidosis is generally one of exclusion and is made by correlation of clinical, radiologic, and pathologic findings.

Pathology

Histology

■ Multiple, noncaseating granulomas that consist of nodules of epithelioid histiocytes surrounded by a mixed inflammatory infiltrate.
■ Langhans type giant cells may be present.
■ Intracytoplasmic inclusions, including star-shaped or calcific laminated bodies, called asteroid and Schaumann bodies, respectively, can be seen.
■ All special stains for microorganisms are negative.

Differential Diagnosis

■ Mycobacterial infection (Chapter 8, #7b).
■ Cat scratch disease (Chapter 8, #7e).
■ Fungal infections.

Treatment and Prognosis

■ Treatment for symptomatic sarcoidosis is with corticosteroid therapy.
■ Prognosis is generally good, with up to 70% of patients improving or remaining stable after therapy.

■ Advanced multisystem disease that leads to extensive pulmonary involvement and respiratory failure may occur but is seen in only a small percentage of cases.

Additional Facts

■ Although the pathologic features are characteristic, they are not specific for sarcoidosis, and the diagnosis of sarcoidosis can only be rendered in the absence of identifying an infectious agent.

References

Lazarus AA: Sarcoidosis. Otolaryngol Clin North Am 15:621–633, 1982.

Miglets AW, Viall JH, Kataria YP: Sarcoidosis of the head and neck. Laryngoscope 87:2038–2048, 1977.

Myerowitz RL: Sarcoidosis. *In:* Barnes L, ed. Surgical pathology of the head and neck. New York: Marcel Dekker, 1985; pp 1809–1811.

Werning JT: Sarcoidosis. *In:* Ellis GL, Auclair PL, Gnepp DR, eds. Surgical pathology of salivary glands. Philadelphia: W.B. Saunders Co., 1991; pp 51–55.

Williams WJ: Aetiology of sarcoidosis. Pathol Res Pract 175:1–12, 1982.

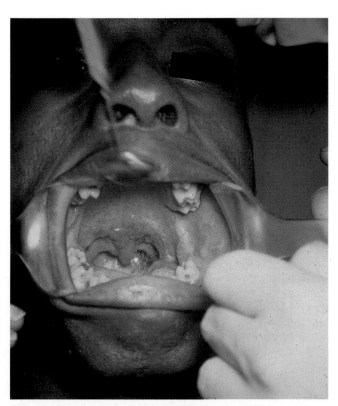

Figure 8–38. Oral cavity (soft palate) sarcoidosis appearing as multiple, irregular nodules with a cobblestone appearance.

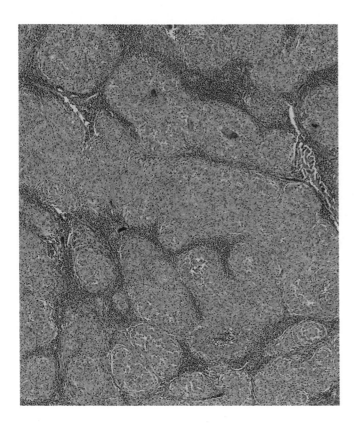

Figure 8–39. Histologic picture of sarcoidosis includes multiple, noncaseating granulomas, consisting of nodules of epithelioid histiocytes surrounded by a mixed inflammatory infiltrate; Langhans-type giant cells are seen in some of the nodules.

d. Cervicofacial Actinomycosis

Definition: Chronic granulomatous and suppurative disease caused by gram-positive, microaerophilic and anaerobic bacteria, the most common isolate causing this disease in humans being *Actinomyces israelii.*

Clinical

■ Actinomyces are endogenous saprophytic organisms in the oral cavity and tonsils that can become pathogenic.
■ Disease is classified according to the anatomic site involved and includes cervicofacial, abdominal, and pulmonary.
■ Cervicofacial actinomycosis is the most common form of disease and is thought to arise secondary to dental manipulation or trauma.
■ No sex predilection; occurs in all age groups.
■ The neck and area around the angle of the mandible are the most common sites of occurrence; however, clinical infection can occur anywhere in the head and neck.
■ Most common symptom is that of a painless, slowly enlarging, indurated mass with or without suppuration; the skin overlying the lesion has a characteristic purple color, from which a draining sinus may be seen.

■ Definitive diagnosis is made bacteriologically; however, the organisms are difficult to culture.

Pathology

Gross

■ Indurated mass with a blue-purple coloration of the overlying skin; fistulization is not uncommon.

Histology

■ Granulomatous reaction with central accumulation of polymorphonuclear leukocytes (abscess formation) and necrosis.
■ Within the abscess and enveloped by the neutrophils, microorganism colonies are seen; the organisms form a characteristic appearance, referred to as "sulfur granules."
■ The granules are lobular, deep purple, and composed of a central meshwork of filaments that typically have eosinophilic, club-shaped ends.
■ Histochemistry: the organisms stain best with Gram and Gomori methenamine silver (GMS) stains.

Differential Diagnosis

■ Nocardia infection.

Treatment and Prognosis

- Intravenous penicillin G followed by oral penicillin is the treatment of choice.
- Patients allergic to penicillin can be given tetracycline.
- Prognosis is good if treated early.
- Osteomyelitis of the jaw is the most common complication; once infection reaches bone, tissue destruction may be extensive and involvement of the cranium, meninges, and brain may occur and may be lethal.

Additional Facts

- Sulfur granules can be identified in pus.
- Actinomyces are often seen within tonsillar crypts, which represent saprophytes and are unaccompanied by an inflammatory response.

References

Kusumi RK: Actinomycosis. *In:* Cummings CW, Frederickson JM, Harker LA, Krause CJ, Schuller DE, eds. Otolaryngology—head and neck surgery. St. Louis: C.V. Mosby Co., 1986; p 1611.

Myerowitz RL: Cervicofacial actinomycosis *In:* Barnes L, ed. Surgical pathology of the head and neck. New York: Marcel Dekker, 1985; p 1780.

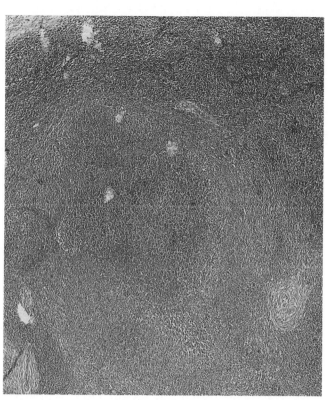

Figure 8-41. Actinomycotic reaction in a cervical lymph node appears as a granulomatous reaction with central accumulation of polymorphonuclear leukocytes (abscess formation) and necrosis.

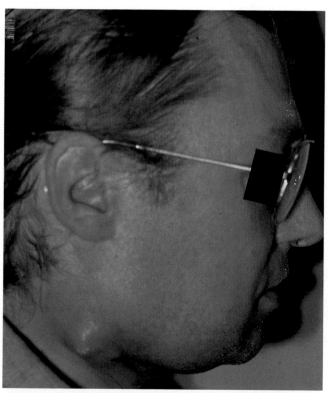

Figure 8-40. Cervicofacial actinomycosis seen as a painless, indurated, suppurative neck mass around the angle of the mandible; the skin overlying the lesion has a characteristic purplish color.

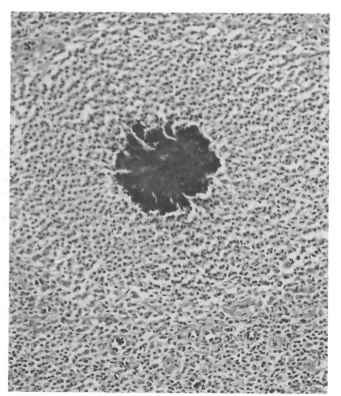

Figure 8-42. Within the abscess and enveloped by the neutrophils, microorganism colonies are seen with a characteristic appearance, referred to as "sulfur granules"; the granules are lobular, deep purple, and composed of a central meshwork of filaments, which typically have eosinophilic, club-shaped ends.

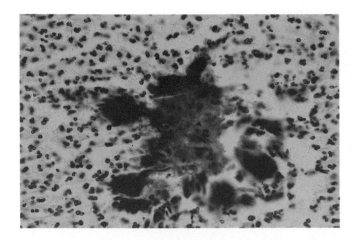

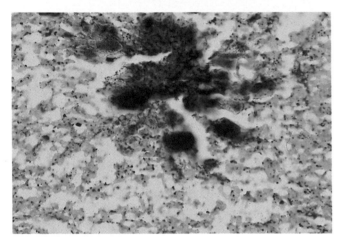

Figure 8-43. The organisms stain best with Gram *(top)* and Gomori methenamine silver (GMS) stains *(bottom)*.

e. Cat Scratch Disease

Definition: Infectious disease caused by a pleomorphic, gram-negative bacillus, resulting in lymphadenopathy.

Clinical

■ No sex predilection or age preference.

■ Mode of transmission is by direct contact from a cat scratch, bite, or lick.

■ In majority of cases, a history of exposure to a cat can be obtained and the primary inoculation site identified; typically seen from 7 to 12 days after contact.

■ Symptoms include:
  Enlarged and often tender lymph nodes with potential involvement of the submental, submandibular, cervical, occipital, and supraclavicular lymph nodes, as well as cervical lymph nodes in both the anterior and posterior triangles of the neck.

Constitutional symptoms include low-grade fever, malaise, myalgias, headaches, and anorexia.
  Obstruction and inflammation may be seen in salivary glands with involved lymph nodes.
  Less common manifestations/complications of cat scratch disease are granulomatous conjunctivitis (Parinaud's oculoglandular syndrome), thrombocytopenic purpura, encephalitis, osteomyelitis, and hepatosplenomegaly.

■ A positive skin test can confirm the diagnosis.

Pathology

Gross

■ Cutaneous lesion is a red papule, which may become crusted or pustular.

Histology

■ Lymph node changes vary with time and include:
  Early: follicular hyperplasia and histiocytic proliferation.

Intermediate: granulomas.
Late: abscess formation.

- The appearance of the abscess suggests the diagnosis; the abscess is composed of a central area of necrosis with a stellate pattern admixed with polymorphonuclear leukocytes, surrounded by palisading of histiocytes.
- Nodal sinuses are packed with monocytoid B cells.
- Skin lesions show necrotic areas within the dermis, surrounded by histiocytes.
- Histochemistry: cat scratch bacilli can be identified by Warthin-Starry stain and appear as extracellular pleomorphic coccobacilli.

Differential Diagnosis

- Toxoplasmosis.
- Lymphogranuloma venereum.

Treatment and Prognosis

- Therapy is supportive and includes analgesics and warm compresses.
- In cases with suppuration, needle aspiration may relieve pain; incision and drainage may produce sinus tract inflammation.
- Antibiotics appear to be of little benefit.

Additional Facts

- There is no evidence to support transmission from human to human.
- The infected cat is not ill and appears to be infectious for only a limited time.

References

Carithers HA: Cat-scratch disease: an overview based on a study of 1200 patients. Am J Dis Child 139:1124–1133, 1985.

English CK, Wear DJ, Margileth AW, Lissner CR, Walsh GP: Cat-scratch disease: isolation and culture of the bacterial agent. JAMA 259:1347–1352, 1988.

Margileth AW, Wear DJ, Hadfield TL, Schlagel CJ, Spigel GT, Muhlbauer JE: Cat-scratch disease: bacteria in skin at the primary inoculation site. JAMA 252:928–931, 1984.

Margileth AW, Wear DJ, English CK: Systemic cat scratch disease: report of 23 patients with prolonged or recurrent severe bacterial infection. J Infect Dis 155:390–402, 1987.

Miller-Catchpole R, Variakojis D, Vardiman JW, Loew JM, Carter J: Cat scratch disease: identification of bacteria in seven cases of lymphadenitis. Am J Surg Pathol 10:276–281, 1986.

Wear DJ, Margileth AW, Hadfield TL, Fisher GW, Schlagel CJ, King FM: Cat scratch disease: a bacterial infection. Science 221:1403–1405, 1983.

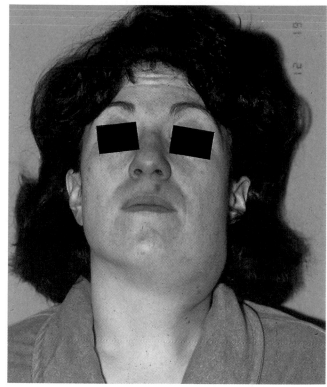

Figure 8–44. Young woman with cat scratch disease, presenting with enlarged and tender left cervical lymph nodes.

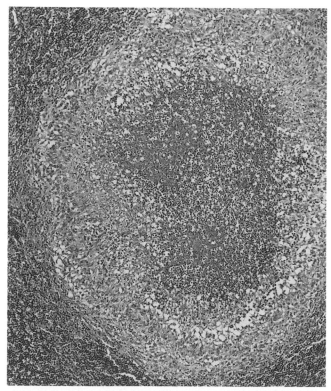

Figure 8–45. Characteristic but not pathognomonic appearance of the abscess seen in cat scratch infection, composed of a central area of necrosis with a stellate pattern admixed with polymorphonuclear leukocytes surrounded by palisading of histiocytes.

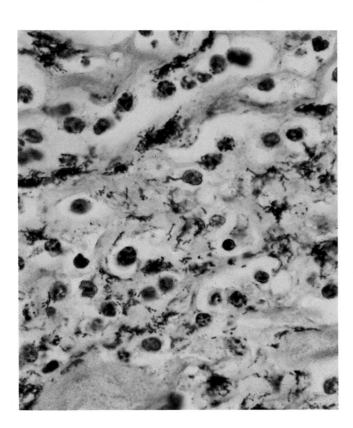

Figure 8-46. Cat scratch bacilli can be identified by Warthin-Starry stain, appearing as extracellular pleomorphic coccobacilli.

f. Otolaryngic Infections and Lymphadenopathies Related to Acquired Immunodeficiency Syndrome (AIDS)

I. Infections

A. VIRUSES

Clinical

- Viral infestation of head and neck sites in human immunodeficiency virus (HIV)–positive patients is common.
- Among the viruses infecting head and neck sites in association with AIDS are cytomegalovirus (CMV) and herpes virus (simplex and zoster).

Cytomegalovirus

- CMV is the most common opportunistic pathogen recognized at autopsy in AIDS patients.
- In general, CMV infection involving the head and neck is not common.
- When it occurs in the head and neck, CMV infection is seen as an ulcerative mucocutaneous lesion.

Herpes Virus

- Two distinct subtypes of herpes simplex virus are identified: type 1 is referred to as the "oral" type and type 2 is referred to as the "genital" type; however, the virus type is not necessarily a reliable indicator of anatomic site affected, especially with changing sexual habits.
- Because of its tendency to infect cells of ectodermal origin (skin or mucous membranes), herpes simplex virus (HSV) is a frequent cause of mucocutaneous disease in the HIV-positive patient.
- Head and neck manifestations are those of an ulcerated lesion with involvement of intraoral sites, nasal cavity, lip, external ear, pharynx, and tonsil; in addition, enlargement and tenderness of cervical and submental lymph nodes may be seen.
- Infection of the pharynx may appear as vesicular lesions that bleed easily and may be covered with a black crust or as shallow tonsillar ulcers covered with a gray exudate.
- Herpes zoster may occur as varicella (chickenpox) or as dermatomal zoster (shingles); the latter, although not specific for HIV infection, appears to be related to HIV infection and may represent an early marker for the immunosuppression associated with HIV infection.
- Herpes zoster can localize to any dermatome, is neurotropic, and can cause unremitting pain.
- Head and neck manifestations include involvement of the eighth nerve or geniculate ganglion *(Ramsay*

Hunt syndrome), producing severe ear pain, hearing loss, vertigo, and facial nerve paralysis.

Pathology

Gross

- Single or multiple, oval, tan-white, ulcerated lesions with a hyperemic rim, with or without an associated exudate.

Histology

Cytomegalovirus

- Mucosal ulceration, necrosis, and cytomegaly.
- Characteristic basophilic intranuclear or intracytoplasmic inclusions.
- Confirmation of CMV infection can be detected by positive anti-CMV immunoreactivity.

Herpes Simplex Virus

- Intraepidermal vesicle marked by acantholysis and balloon degeneration of epithelial cells.
- Intranuclear inclusions may be identified within the degenerating epithelial cells.
- Multinucleated giant cells may be numerous.
- Positive identification of herpetic lesions can be seen by its positive anti-HSV immunoreactivity.
- Herpes zoster virus: intranuclear inclusions indistinguishable from those seen in herpes simplex are identified.

Treatment

- Antiviral chemotherapy, including acyclovir, ganciclovir, and foscarnet.

B. Fungi

- In the upper aerodigestive tract, *Candida* species normally reside in the mouth; however, under conditions where the immune system is compromised, invasion of oral mucosal surfaces can occur.
- Many fungi are implicated in causing disease in the HIV-infected patient.
- In the head and neck, the single most important fungal pathogen is the *Candida* species.
- Oral candidiasis (thrush) frequently occurs in AIDS patients, and its presence is a strong indication for the subsequent development of AIDS.
- Identification of the organism can be accomplished by culture on Sabouraud's agar.
- *Candida* is seen in association with *oral hairy leukoplakia,* where it is identified on the surface of the lesion; this form of *Candida* infection is unrelated to AIDS.

Pathology

Gross

- The most common form of oral candidiasis (thrush) appears as a "cheesy" or creamy appearing mucosal plaque.

Histology

- Budding yeasts and pseudohyphae typically are identified and are easily identifiable after staining with periodic acid–Schiff or silver stains.

Treatment

- Candidiasis limited to the oral cavity or pharynx is treated with topical nystatin or oral ketoconazole and its derivatives; however, if oral or pharyngeal infection represents part of systemic involvement, amphotericin B is the drug of choice.

C. Protozoa

- *Pneumocystis carinii* is an opportunistic organism that is usually associated with pneumonia in the immunodeficient host; it is the most common life-threatening infection in AIDS patients.
- It is unusual for *Pneumocystis* to cause clinical manifestations outside of the pulmonary system.
- In the head and neck, *Pneumocystis* infection has been identified involving the external auditory canal and the middle ear.
- Clinical manifestations differ according to the site of infection and include ear pain, hypomobility of the tympanic membrane, and otitis media, as well as conductive and sensorineural hearing losses.
- The presumed mode of dissemination from the lung to extrapulmonary sites is via vascular channels; typically, the pulmonary manifestations of *Pneumocystis* infection precede those of extrapulmonary involvement; however, on occasion the initial diagnosis of AIDS has been made after identification of its associated pathology in extrapulmonary locations.

Pathology

Gross

- May appear as a polypoid mass arising from the external or middle ear.

Histology

- Findings are similar to those seen in the lung and include a submucosal foamy exudate within which the organism can be identified by Gomori methenamine silver (GMS) stain.
- Overlying epithelium can be ulcerated.

Treatment

- Treatment of otologic pneumocystosis should be directed at systemic pneumocystosis, even in the face of subclinical pulmonary manifestations.

D. Bacteria and Spirochetes

- AIDS patients may experience an increased incidence of otolaryngic gonorrhea and syphilis.

Gonorrhea

Caused by *Neisseria gonorrhoeae,* a pyogenic, gram-negative diplococcus.

Otolaryngic manifestations include gonococcal pharyngitis, which generally is asymptomatic but may present with sore throat, tonsillar hypertrophy, or cervical adenopathy.

■ The organism infects mucosal and glandular structures.

■ Gram stain smears from the pharynx are unreliable due to the presence of other organisms, so samples must be cultured on appropriate media (chocolate agar) for identification.

Syphilis

■ Systemic venereal disease caused by *Treponema pallidum,* a member of the family Spirochaetaceae, which includes *T. pertenue* (yaws) and *T. carateum* (pinta).

■ Clinical stages of syphilis are primary, secondary, tertiary, and congenital, any of which can affect virtually any site in the head and neck.

■ Protean clinical manifestations include involvement of the head and neck, including:

Tonsillar involvement manifests as a painless solitary chancre, which appears at the site of inoculation in the primary stage; chancres may clinically mimic a neoplasm.

Skin lesions and lymphadenopathy (seen in 90% of the patients in the secondary or disseminated stage); pharyngotonsillitis may be a presenting symptom in secondary syphilis, and mucosal involvement produces so-called "mucous patches," which are highly contagious.

Other head and neck symptoms in the secondary stage include rhinitis, laryngitis, pharyngitis, cranial nerve deficits, sensorineural deafness, labyrinthitis, and glossitis.

Tertiary stage typically involves the central nervous system (neurosyphilis) and aorta (cardiovascular syphilis); however, localized, nonprogressive lesions may develop in mucosal otolaryngic sites, termed "benign tertiary syphilis" or "gummas"; the gummatous reaction represents a pronounced immunologic reaction of the host.

■ Laboratory evaluation includes two types of serologic tests for syphilis, the nontreponemal (nonspecific) antibody tests and the treponemal (specific) antibody tests; these tests are most reactive in the secondary stage of disease.

Pathology

Histology

Syphilis

■ An inflammatory infiltrate can be seen that is predominantly composed of plasma cells with scattered histiocytes, lymphocytes, and polymorphonuclear leukocytes.

■ This infiltrate has a tendency to involve small blood vessels that display endothelial cell proliferation; concentric layers are produced that markedly narrow the affected vessel's lumen, resulting in obliterative endarteritis.

■ The obliterative endarteritis coupled with the inflammatory infiltrate produced by the spirochetes represents the histologic hallmarks of the disease.

■ Organisms can be demonstrated in the chancre by Warthin-Starry staining and appear as elongated, thin, rod-like structures.

Differential Diagnosis

■ Non-specific inflammatory reactions.

Treatment and Prognosis

■ Pencillin remains the treatment of choice for both gonorrhea and syphilis; penicillin G or procaine is administered parenterally.

■ For those persons allergic to penicillin, either tetracycline or erythromycin is an effective alternative.

■ For penicillinase-producing strains, spectinomycin hydrochloride, cefoxitin sodium, or ampicillin have been used.

Additional Facts

■ A variety of techniques, including darkfield examination of smears and immunohistochemistry, may be used to detect organisms.

■ Although unproved, syphilitic involvement of the oral mucosa has been considered a precancerous lesion.

■ *Congenital syphilis*

Develops via transplacental infection.

Primarily occurs with mucocutaneous and osseous manifestations, including, in decreasing percentage, frontal boss > short maxilla > high palatal arch > saddle nose > mulberry molars > Hutchinson's incisors > sternoclavicular thickening > interstitial keratitis > rhagades > VIII nerve deafness.

References

Drew WL: Diagnosis of cytomegalovirus infection. Rev Infect Dis 10:S468–S476, 1988.

Jacobsen MA, Mills J: Serious cytomegalovirus disease in acquired immunodeficiency syndrome (AIDS). Ann Intern Med 108:585–594, 1988.

Kovacs JA, Masur H: Opportunistic infections. *In:* DeVita VT, Hellman S, Rosenberg SA, eds. AIDS: etiology, diagnosis, treatment and prevention, 2nd ed. Philadelphia: J.B. Lippincott Co., 1988; pp 199–225.

Lalwani AK, Snyderman NL: Pharyngeal ulceration in AIDS patients secondary to cytomegalovirus infection. Ann Otol Rhinol Laryngol 100:484–487, 1991.

Tramont EC: *Treponema pallidum* (syphilis). *In:* Mandell GL, Douglas RG, Bennett JE, eds. Principles and practice of infectious diseases. New York: Wiley, 1985; pp 1323–1333.

Sandler ED, Sandler JM, Leboit P, Wenig BM, Mortensen N: *Pneumocystis carinii* otitis media in AIDS: a case report and review of the literature regarding extrapulmonary pneumocystosis. Otolaryngol Head Neck Surg 103:817–821, 1990.

Scully C, Laskaris G, Pindborg J, Porter SR: Oral manifestations of HIV infection and their management: I. More common lesions. Oral Surg Oral Med Oral Pathol 71:158–166, 1991.

Scully C, Laskaris G, Pindborg J, Porter SR: Oral manifestations of HIV infection and their management: II. Less common lesions. Oral Surg Oral Med Oral Pathol 71:167–171, 1991.

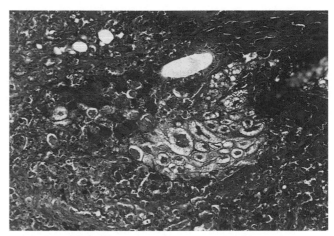

Figure 8–49. Histologic appearance of herpes simplex virus, with cutaneous ulceration and degeneration of epithelial cells with enlarged nuclei characterized by intranuclear eosinophilic inclusions.

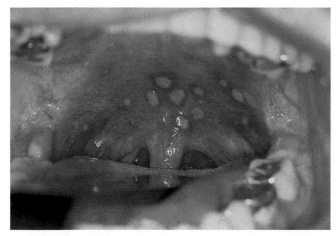

Figure 8-47. Cytomegalovirus (CMV) pharyngitis, appearing as multiple, discrete, oval mucosal lesions.

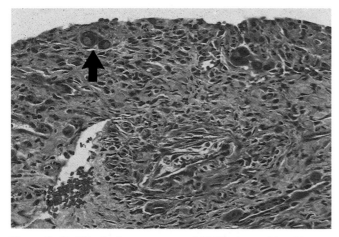

Figure 8–48. Histologic appearance of CMV pharyngitis with mucosal ulceration, necrosis, and cytomegaly and characteristic intranuclear basophilic inclusions *(arrow).*

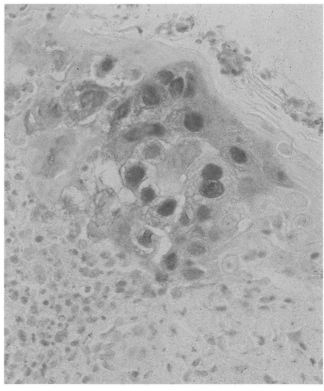

Figure 8–50. Herpetic lesions are positively identified by anti-HSV immunoreactivity.

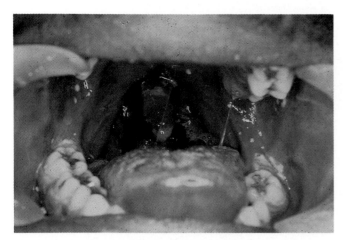

Figure 8–51. Oral candidiasis (thrush) in this AIDS patient appears as a "cheesy" or creamy-appearing plaque, seen coating the tongue.

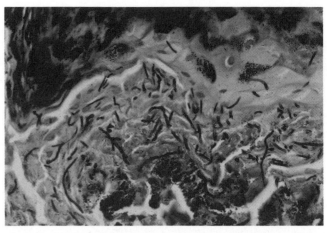

Figure 8–52. *Candida* budding yeasts and pseudohyphae are identified by periodic acid–Schiff stain.

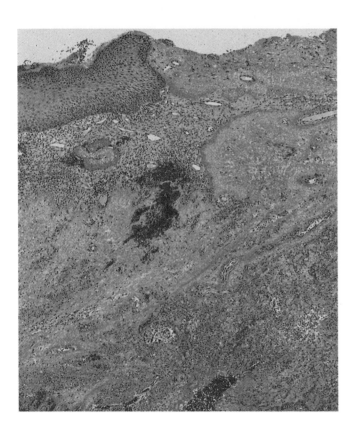

Figure 8–53. AIDS patient who presented with persistent otitis media and decreased hearing had a polypoid mass removed from his ear. The histologic appearance revealed an ulcerated epithelium with a submucosal foamy exudate.

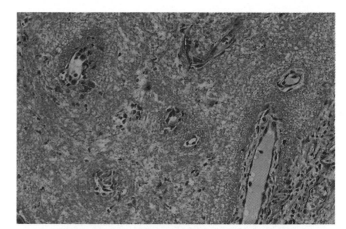

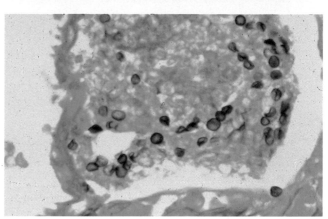

Figure 8–54. *(Top)* Submucosal foamy exudate, also identified adjacent to vascular spaces within which *Pneumocystis* organisms were identified. *(Bottom)* Gomori methenamine silver stain showing *Pneumocystis carinii* organisms appearing black with a round to oval shape and a linear groove in the center of some of the organisms.

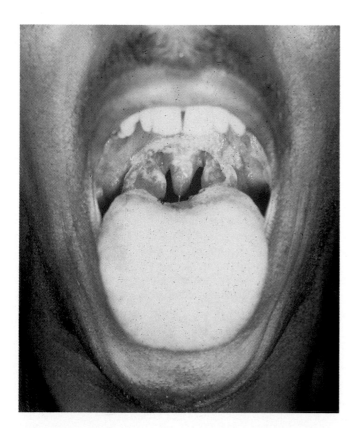

Figure 8–55. Syphilitic pharyngotonsillitis with diffuse white exudate overlying the soft palate, uvula, and tonsils.

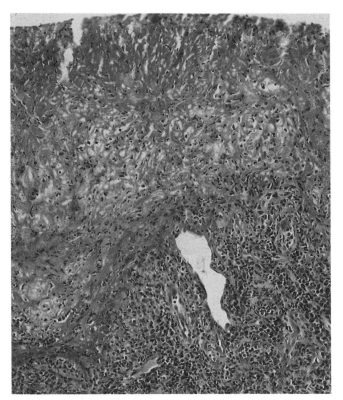

Figure 8-56. Surface ulceration and an inflammatory infiltrate predominantly composed of plasma cells with scattered histiocytes, lymphocytes, and polymorphonuclear leukocytes depict the histologic appearance of syphilis. The inflammatory infiltrate has a tendency to involve small blood vessels, which may result in an obliterative endarteritis.

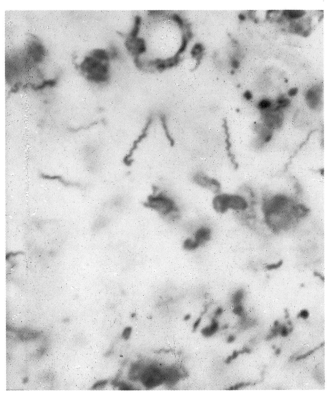

Figure 8-57. Organisms can be demonstrated by Warthin-Starry staining, appearing as elongated, thin, rod-like or corkscrew-shaped structures.

II. AIDS-Related Lymphadenopathies

Clinical

■ A spectrum of AIDS-related lymph node abnormalities can be seen, including:
Opportunistic infections.
Lymphomas (non-Hodgkin's and Hodgkin's).
Kaposi's sarcoma.
Persistent generalized lymphadenopathy (PGL), also referred to as *lymphadenopathy syndrome (LAS),* commonly found in patients with early HIV infection, and *generalized lymphadenopathy,* found in patients with AIDS-related complex (ARC) and those with frank AIDS; the common histologic pattern identified in these lymph nodes is that of florid reactive lymphoid hyperplasia.

Pathology

Histology

■ Florid reactive lymphoid hyperplasia consists of:
Enlarged, hyperplastic, and irregularly shaped germinal centers (GCs); GC enlargement may be so pronounced as to suggest confluence with other GCs.
GCs display increased mitotic activity and demonstrate prominent tingible body macrophages.
Attenuation or effacement of the mantle zones ("naked" GCs) is seen.
Invagination of the mantle zone lymphocytes into the GCs with disruption of the GCs can be seen and is termed follicle lysis; this feature creates a "moth-eaten" appearance to the lymph node.
Presence of sinusoidal or parasinusoidal monocytoid B-cell hyperplasia, which may be accompanied by neutrophils; monocytoid B cells consist of cells with distinct cell borders, moderate amounts of clear cytoplasm, and indented or angulated nuclei.
Increased numbers of histiocytes and immunoblasts and scattered eosinophils, mast cells, and plasma cells in the lymph node parenchyma.
Occasionally, multinucleated giant cells are seen; GC hemorrhage can be identified.

A prominent feature is the interfollicular proliferation of blood vessels with plump endothelial cells, showing rare mitoses.

- With progression of disease, the following features can be seen:

  Effacement of the lymph node architecture by diffuse lymphoid hyperplasia, eventually progressing to marked lymphoid depletion with atrophic or completely absent GCs; the latter findings often reflect the profound immunodeficiency characteristic of terminal AIDS.

Differential Diagnosis

- Other causes of reactive lymphoid hyperplasia.
- Castleman's disease.
- Vascular transformation of sinuses.

Additional Facts

- The histomorphologic changes detailed above appear to represent a continuum in the progression of disease.
- Erythrophagocytosis can be identified in all phases of disease but is most frequently identified in the advanced (profoundly immunodeficient) state.
- *Salivary gland (parotid) lymphoepithelial cysts* may represent a manifestation of AIDS or ARC patients and have the following features:

  To date, have exclusively occurred in men ranging in age from 29 to 47 years.

  Parotid swelling is uni- or bilateral.

  CT findings reveal the presence of multiple, frequently bilateral, parotid cysts; and, in association with diffuse cervical adenopathy, may represent specific CT findings in HIV-positive patients.

  Histologically, the cysts have a lymphoepithelial lining composed of squamous epithelium; epimyoepithelial islands may be seen, reminiscent of Sjögren's syndrome.

References

Burns BF, Wood GS, Dorfman RF: The varied histopathology of lymphadenopathy in homosexual men. Am J Surg Pathol 9:287-297, 1985.

Ewing EP, Chandler FW, Spira TJ, Byrnes RK, Chan WC: Primary lymph node pathology in AIDS and AIDS-related lymphadenopathy. Arch Pathol Lab Med 109:977–981, 1985.

Holliday RA, Cohen WA, Schinella RA, Rothstein SG, Persky MS, Jacobs JM, Som PM: Benign lymphoepithelial parotid cysts and hyperplastic cervical adenopathy in AIDS-risk patients: a new CT appearance. Radiology 168:439–441, 1988.

Schuurman HJ, Kluin PM, Gmelig Meijling FHJ, Van Unnik JAM, Kater L: Lymphocyte status of lymph node and blood in acquired immunodeficiency syndrome (AIDS) and AIDS-related complex disease. J Pathol 147:269–280, 1985.

Smith FB, Rajdeo H, Panesar N, Bhuta K, Stahl R: Benign lymphoepithelial lesion of the parotid gland in intravenous drug users. Arch Pathol Lab Med 112:742–745, 1988.

Stanley MW, Frizzera G: Diagnostic specificity of histologic features in lymph nodes biopsy from patients at risk for the acquired immunodeficiency syndrome. Hum Pathol 17:1231–1239, 1986.

Ulirisch RC, Jaffe ES: Sjögren's syndrome-like illness associated with the acquired immunodeficiency syndrome-related complex. Hum Pathol 18:1063–1068, 1987.

Wood GS, Garcia CF, Dorfman RF, Warnke RA: The immunohistology of follicle lysis in lymph node biopsies from homosexual men. Blood 66:1092–1097, 1985.

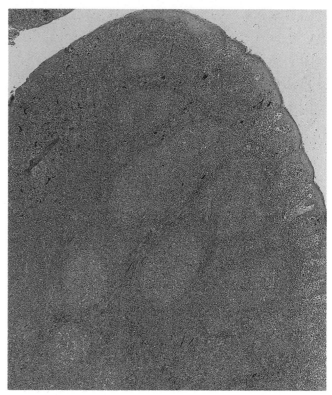

Figure 8–58. Tonsillar biopsy specimen in AIDS-related complex (ARC) showing florid reactive lymphoid hyperplasia with enlarged, hyperplastic, irregularly shaped and focally confluent germinal centers (GC).

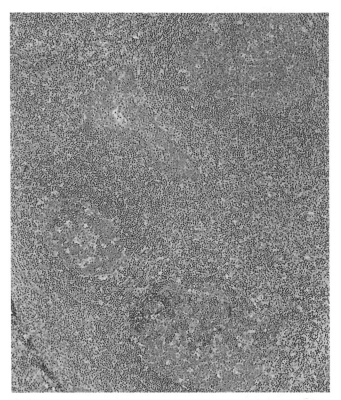

Figure 8–59. ARC: attenuation of the mantle zones ("naked" GC) is seen, with invagination of the mantle zone lymphocytes into the GC with disruption of the GC (follicle lysis), creating a "moth-eaten" appearance.

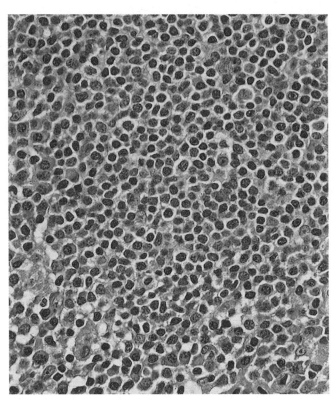

Figure 8–61. Monocytoid B-cell hyperplasia, consisting of cells with distinct cell borders, moderate amounts of clear cytoplasm, and indented or angulated nuclei, seen in sinusoidal or parasinusoidal areas.

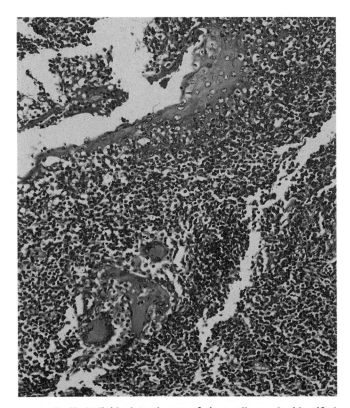

Figure 8–60. Individual or clusters of giant cells can be identified in proximity to crypt epithelium or within GC (not shown).

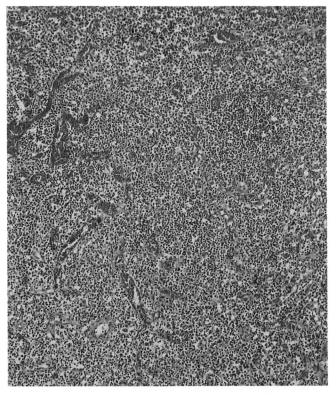

Figure 8–62. Lymph node from a preterminal AIDS patient, showing marked progression of disease with effacement of the lymph node architecture, lymphoid depletion with completely absent GC, and proliferation of blood vessels.

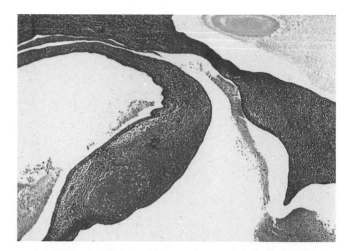

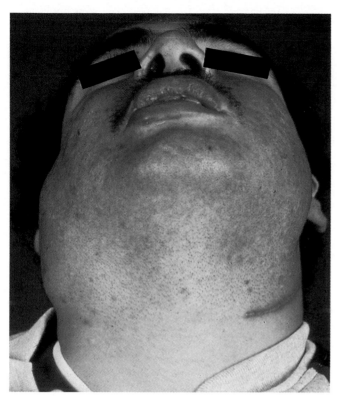

Figure 8–63. AIDS patient with unilateral swelling in the right parotid gland area, representing the clinical presentation of parotid lymphoepithelial cysts associated with AIDS.

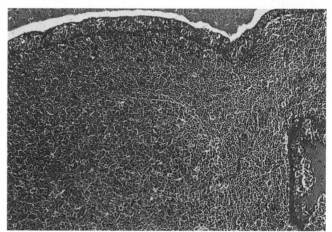

Figure 8–64. Lymphoepithelial cyst in association with AIDS. (*Top*) Multiloculated-appearing parotid cyst composed of an epithelial lining and a dense lymphoid cellular infiltrate with a germinal center in the cyst wall. (*Bottom*) Lymphoepithelial lining is seen toward the upper portion and is composed of squamous epithelium permeated by lymphocytes; the cyst wall contains a germinal center associated with a mature lymphocytic cell infiltrate, and toward the lower right portion of the illustration is an epimyoepithelial island reminiscent of those seen in Sjögren's syndrome.

CHAPTER 9

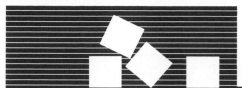

Neoplasms of the Oral Cavity, Nasopharynx, Tonsils, and Neck

A. BENIGN NEOPLASMS

1. Squamous Papillomas

Definition: Benign, exophytic epithelial neoplastic growth, composed of branching fronds of squamous epithelium with fibrovascular cores.

Clinical

- Most common benign neoplasm of the oral cavity; papillomas involving the nasopharynx are uncommon.
- Affects men more than women; most commonly seen in the third to sixth decades of life.
- Any site can be affected, but is most frequently identified involving the tongue, lips, palate, buccal mucosa, tonsil, and uvula.
- Symptoms relate to a painless mass; majority are solitary, but may be multiple.
- Viral etiology has been proposed but still remains unproven.

Pathology

Gross

- Exophytic, pink to tan-white lesion with a warty or cauliflower-like appearance; variation in size from a few millimeters up to 3.0 cm in greatest dimension.

Histology

- Hyperplastic squamous epithelium arranged in multiple, finger-like projections; squamous cell component generally is free of any dysplastic change.
- Prominent fibrovascular cores.
- Variable amount of hyper-, para-, and orthokeratosis may be seen.
- On rare occasions, an "inverted" growth may be seen.

Differential Diagnosis

- Verruca vulgaris (Chapter 14A, #1).

- Syringocystadenoma papilliferum (Chapter 19, #3a)
- Verrucous carcinoma (Chapter 14B, #3).
- Exophytic squamous cell carcinoma (Chapter 14B, #1).

Treatment and Prognosis

- Complete surgical excision.
- Recurrences occur infrequently and relate to inadequate excision.
- Malignant transformation does not occur.

Additional Facts

- In contrast to the sinonasal papillomas, those occurring in the oral cavity and nasopharynx are endodermally derived.
- Multiple papillomas may occur in association with focal dermal hypoplasia syndrome or focal epithelial hyperplasia (Heck's syndrome).
- Oral papillomatous lesions may also be a component of Cowden's syndrome, an autosomal dominant disease characterized by facial trichilemmomas associated with gastrointestinal tract (GIT), central nervous system (CNS), musculoskeletal and thyroid abnormalities.

References

Abbey LM, Page DG, Sawyer DR: The clinical and histopathologic features of a series of 464 oral squamous cell papillomas. Oral Surg Oral Med Oral Pathol 49:419–428, 1980.

Archard HO, Heck JW, Stanley HR: Focal epithelial hyperplasia: an unusual oral mucosal lesion found in Indian children. Oral Surg Oral Med Oral Pathol 20:201–212, 1965.

Eversole LR, Laipis PJ: Oral squamous papillomas: detection of HPV DNA by in situ hybridization. Oral Surg Oral Med Oral Pathol 65:545–550, 1988.

Goltz RW, Peterson WC, Gorlin RJ, Ravitis HG: Focal dermal hypoplasia syndrome. Acta Dermatol 86:708–717, 1962.

Greer RO, Goldman HM: Oral papillomas. Oral Surg Oral Med Oral Pathol 38:435–440, 1974.

Swart JGN, Lekkas C, Allard RHB: Oral manifestations in Cowden's syndrome: report of four cases. Oral Surg Oral Med Oral Pathol 59:264–268, 1985.

Young SK, Min KW: In situ hybridization analysis of oral papillomas, leukoplakias, and carcinomas for human papillomavirus. Oral Surg Oral Med Oral Pathol 71:726–729, 1991.

Zeuss MS, Miller CS, White DK: In situ hybridization analysis of human papillomavirus DNA in oral mucosal lesions. Oral Surg Oral Med Oral Pathol 71:714–720, 1991.

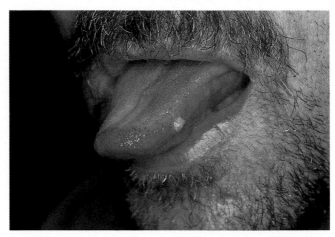

Figure 9-1. Squamous papilloma of the tongue: exophytic, tan-white lesion with a warty or cauliflower-like appearance.

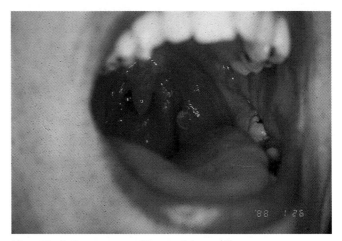

Figure 9-2. Squamous papilloma of the tonsil.

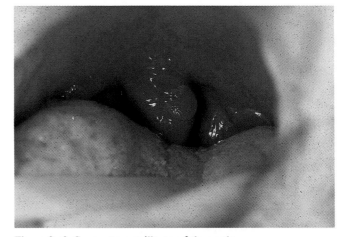

Figure 9-3. Squamous papilloma of the uvula.

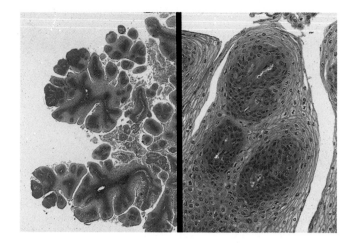

Figure 9-4. Squamous papilloma. (*Left*) Characteristic histologic appearance composed of hyperplastic squamous epithelium arranged in multiple fingerlike projections with fibrovascular cores. (*Right*) Papillary growth of hyperplastic epithelium with associated fibrovascular cores; the epithelial component matures (becomes less cellular) toward the surface, which generally has absent surface keratinization.

2. Nasopharyngeal Angiofibroma

Definition: Benign neoplasm, composed of an admixture of mature vascular and fibrous tissue with locally destructive properties.

Synonym: Juvenile angiofibroma.

Clinical

■ Relatively rare neoplasm, accounting for less than 1% of all head and neck tumors.
■ This tumor occurs almost exclusively in men, and some believe that it is a tumor exclusively limited to the male population.
■ May occur over a wide age range, but is most common in the second decade of life; uncommon over the age of 25 years.
■ Typically occurs along the lateral or upper posterior nasopharyngeal wall; rare examples have been reported to occur within the paranasal sinuses or the pterygomaxillary fossa.
■ The most common symptoms are unilateral nasal obstruction and epistaxis; less common symptoms include facial swelling or deformity (swelling of the cheek), nasal discharge, proptosis, diplopia, headache, sinusitis, and anosmia; pain may occur but is considered an unusual finding.
■ Typically, symptoms have been present for more than 1 year prior to diagnosis.

Radiology

■ Computed tomography (CT) scan with contrast enhancement demonstrates the mass and its extension into other areas.
■ Arteriography: marked vascular hypertrophy with increased number of arteries without beading, dilatation, segmental narrowing, or aneurysmal dilatation.

The blood supply may be unilateral or bilateral and typically comes from branches of the external carotid artery (internal maxillary or ascending pharyngeal).

Intracranial extension should be considered in cases where the internal carotid artery is the dominant vascular supply.

Pathology

Gross

■ Sessile, lobulated, rubbery, red-pink to tan-gray mass that can attain a large size, completely filling the nasopharynx.
■ Mucosal ulceration is uncommonly seen.
■ In general, angiofibromas are sessile but may be polypoid or pedunculated.

Histology

■ The tumor is unencapsulated and is composed of an admixture of vascular tissue and fibrous stroma.
■ The vascular component is made up of thin-walled, small to large vessels, varying in appearance from stellate or staghorn to barely conspicuous due to marked compression from the stromal component.
■ The endothelial cells form a single layer and are flat or plump in appearance.
■ The vessel walls lack elastic fibers and have incomplete or absent smooth muscle.
■ The stroma is composed of fibrous tissue with fine or coarse collagen fibers.
■ Stromal cells are stellate-appearing with plump nuclei and tend to radiate around vessels.
■ Mast cells are common; however, other inflammatory cells are absent, except near areas of surface ulceration.

- The stroma may have myxomatous change, which when present is focal in distribution.
- Nuclear pleomorphism and mitoses may be seen.

Differential Diagnosis

- Inflammatory nasal polyps (Chapter 3, #1).
- Antrochoanal polyp (Chapter 3, #2).

Treatment and Prognosis

- In uncomplicated cases with tumor limited to the nasopharynx, surgical excision via a transverse palatal approach is the treatment of choice.
- In order to control bleeding, vascular embolization should precede surgical intervention; furthermore, because of the vascularity of the tumor, biopsies should be performed with caution.
- Nonsurgical management has been proposed and includes estrogen therapy or irradiation; both of these treatment modalities reduce the angiomatous component of the tumor; however, although advocated, particularly with extension to the cranial cavity, surgical intervention remains the definitive mode of treatment.
- Complications associated with angiofibromas relate to extension of the tumor and to recurrence.
- Extension can occur in all directions, including:
  Anterior, with extension to the sinonasal cavities, oropharynx, pterygomaxillary fossa, superior buccal sulcus.
  Lateral, superior, and posterior, with extension into the orbit, infratemporal fossa, and cranial fossae (middle > anterior), and intracranially.
  Medial, with extension to the opposite side.
- Recurrence in cases without intracranial extension is low and usually occurs within 2 years of treatment; recurrence rates increase in cases with intracranial extension.
- In general, prognosis is excellent after surgical removal; mortality rates are around 5%.
- Rare cases have been reported to:
  Spontaneously regress.
  Undergo malignant (sarcomatous) transformation (related to radiotherapy).

Additional Facts

- Pathogenesis remains controversial and most probably arises from the nasopharyngeal fibrovascular tissue.
- As a result of the overwhelming occurrence in males, this tumor is thought to be hormonally driven, being dependent on testosterone and inhibited by estrogen; however, there is no definitive evidence confirming a hormonal imbalance in the development of this neoplasm.

References

Barnes L: Nasopharyngeal angiofibroma. *In*: Barnes L, ed. Surgical pathology of the head and neck. New York: Marcel Dekker, 1985; pp 416-420.

Bremer JW, Neel HB, DeSanto LW, Jones GC: Angiofibroma: treatment trends in 150 patients during 40 years. Laryngoscope 96:1321-1329, 1986.

Fu YS, Perzin KH: Non-epithelial tumors of the nasal cavity, paranasal sinuses, and nasopharynx: a clinical study, I. General features and vascular tumors. Cancer 33:1275-1288, 1974.

Heffner DK: Problems in pediatric otorhinolaryngic pathology: II. Vascular tumors and lesions of the sinonasal tract and nasopharynx. Int J Pediatr Otorhinolaryngol 5:125-138, 1983.

Hyams VJ, Batsakis JG, Michaels L: Angiofibroma. *In*: Hyams VJ, Batsakis JG, Michaels L, eds. Tumors of the upper respiratory tract and ear. Fascicle 25, second series. Washington, D.C.: Armed Forces Institute of Pathology, 1988; pp 130-134.

Kumagami H: Testosterone and estradiol in juvenile nasopharyngeal angiofibroma tissue. Acta Otolaryngol (Stockh) 111:569-573, 1991.

Neel HB, Whicker JH, Devine KD, Weiland LH: Juvenile angiofibroma: review of 120 cases. Am J Surg 126:547-556, 1973.

Sternberg SS: Pathology of juvenile nasopharyngeal angiofibroma—a lesion of adolescent males. Cancer 7:15-28, 1954.

Weprin LS, Siemers PT: Spontaneous regression of juvenile nasopharyngeal angiofibroma. Arch Otolaryngol Head Neck Surg 117:796-799, 1991.

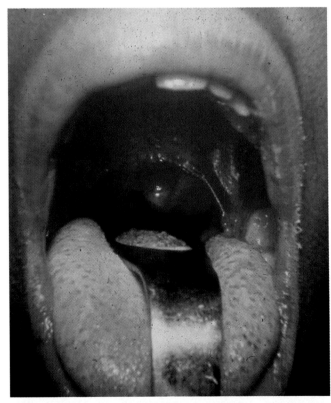

Figure 9-5. Juvenile nasopharyngeal angiofibroma (JNAF), clinically presenting as a lobulated, red-pink mass that completely fills the nasopharynx and protrudes down into the oropharynx.

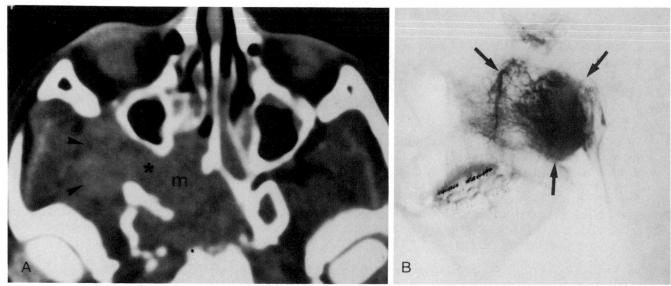

Figure 9-6. JNAF: axial CT. *(A)* Soft tissue mass (m) extending from the nasopharynx into the right pterygopalatine fossa *(asterisk)* and infratemporal fossa *(arrowheads)*. The posterior wall of the right maxillary antrum is remodeled and displaced anteriorly. *(B)* Lateral right external carotid angiogram: the tumor *(arrows)* is mainly supplied by the internal maxillary artery and densely stains during the capillary phase. (Courtesy of Franz J. Wippold II, M.D., Mallinckrodt Institute of Radiology, St. Louis, MO.)

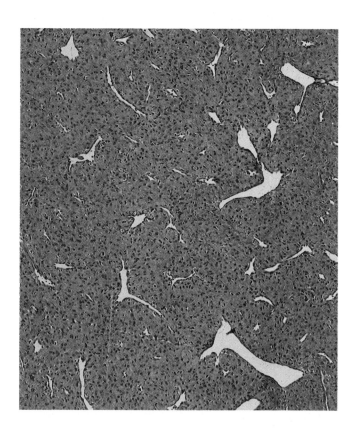

Figure 9-7. JNAF is composed of an admixture of vascular tissue and fibrous stroma. The vascular component is made up of thin-walled, small to large vessels varying in appearance from stellate or staghorn to barely conspicuous due to marked compression from the stromal component. Vascular spaces are lined by a single layer of flattened or plump endothelial cells; vascular walls demonstrate an absence of elastic fibers and incomplete or absent smooth muscle in the vascular walls. The stroma is composed of fibrous tissue, with fine or course collagen fibers and stellate-appearing fibroblasts with plump nuclei having a tendency to radiate around vessels.

3. Lymphangioma of the Cystic Hygroma Type

Definition: Benign, congenital malformations of lymphatic spaces that are divided into three types, including capillary (lymphangioma simplex), cavernous, and cystic; the latter is termed *cystic hygroma.*

Clinical

- No sex predilection; usually present at birth; from 80% to 90% of all cystic hygromas are identified by 2 years of age; less than 10% occur in adults.
- May occur anywhere in the body, but most commonly are seen in the head and neck region.
- In the head and neck, the overwhelming majority are identified in the lateral neck (posterior and anterior triangles) and are rarely seen in the midline.
- Presentation is usually as a painless, soft neck mass that can attain large sizes, filling the entire side of the neck; large lesions compress adjacent structures, potentially causing dysphagia, dyspnea, and stridor; pain is not commonly seen unless infection is present.
- Presumed to arise as congenital anomalies of the jugular lymphatic sac.
- Commonly seen in patients with Turner's syndrome; can be associated with other congenital anomalies, including thyroglossal duct cysts, harelip, congenital heart anomalies, hand and foot deformities, and in Down syndrome.

Radiology

- CT scan: well-circumscribed, solitary or multicystic masses varying in density, based on the presence or absence of intracystic hemorrhage or infection.

Pathology

Gross

- Soft, single or multiloculated, compressible mass varying in size from a few centimeters to more than 30 cm.
- Overlying skin may appear unremarkable or atrophic and may have a blue hue.
- In cases uncomplicated by hemorrhage or infection, the cysts contain clear to lightly pink-colored, watery fluid.

Histology

- Large, irregularly shaped spaces lined by a single layer of endothelial cells and containing proteinaceous fluid and lymphocytes.

- Intervening stroma contains small amounts of fibrous connective tissue and muscle with lymphoid aggregates; however, the stroma may become inflamed and fibrotic after repeated infections.

Differential Diagnosis

- Branchial cleft cyst (Chapter 8, #1).
- Thyroglossal duct cyst (Chapter 8, #1).
- Teratoma (Chapter 8, #2).
- Ranula (Chapter 8, #3).

Treatment and Prognosis

- Surgical excision is the treatment of choice.
- Some lymphangiomas may undergo spontaneous regression, and, in infants with uncomplicated cystic hygromas, surgery should be postponed until 3 to 4 years of age to allow for regression of the lesion; recurrent infections and symptoms of compression necessitate surgical intervention at younger ages.
- Lesions may extend extensively through soft tissue structures and can extend to the base of the skull and floor of the mouth and into the thoracic cavity.
- Recurrence rates after surgery range from 5% to 10% and may represent persistence rather than true recurrence of the lesion.
- Cystic hygromas have no malignant potential.
- Other therapeutic modalities (radiation, injection of sclerosing agents) have little if any benefit.

Additional Facts

- Due to the potential for extension of the lesion away from the neck, appropriate clinical evaluation should include complete radiographic evaluation including chest radiographs.
- Elevation of serum alpha-fetoprotein may be seen with in utero cases of cystic hygromas.

References

Barnes L: Lymphangioma. *In:* Barnes L, ed. Surgical pathology of the head and neck. New York: Marcel Dekker, 1985; pp 734–740.

Bill AH, Sumner DS: A unified concept of lymphangioma and cystic hygroma. Surg Gynecol Obstet 120:79–89, 1965.

Emery PJ, Bailey CM, Evans JNG: Cystic hygroma of the head and neck: a review of 37 cases. J Laryngol Otol 98:613–619, 1984.

Ricciardelli E, Richardson MA: Cervicofacial cystic hygroma: patterns of recurrence and management of difficult cases. Arch Otolaryngol Head Neck Surg 117:546–553, 1991.

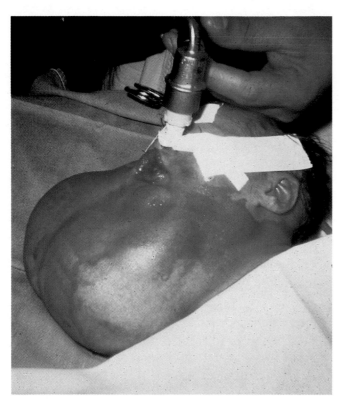

Figure 9-8. Cystic hygroma presenting as an enormous neck mass that completely obliterates the normal appearance of this infant's neck and lower face, bilaterally.

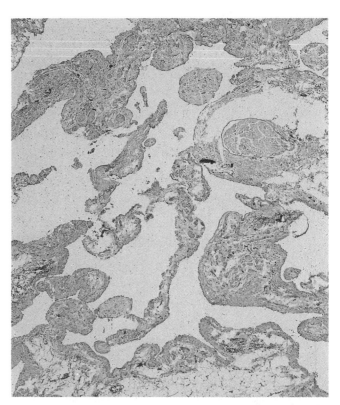

Figure 9-10. Histology of the lymphangioma, characterized by large, irregularly shaped spaces lined by a single layer of endothelial cells and containing proteinaceous fluid and lymphocytes. The intervening stroma contains small amounts of fibrous connective tissue and muscle, and adipose tissue is seen in the lower portion of the illustration.

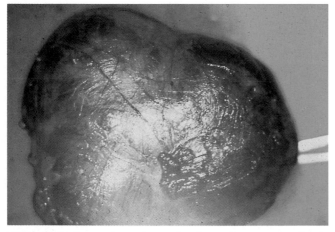

Figure 9-9. Resected specimen showing a large, encapsulated, fluid-filled cystic structure.

4. Carotid Body Paraganglioma

Definition: Benign tumor arising from the neural crest-derived paraganglia of the autonomic nervous system.

Synonym: Chemodectoma.

Clinical

- Extra-adrenal paraganglia are identified in the abdomen, retroperitoneum, chest, and mediastinum and in various head and neck sites; adrenal-derived paraganglioma arises from the adrenal medulla and is called a pheochromocytoma.
- Classification of paragangliomas is based on the anatomic site of occurrence and in the head and neck region includes carotid body, jugulotympanic, vagal, laryngeal, nasal, and orbital paragangliomas.
- The most common site of occurrence in the head and neck is the carotid body; the jugulotympanic paragangliomas represent the second most common site of occurrence.
- The carotid body is identified in the medial aspect of the common carotid artery and its bifurcation and, similar to the aortic body, functions as a chemoreceptor.
- No sex predilection; occurs over a wide age range but is most common in the fifth decade of life.
- The most common symptom is a painless neck mass, and often the mass has been present for years prior to the patient seeking medical attention.
- In general, this a slow-growing tumor, but it can attain a large size, leading to additional symptoms, including para- or hypopharyngeal mass, hoarseness, cranial nerve deficits, pain, vocal cord paralysis, and Horner's syndrome.
- Rarely, carotid body paragangliomas may be functional but, in general, paragangliomas of the head and neck are nonfunctional.
- May be familial or multicentric.

Radiology

- Carotid arteriogram: demonstrates a vascular tumor mass at the bifurcation of the common carotid artery.
- The tumor may extend superiorly and involve the parapharyngeal space.

Pathology

Gross

- Encapsulated, ovoid, rubbery, red-pink to tan-gray tumor of varying size.

Histology

- Cell nest or "zellballen" pattern is characteristic of paragangliomas.
- The stroma surrounding and separating the nests is composed of a prominent fibrovascular tissue.

- The neoplasm is composed predominantly of chief cells, which are round or oval with uniform nuclei, dispersed chromatin pattern, and abundant eosinophilic, granular, or vacuolated cytoplasm.
- Sustentacular cells may be seen; these cells represent modified Schwann cells and are seen at the periphery of the cell nests as spindle-shaped, basophilic appearing cells.
- No glandular or alveolar differentiation is seen.
- Cellular pleomorphism can be seen; mitoses and necrosis are infrequently identified.
- Spindling of the chief cells may be seen and infrequently may predominate.
- Histochemistry: tumor cells are argyrophilic and the presence of reticulin staining delineates the cell nests; argentaffin, mucin, and periodic acid–Schiff stains are negative.
- Immunohistochemistry:
  Chief cells: chromogranin, synaptophysin, neuron specific enolase positive.
  Sustentacular cells: S-100 protein positive.
- Electronmicroscopic: the hallmark of electronmicroscopic findings is the presence of neurosecretory granules.

Differential Diagnosis

- Hemangiopericytoma (Chapter 3, #8).
- Neuroendocrine carcinomas (Chapter 14B, #6).
- Alveolar soft part sarcoma (see below).
- Metastatic medullary carcinoma of the thyroid.
- Metastatic renal cell carcinoma.

Treatment and Prognosis

- Surgical excision is the treatment of choice.
- Prognosis is excellent after complete resection.
- Although these tumors are benign and behave in an indolent manner, approximately 10% may be malignant, as manifested by local invasion or metastases to regional lymph nodes or to the lung.
- Histologic criteria for malignancy include:
  Increased mitotic activity.
  Necrosis usually seen within the center of the cell nests.
  Vascular invasion.
  Extensive local infiltration or metastases.

Additional Facts

- Irrespective of the site of origin, the histologic appearance of all extra-adrenal paragangliomas is the same.
- Carotid body paragangliomas are much more common in people living at high altitudes than in those living at sea level.
- The histologic criteria for malignancy can also be identified in benign paragangliomas and, therefore, invasiveness or metastasis, or both, may be the only true criteria for malignant paraganglioma.
- The estimated 10% malignancy rate associated with carotid body paragangliomas may be high and may

represent multicentrically occurring paragangliomas.

■ Alveolar soft part sarcoma:

Rare, slow-growing, but highly malignant neoplasm of uncertain histogenesis.

Affects women more than men; occurs most frequently in the second to fourth decades of life.

Most common sites of occurrence are the soft tissues of the extremities; rare in the head and neck (orbit and tongue).

Histopathologic appearance characterized by an alveolar, organoid, or nest-like growth separated by thin-walled, fibrovascular septae; cells are large and round to polygonal with large, vesicular nuclei, one or more nucleoli, and abundant granular, eosinophilic cytoplasm; mitoses are uncommon.

Histochemistry: intracytoplasmic diastase-resistant, PAS-positive crystalline material is diagnostic for this tumor; immunohistochemistry is essentially noncontributory.

Expression of MyoD1, a regulatory gene in the control of myogenic differentiation, strongly suggests skeletal muscle differentiation for alveolar soft part sarcoma.

Surgery is the treatment of choice; however, local recurrence and metastatic disease (lung, bone, brain) commonly occur.

References

Auerbach HE, Brooks JJ: Alveolar soft part sarcoma: a clinicopathologic and immunohistochemical study. Cancer 60:66–73, 1987.

Barnes L, Taylor SR: Carotid body paragangliomas: a clinicopathologic and DNA analysis of 13 cases. Arch Otolaryngol Head Neck Surg 116:447–453, 1990.

Lack EE, Cubilla AL, Woodruff JM: Paragangliomas of the head and neck region: a pathologic study of tumors from 71 patients. Hum Pathol 10:191–218, 1979.

Lieberman PH, Brennan MF, Kimmel M, Erlandson RA, Garin-Chesa P, Flehinger BY: Alveolar soft part sarcoma: a clinicopathologic study of half a century. Cancer 63:1–13, 1989.

Peel RL: Tumors of the paraganglionic nervous system. In: Barnes L, ed. Surgical pathology of the head and neck. New York: Marcel Dekker, 1985; pp 684–695.

Rosai J, Dias P, Parham DM, Shapiro DN, Houghton P: MyoD1 protein expression in alveolar soft part sarcoma as confirmatory evidence of its skeletal muscle nature. Am J Surg Pathol 15:974–981, 1991.

Zak FG, Lawson W (eds.): The paraganglionic chemoreceptor system: physiology, pathology and clinical medicine. New York: Springer-Verlag, 1982.

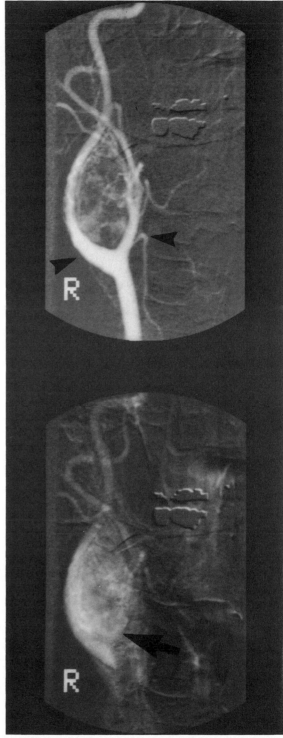

Figure 9–11. Right common carotid arteriogram demonstrating a carotid body paraganglioma. (*Top*) Splaying of the internal and external carotid arteries (*arrowheads*) by a vascular lesion. (*Bottom*) Slightly later in the arteriography the full extent of the vascular tumor mass can be appreciated (*arrow*).

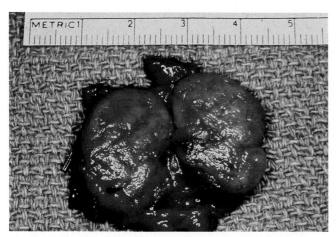

Figure 9-12. Carotid body tumor (paraganglioma)—encapsulated, ovoid, rubbery, red-brown mass.

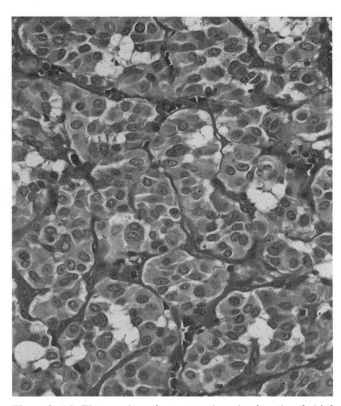

Figure 9-14. The neoplasm is composed predominantly of chief cells, which are round or oval with uniform nuclei, dispersed chromatin pattern, and abundant eosinophilic, granular, or vacuolated cytoplasm, peripherally surrounded by sustentacular cells, which are often difficult to identify by light microscopy and appear as spindle-shaped, basophilic cells.

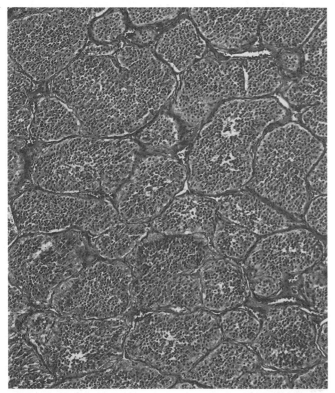

Figure 9-13. Characteristic histologic picture of paraganglioma, consisting of a cell nest or "zellballen" pattern, with a prominent fibrovascular connective tissue stroma surrounding and separating the nests.

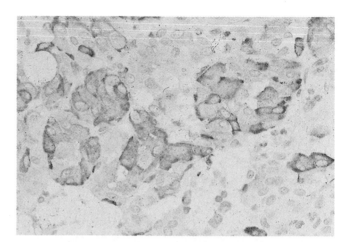

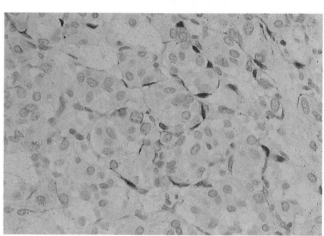

Figure 9-15. Immunohistochemistry of paragangliomas. *(Top)* Chief cells are diffusely reactive with chromogranin. *(Bottom)* Characteristic immunohistochemical staining pattern of the peripherally located sustentacular cells, as seen by their reactivity with S-100 protein, which is not identified in the chief cells.

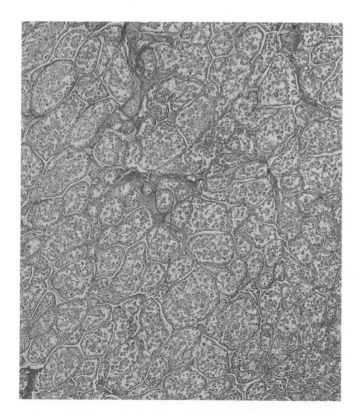

Figure 9-16. Alveolar soft part sarcoma (ASPS), characterized by an alveolar, organoid, or nestlike growth separated by thin-walled fibrovascular septae.

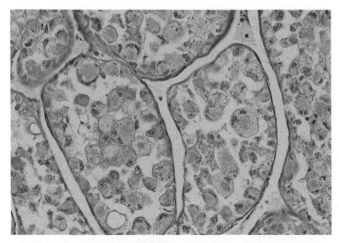

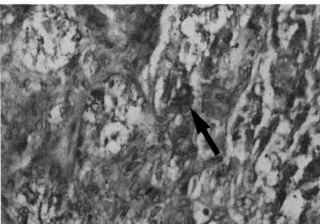

Figure 9-17. ASPS. *(Top)* Neoplasm is composed of large, round to polygonal-shaped cells with large, vesicular nuclei, one or more eosinophilic nucleoli, and abundant granular, eosinophilic cytoplasm. *(Bottom)* PAS-positive, intracytoplasmic, crystalline-like material is characteristically found *(arrow)*.

5. Lipoma

Definition: Benign tumor of mature adipose tissue.

Clinical

- Overall, lipomas represent the most common tumor of mesenchymal origin.
- Approximately 13% of all lipomas occur in the head and neck region.
- Lipomas can be seen in all areas of the head and neck, but the most common site of occurrence is the neck area; other sites in which lipomas are seen include the parotid gland, oral cavity (buccal mucosa), pharyngeal region (hypo- and retropharynx), and larynx.
- No sex predilection; occur in all age groups but most commonly seen in the fifth to sixth decades of life.
- Symptoms are generally related to a painless mass; pain or sensory and motor nerve disturbances are rarely seen, but may occur because of compression of nerves by large tumors.
- Upper respiratory tract lipomas present with symptoms related to airway obstruction, problems with deglutition, or voice disturbances (hoarseness, voice changes); often, symptoms manifest only after the tumor has reached a considerably large size.

Pathology

Gross

- Subcutaneous lipomas are encapsulated, soft, and round, varying in size and measuring from a few millimeters to more than 20 cm.
- Upper respiratory tract lipomas are encapsulated, soft, polypoid, and can grow to large sizes.
- Cut section shows an irregular, lobular pattern with a yellow color and a soft, greasy consistency.

Histology

- Thin capsule surrounding a tumor, arranged in a lobular growth pattern.
- The tumor is composed of mature fat cells (adipocytes), consisting of a vacuolated cell with compression and peripheral placement of the nucleus; little variation in size and shape of the adipocytes.

■ Lipoblasts are not seen.
■ Lipomas are richly vascular, but typically the vascular network is difficult to identify due to compression by distended lipocytes.
■ Secondary changes due to trauma or vascular compromise include necrosis, hemorrhage, infarction, calcification, and cyst formation.
■ A variety of histologic changes can be seen in lipomas, with subclassification based on the presence of these changes:
Myxoid stroma = myxolipoma.
Fibrous stroma = fibrolipoma.
Pleomorphic cells = pleomorphic or atypical lipoma.
Spindle cells = spindle cell lipoma.
Prominent vascular or smooth muscle component = angio- or angiomyolipoma.
Bone marrow elements = myelolipoma.
Chondroid or osseous metaplasia = chondro- or osteolipoma.

Differential Diagnosis

■ Well-differentiated liposarcoma (Chapter 9B, #8).

Treatment and Prognosis

■ Complete surgical excision is the treatment of choice.
■ Prognosis is excellent after surgical removal.
■ Local recurrence may be seen and occurs in approximately 5% of cases.

Additional Facts

■ Lipomas can arise within or between muscle fibers (intra- and intermuscular lipoma); these have also been called infiltrating lipomas.
■ Tumors arising from brown (immature or fetal) fat are called hibernomas, which are benign and are most often subcutaneous.
■ A rare, idiopathic condition of massive symmetric enlargement of the neck as a result of fat deposition is seen in middle-aged men and is termed *benign symmetric lipomatosis* or *Madelung's disease.*

References

Enzinger FW, Weiss SW: Benign lipomatous tumors. *In*: Enzinger FW, Weiss SW, eds. Soft tissue tumors, 2nd ed. St. Louis: C.V. Mosby, 1988; pp 301–345.
Evans HL, Soule EH, Winkelmann RK: Atypical lipoma, atypical intramuscular lipoma, and well differentiated retroperitoneal liposarcoma: a reappraisal of 30 cases formerly classified as well differentiated liposarcoma. Cancer 43:574–584, 1979.
Fu YS, Perzin KH: Non-epithelial tumors of the nasal cavity, paranasal sinuses, and nasopharynx: a clinical study. VIII. Adipose tissue tumors (lipoma and liposarcoma). Cancer 40:1314–1317, 1977.
Shmookler BM, Enzinger FM: Pleomorphic lipoma: a benign tumor simulating liposarcoma. A clinicopathologic analysis of 48 cases. Cancer 47:126–133, 1981.

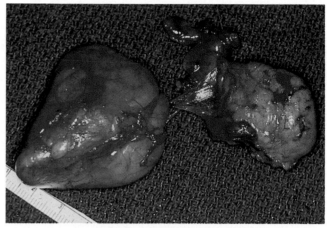

Figure 9–18. Encapsulated, irregularly shaped lipoma with a yellow color attached to the submandibular gland.

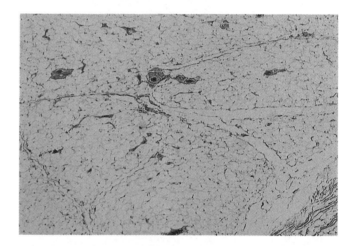

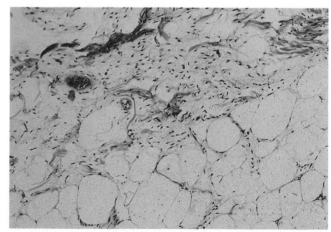

Figure 9–19. *(Top)* Characteristic histologic appearance of a lipoma composed of mature fat cells (adipocytes), consisting of a vacuolated cell with compression and peripheral placement of the nucleus, with little variation in size and shape of the adipocytes. *(Bottom)* Spindle cell lipoma characterized by an admixture of small, uniform, spindle-shaped cells with mature fat cells.

6. Benign Peripheral Nerve Sheath Neoplasms (Table 9–1)

a. Neurilemmoma or Benign Schwannoma

Definition: Benign tumor of Schwann cell origin.
Synonyms: Neuroma; acoustic neuroma.

Clinical

- Neurilemmomas can arise anywhere in the body, but have a predilection for the head and neck region and the extremities.
- Affect women more than men; occur in all ages, but most common in the third to sixth decades of life.
- In the head and neck, the most common site of occurrence is the neck (lateral aspect); other sites include middle ear (acoustic neuroma) and sinonasal cavity.
- Symptoms vary according to site, but most typically present as a solitary, painless neck mass; other symptoms may include airway obstruction, dysphagia, and voice changes.
- Pain, paresthesia, or other neurologic symptoms are uncommon.

Pathology

Gross

- Encapsulated mass, often seen attached to an identifiable nerve, with a tan-white color, rubbery to firm consistency, and a solid to partly cystic appearance.
- Neurilemmomas vary in size, but generally are less than 5 cm in diameter.
- Myxoid change may be prominent.

Histology

- Tumors are composed of alternating regions consisting of compact spindle cells called Antoni A areas, and loose, hypocellular zones called Antoni B areas; in a given tumor, the proportion of these components varies.
- Nuclei are vesicular to hyperchromatic, elongated and twisted, with indistinct cytoplasmic borders.
- Cells are arranged in short, interlacing fascicles, and whorling or palisading of nuclei may be seen; nuclear palisading with nuclear alignment in rows are called Verocay bodies.
- Antoni B areas display a disorderly cellular arrangement, myxoid stroma, and a chronic inflammatory cell infiltrate.
- Increased vascularity is prominent, composed of large vessels with thickened (hyalinized) walls.
- Mitoses, usually sparse in number, and cellular pleomorphism with hyperchromasia can be identified, but are not evidence of malignancy.
- Cellularity may vary; and some benign schwannomas can be very cellular, conferring the name cellular schwannoma.

- Retrogressive changes, including cystic degeneration, necrosis, hyalinization, calcification, and hemorrhage may be seen; pronounced degenerative changes in a neurilemmoma collectively are termed *ancient schwannomas.*
- Immunohistochemistry: S-100 protein is uniformly and intensely positive.

Differential Diagnosis

- Neurofibroma (see below).

Treatment and Prognosis

- Surgical excision is the treatment of choice, and every effort should be made to preserve the integrity of the nerve from which the tumor arises.
- In cases where the complete excision would result in damage or sacrifice of the parent nerve, incomplete excision can be performed.
- Local recurrences are infrequent.
- Prognosis is excellent after surgical removal; malignant transformation is extremely rare.

Additional Facts

- As a result of these tumors arising in the nerve sheath, the epi- or perineurium envelops the tumor, creating a true capsule.
- Occurrence in neurofibromatosis (von Recklinghausen's disease) is uncommon.
- The neural crest is thought to be the origin of the Schwann cell, although there is still controversy regarding this issue.

b. Solitary Neurofibroma

Definition: Localized, benign peripheral nerve sheath neoplasm, principally composed of Schwann cells.

Clinical

- By definition, the solitary or localized neurofibroma occurs in patients who do not have von Recklinghausen's disease.
- No sex predilection; most commonly occurs in the third and fourth decades of life.
- May affect any part of the body and are by far most commonly seen in the skin and subcutaneous tissue; can be seen in all upper respiratory tract sites.
- Symptoms vary according to site of occurrence and most commonly present as a painless mass.

Pathology

Gross

- Circumscribed but unencapsulated tan-white to gray mass.
- Involved nerve may be identified entering and exiting from the tumor, which expands the nerve in a fusiform manner.

Table 9-1

CLINICOPATHOLOGIC COMPARISON BETWEEN BENIGN PERIPHERAL
NERVE SHEATH TUMORS

	Benign Schwannoma	Solitary Neurofibroma	Neurofibroma in Association with VRD
Sex/age	♀ > ♂; 3rd–6th decades	♂ = ♀; 3rd–4th decades	Occurs at much younger ages
Common site(s) in head and neck	Lateral neck; middle ear	Cutaneous	Cutaneous, deep nerves and viscera
Gross	Encapsulated; often seen attached to parent nerve	Unencapsulated; associated nerve infrequently identified	Unencapsulated; marked distortion of nerve may occur
Histology	1. Spindle cells seen in cellular (Antoni A) and hypocellular (Antoni B) areas 2. Palisading nuclei (Verocay bodies) 3. Prominent thick-walled vessels 4. Degenerative changes are common	Interlacing bundles of spindle cells with wavy or buckled nuclei associated with collagen strands and separated by a myxomatous stroma containing mast cells and lymphocytes	Proliferation of spindle cells with increase in the endoneurial matrix and separation of the nerve fascicles with associated thick collagen fibers
Immunohistochemistry	Diffuse and intense S-100 protein positive	Variable S-100 protein staining	Variable S-100 protein staining
Association with VRD	Uncommon	Uncommon	Multiple or plexiform types are typical of the disease
Malignant transformation	Rare	Rare	More common ranging from 2%–15% of cases

VRD—von Recklinghausen's Disease

Histology

- Interlacing bundles of spindle-shaped cells.
- Nuclei are hyperchromatic, with a wavy or buckled appearance.
- The cells are associated with collagen strands and are separated by a myxomatous stroma that contains mast cells and lymphocytes.
- Cellularity can vary, including hypercellular tumors and hypocellular tumors with a prominent myxoid change.
- Immunohistochemistry: S-100 protein positive, but less striking as compared with benign schwannomas.

Differential Diagnosis

- Benign schwannoma (see above).
- Myxoma (Chapter 4A, #9).

Treatment and Prognosis

- Simple surgical excision is the treatment of choice and is curative.

Additional Facts

- Neurofibromas result from a diffuse increase in the endoneurial matrix, with proliferation and distortion of Schwann cells and axons resulting in an unencapsulated neoplasm.

c. Neurofibromatosis or von Recklinghausen's Disease

Definition: Autosomal dominant, neurocutaneous phakomatosis characterized by formation of multiple nerve sheath tumors or marked nerve sheath distortion (plexiform neurofibroma), and by changes affecting the skin, bones, joints, and central nervous system.

Clinical

- Affects men more than women; more than 40% of patients have the onset of disease before the first year of life; onset of disease is uncommon after 25 years of age.
- The syndrome may be expressed in four clinical types:
  1. Neurofibromatosis 1 (NF-1) or peripheral neurofibromatosis:
     Most common type; incidence is reported to be 1/4000 live births.
     Autosomal dominant; NF-1 gene localized to chromosome 17.
     Characterized by multiple cutaneous hyperpigmented areas (café au lait macules) and neurofibromas.
  2. Neurofibromatosis 2 (NF-2) or central neurofibromatosis:
     Autosomal dominant; NF-2 gene probably on chromosome 22.
     Primarily affects the central nervous system, as manifested by a varying combination of intracranial or intraspinal tumors, including neurofibroma, neurilemmoma (acoustic neuroma), meningioma, astrocytoma, and ependymoma.
  3. Visceral: multiple autonomic nervous system or visceral neural tumors.
  4. Forme fruste: incomplete development of the

syndrome (*café au lait* spots, plexiform neurofibroma, or nerve sheath tumor).

■ *Café au lait* spots are usually the first sign of disease, and the presence of six or more spots of more than 1.5 cm in size is presumptive evidence for diagnosis; patients who have less than six spots are at increased risk of developing the disease.

■ Involvement of the head and neck region is seen in up to 35% of the cases, primarily occurring as peripheral nerve sheath tumors involving the neck, cerebellopontine angle, oral cavity, larynx, and nasopharynx.

■ 50% of the patients have a family member affected by the syndrome; somatic mutation rate is among the highest for a dominantly inherited trait; degree of penetrance is high.

Plexiform Neurofibroma

■ Considered pathognomonic for the diagnosis of neurofibromatosis.

■ Involvement of major nerves, leading to the characteristic appearance termed "bag of worms."

■ Involvement of the entire extremity, termed "elephantiasis neuromatosa."

■ Involvement of the tongue, producing macroglossia.

Pathology

Gross

■ Ill-defined nodular growth or cylindrical enlargement of the involved nerve.

Histology

■ Increase in the endoneurial matrix, with separation of the nerve fascicles.

■ Proliferation of Schwann cells, with associated thick collagen fibers.

■ Perineurial thickening.

■ Hypercellularity, cellular pleomorphism, and mitoses may be seen; among these findings, the presence of increased mitotic activity is the essential factor, indicating malignant transformation.

Differential Diagnosis

■ Nerve sheath myxoma (see below).

Treatment and Prognosis

■ There are no treatment modalities that will alter the course of neurofibromatosis.

■ Surgery is indicated for:
Tumors located in areas where compromise of function or involvement of vital structures may occur.
Large tumors.
Painful tumors.
Tumors that have become malignant.

■ Complete surgical excision is problematic, given the infiltrative and ill-defined growth of the tumor.

■ The most serious complication is malignant transformation, which:
Is estimated to occur in 2% to 15% of cases.
Is usually seen in long-standing cases of neurofibromatosis.
Presents with a rapidly enlarging or painful (preexisting) neurofibroma.
Should always be biopsied.
Requires radical excision or amputation.
May benefit from radiotherapy.
Is associated with a poor prognosis with less than 20% 5-year survival rates.

Additional Facts

■ Diagnostic criteria for NF-1 include two or more of the following:
Six or more *café au lait* macules larger than 5 mm in prepubertal individuals and larger than 15 mm in postpubertal individuals.
Two or more neurofibromas of any type and one plexiform neurofibroma.
Freckling in the axillary or inguinal regions.
Optic gliomas.
Two or more Lisch nodules (optic hamartomas).
Distinctive osseous lesion (sphenoid dysplasia or thinning of long bone cortex).
First-degree relative (parent, sibling, offspring) with NF-1.

■ Diagnostic criteria for NF-2 include:
Bilateral VIIIth nerve masses seen by image analysis (CT, MRI).
First-degree relative with NF-2.
Either unilateral VIIIth nerve mass or two of the following: neurofibroma, meningioma, glioma, schwannoma, or juvenile posterior subcapsular lenticular opacity.

■ In addition to malignant transformation of a neurofibroma, other sarcomas may be associated with neurofibromatosis.

■ *Diffuse neurofibroma,* an uncommon form of neurofibroma, may be seen in neurofibromatosis; features of this tumor include:
Principally occurs in children and young adults.
Primarily occurs in the skin of the head and neck.
Presents as an ill-defined, plaque-like, subcutaneous mass.
Shares histologic features of conventional neurofibroma, but differs in that the Schwann cells are less elongated with fusiform or round contours, have a more uniform collagenous matrix, and have numerous Meissner bodies.
Rarely undergoes malignant transformation.
Infiltrates along connective tissue septa and envelops rather than destroys normal structures.
Is difficult to treat and has a tendency to recur.
Not pathognomonic of neurofibromatosis.

■ *Neurothekeoma:*

Benign nerve sheath myxoma.

Occurs primarily in children and young adults.

Predilection for the cutaneous (dermal and subcutaneous) sites of the head and neck.

Characterized histologically by a lobular growth, spindled, or rounded cells in a myxoid matrix and variable presence of S-100 protein immunoreactivity.

Treated by local excision.

References

Barnes L: Tumors and tumorlike lesions of peripheral nerves. *In*: Barnes L, ed. Surgical pathology of the head and neck. New York: Marcel Dekker, 1985; pp 660–671.

Enzinger FW, Weiss SW: Benign tumors of peripheral nerves. *In*: Enzinger FW, Weiss SW, eds. Soft tissue tumors, 2nd ed. St. Louis: C.V. Mosby, 1988; pp 719–780.

Neurofibromatosis: Conference statement. National Institutes of Health Concensus Development Conference. Arch Neurol 45:575–578, 1988.

Ross C, Wright E, Moseley J, Rees R: Massive schwannoma of the nose and paranasal sinuses. South Med J 81:1588–1591, 1988.

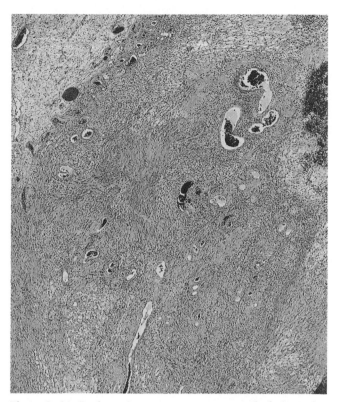

Figure 9–21. Benign schwannomas are composed of alternating regions that consist of compact spindle cells (Antoni A areas), and loose, hypocellular zones (Antoni B areas). Cells are arranged in short, interlacing fascicles with nuclear whorling, palisading, or alignment in rows (Verocay bodies). Increased vascularity is prominently seen, composed of large vessels with thickened (hyalinized) walls.

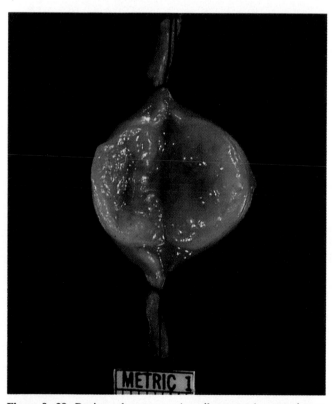

Figure 9–20. Benign schwannoma (neurilemmoma), appearing as an encapsulated, tan-white, solid to partly cystic mass attached to an identifiable nerve.

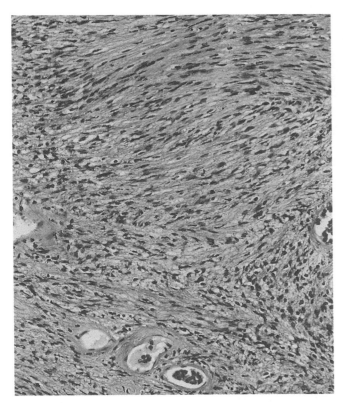

Figure 9–22. Cellular component of benign schwannoma, composed of vesicular to hyperchromatic nuclei with an elongated and twisted appearance and with indistinct cytoplasmic borders.

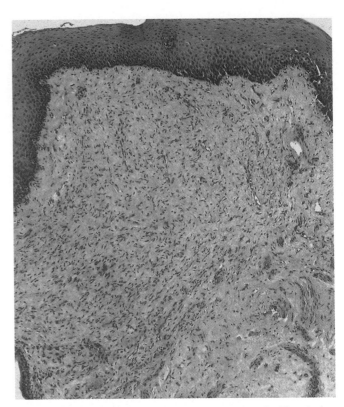

Figure 9–24. Neurofibroma, histologically composed of interlacing bundles and haphazardly arranged spindle-shaped cells.

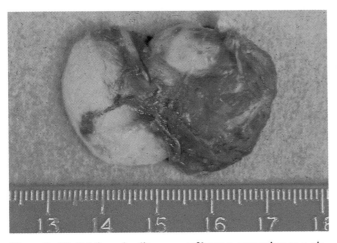

Figure 9–23. Sublingual solitary neurofibroma, appearing as a circumscribed but unencapsulated tan-white to gray mass.

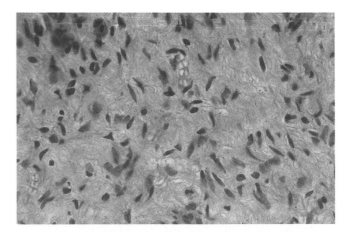

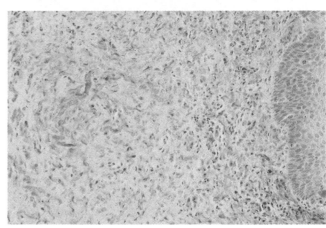

Figure 9–25. *(Top)* Nuclei are hyperchromatic, with a wavy or buckled appearance associated with collagen strands, and are separated by a myxomatous stroma. *(Bottom)* Immunohistochemistry shows diffuse S-100 protein reactivity.

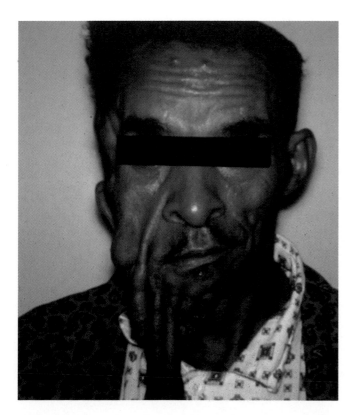

Figure 9–26. Clinical presentation of plexiform neurofibromas in this man with neurofibromatosis.

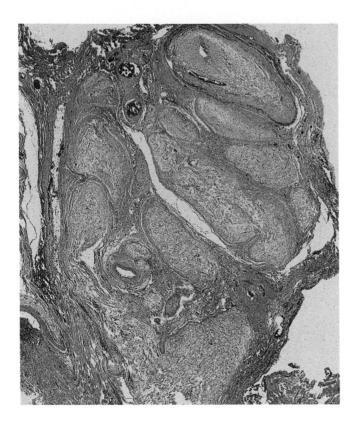

Figure 9–27. Histologic appearance of plexiform neurofibroma, showing an increase in the endoneurial matrix with separation of the nerve fascicles by mucinous-appearing material and proliferation of Schwann cells with associated thick collagen fibers and perineurial thickening.

B. MALIGNANT NEOPLASMS

1. Squamous Cell Carcinoma of the Oral Cavity and Tonsils

Clinical

■ Oral carcinomas represent approximately 4% of all malignant tumors occurring in humans.
■ Squamous cell carcinoma is the most common malignant tumor of the oral cavity, accounting for over 90% of the malignant neoplasms of this area.
■ Affects men more than women; age of onset of carcinoma is in the fifth to ninth decades of life and is unusual prior to 40 years of age.
■ The order of frequency of squamous cell carcinoma in the oral cavity is lower lip > tongue > floor of mouth > gingiva > palate > tonsil > upper lip > buccal mucosa > uvula.
■ Etiologic factors clearly linked to the development of oral squamous carcinoma include tobacco (smoking or chewing) or alcohol and sunlight (for carcinoma of the lip).
■ Other factors cited as potentially but not definitively linked to the development of oral carcinoma include syphilis, nutritional deficiency (Plummer-Vinson syndrome; cirrhosis), trauma and dental irritation, poor oral hygiene, and viruses (herpes virus, CMV).
■ The incidence of developing a second primary tumor in patients with oral carcinoma is increased four-fold; 50% to 75% of these second malignancies occur in the same or other upper aerodigestive tract sites, occur synchronously or metachronously, and probably are associated with the effects of tobacco and alcohol abuse.
■ Prognosis is influenced by a variety of factors, the most important being the clinical stage (TNM, classification, Chapter 10) of the neoplasm.
■ Because of the differences in the clinicopathologic and prognostic findings, site-specific oral squamous carcinoma is addressed separately.

I. SQUAMOUS CARCINOMA OF THE LIP

■ Accounts for over 40% of all oral carcinomas.
■ Over 90% of the squamous carcinomas affecting the lip occur on the lower lip.
■ Affects men more than women; most frequently identified in the fifth to eighth decades of life.
■ The most common site of occurrence on the lower lip is the vermillion border lateral to the midline.

- The most common clinical appearance is that of an ulcerated and indurated lesion.
- Conventional, well- to moderately differentiated squamous carcinoma accounts for the majority of the carcinomas; other histologic variants of squamous carcinoma, including spindle cell and adenoid squamous carcinoma, can occur.
- Complete surgical excision and radiotherapy are the treatments of choice.
- Carcinomas of the lower lip are slow growing but eventually spread to adjacent structures; metastases occur late in the disease course, involving the submandibular and submental lymph nodes first.
- Carcinomas of the upper lip metastasize to regional lymph nodes (periparotid) relatively early in the course of disease.
- Factors influencing prognosis include age of the patient, size and histologic grade of the tumor, and presence of metastatic disease.
- Overall 5-year survival rate is more than 75%.
- Etiology linked to sunlight and pipe smoking.

II. SQUAMOUS CARCINOMA OF THE TONGUE

- Accounts for approximately 25% of all oral carcinomas; excluding the lips, lingual carcinomas comprise more than 50% of all intraoral carcinomas.
- Affects men more than women; most frequently identified in the fifth to ninth decades of life.
- The most common site of occurrence is the lateral or ventral aspect of the anterior two thirds of the tongue (mobile portion).
- The most common clinical appearance is that of painless ulcerated or exophytic mass.
- Conventional well- to moderately differentiated squamous carcinoma accounts for the majority of the carcinomas; other histologic variants of squamous carcinoma, including spindle cell and adenoid squamous carcinoma, can occur.
- Complete surgical excision and radiotherapy are the treatments of choice.
- Metastases initially seed to the ipsilateral subdigastric lymph nodes, followed by the submaxillary region, and then to the mid-jugular chain.
- Overall 5-year survival is less than 30%.
- Factors influencing prognosis include size, location, sex, histologic grade of the tumor, and presence of metastases.
- Etiologic causes include tobacco and alcohol; syphilis, nutritional deficiency, trauma, dental irritation, and poor oral hygiene have been implicated.
- Carcinoma of the base of the tongue may be clinically silent, presenting as an (occult) metastatic carcinoma in a cervical lymph node.

III. SQUAMOUS CARCINOMA OF THE FLOOR OF THE MOUTH

- Accounts for approximately 20% of all oral carcinomas.

- Affects men more than women; most frequently identified in the sixth and seventh decades of life.
- The most common site of occurrence is along the anterior aspect of the floor of mouth rather than the posterior portion.
- The most common clinical appearance is that of ulcerated mass.
- Conventional well- to moderately differentiated squamous carcinoma is the most common histologic type.
- Complete surgical excision and radiotherapy are the treatments of choice.
- Irrespective of size, a large percentage of carcinomas of the floor of the mouth have spread to adjacent structures at the time of diagnosis.
- Metastases to regional lymph nodes occur to the submandibular triangle and upper jugular chain.
- Overall 5-year survival rates vary from 21% to 66%.
- Factors influencing prognosis include size of the tumor and the presence of metastases.
- Etiologic causes include tobacco and alcohol.

IV. SQUAMOUS CARCINOMA OF THE GINGIVA

- Accounts for approximately 6% of all oral carcinomas.
- Affects men more than women; most frequently identified in the sixth and seventh decades of life.
- The mandibular gingiva is more commonly affected than the maxillary gingiva, and the most common area of gingival carcinoma occurs posterior to the canine teeth; edentulous areas are more commonly affected than those areas in which teeth are present.
- Initial manifestations of cancer mimic common dental infections, delaying diagnosis; the most common clinical appearance is that of ulcerated or exophytic mass.
- As a result of the proximity of the periosteum and underlying bone, invasion of these structures occurs early in the course of disease.
- Conventional well- to moderately differentiated squamous carcinoma is the most common histologic type.
- Treatment of gingival carcinoma is by surgical excision or radiotherapy; segmental mandibulectomy is indicated for those carcinomas invading bone; radical neck dissection is performed in the face of overt neck disease and in conjunction with a segmental mandibulectomy.
- Metastases to submandibular and cervical lymph nodes occur commonly and in a high percentage of patients, especially with carcinomas of the mandibular gingiva.
- Overall 5-year survival rate is aprroximately 26%.
- Factors influencing prognosis include size and site of the tumor, presence of bone involvement, and presence of metastases.
- Etiologic causes include tobacco, alcohol, and poor oral hygiene.

V. Squamous Carcinoma of the Palate (Including Hard and Soft Palate, and the Uvula)

- Accounts for approximately 5% to 6% of all oral carcinomas; less than 1% involve the uvula.
- Although minor salivary gland malignant tumors occur frequently in this area, squamous cell carcinoma remains the most common malignancy affecting the palate.
- Affects men more than women; most frequently occurs in patients in the sixth decade of life and older.
- Palate squamous cell carcinomas are generally ulcerative tumors, but may be exophytic or papillary.
- Carcinomas of the hard palate may invade into bone early in the disease course, and occasionally invade into the nasal cavity; soft palate carcinomas may invade into the nasopharynx.
- Conventional, moderately differentiated squamous carcinoma is the most common histologic type.
- Treatment of palatal carcinoma includes wide surgical excision and radiotherapy; large soft palate carcinomas can be treated by radiotherapy alone.
- Some advocate not using radiotherapy for hard palate cancers because of the risk involved to the underlying bone (osteoradionecrosis) and because of the limited loss of function to this site after surgery.
- Radical neck dissection or radiotherapy is performed in the face of overt neck disease.
- Metastases occur most frequently to the subdigastric lymph nodes.
- Overall 5-year survival rate is approximately 35%.
- Factors influencing prognosis include size of the tumor, presence of metastases, age of the patient, and histologic grade of the tumor.
- Etiologic causes include tobacco and alcohol.

VI. Squamous Carcinoma of the Tonsil

- Accounts for approximately 5% of all oral carcinomas.
- Majority of tonsillar cancers arise from the tonsillar fossa or faucial pillars.
- Overwhelming majority of tonsillar cancers are epithelial tumors originating from the surface or crypt epithelium.
- Affects men more than women; most frequently occurs in the sixth to eighth decades of life; infrequently (less than 3%) occurs in younger individuals, in whom the prognosis is decidedly worse.
- Tonsillar squamous cell carcinomas are generally large, indurated, fungating, or ulcerative tumors.
- Tonsillar carcinomas may spread to adjacent structures, including the base of the tongue, soft palate, retromolar trigone, or the pharyngeal wall.
- Conventional, moderately differentiated keratinizing squamous carcinoma is the most common histologic type; other histologic types include nonkeratinizing or transitional carcinoma and undifferentiated carcinoma.

- Treatment of tonsillar carcinoma includes surgical excision and radiotherapy.
- Metastases occur most frequently to the subdigastric lymph nodes, are seen in a large percentage of patients at the time of diagnosis and correlate to the histology of the tumor.
- Overall 5-year survival rates vary and have been reported to be as low as 12% and as high as 48%.
- Factors influencing prognosis include size of the tumor, presence of metastases, age of the patient, and histologic grade of the tumor.
- Etiologic causes, as compared with other oral cancers, have not been clearly delineated.
- Similar to the carcinoma of the base of the tongue, tonsillar carcinomas may be clinically silent, initially presenting as an (occult) metastatic carcinoma in a cervical lymph node.

VII. Squamous Carcinoma of the Buccal Mucosa

- Accounts for approximately 2% of all oral carcinomas.
- Majority of buccal mucosal carcinomas arise inferior to or along a line opposite the plane of occlusion.
- Affects men more than women; most frequently occurs in the sixth to eighth decades of life.
- Buccal mucosal carcinomas are generally painful and appear as ulcerated, exophytic, or verrucoid tumors.
- Buccal mucosal carcinomas often present with tumor invasion into the cheek; spread to other adjacent structures, including the jaws (upper and lower), mandibular ramus mucosa, lips, pharynx, tonsil, palate, retromolar trigone, and, in advanced disease, to the mandible and maxilla.
- Conventional, moderately differentiated keratinizing squamous carcinoma is the most common histologic type; verrucous carcinoma also involves the buccal mucosa.
- Treatment of buccal mucosal carcinoma includes surgical excision and radiotherapy.
- Metastases occur most frequently to the submaxillary lymph nodes and are seen in a large percentage of patients.
- Overall 5-year survival rates vary and have been reported to be as low as 16% and as high as 89%.
- Factors influencing prognosis include location of the tumor and the presence of metastases.
- Etiologic causes include tobacco smoking or chewing, snuff dipping, and alcohol.

References

Krutchkoff DJ, Chen J, Katz RV: Oral cancer: a survey of 566 cases from the University of Connecticut oral pathology biopsy service, 1975–1986. Oral Surg Oral Med Oral Pathol 70:192–198, 1990.

Verbin RS, Bouquot JE, Guggenheimer J, Barnes L, Peel RL: Cancer of the oral cavity and oropharynx. In: Barnes L, ed. Surgical pathology of the head and neck. New York: Marcel Dekker, 1985; pp 330–401.

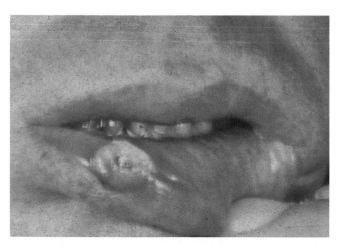

Figure 9–28. Squamous cell carcinoma of the lower lip presenting as a delineated, oval, tan-white indurated lesion.

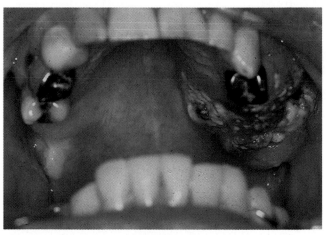

Figure 9–31. Squamous cell carcinoma of the alveolar ridge presenting as a large, infiltrative mass.

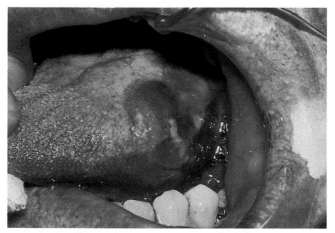

Figure 9–29. Squamous cell carcinoma of the lateral aspect of the left side of the tongue presenting as an ill-defined, ulcerated and indurated lesion.

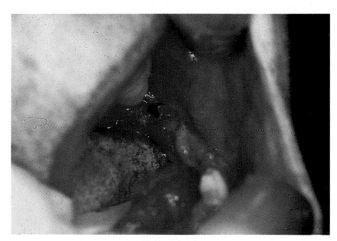

Figure 9–32. Squamous cell carcinoma of the retromolar trigone presenting as a semilunar-appearing white lesion.

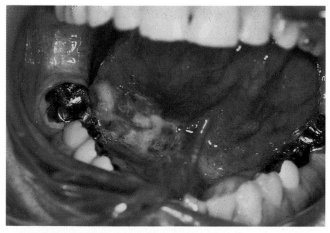

Figure 9–30. Squamous cell carcinoma of the floor of the mouth presenting as an ill-defined, tan-white indurated lesion.

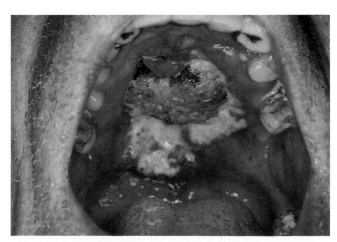

Figure 9–33. Squamous cell carcinoma of the hard palate with involvement of the uvula.

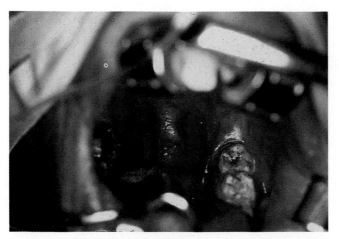

Figure 9–34. Squamous cell carcinoma of the tonsil presenting with enlargement of the tonsil, which has an erythroplakic appearance.

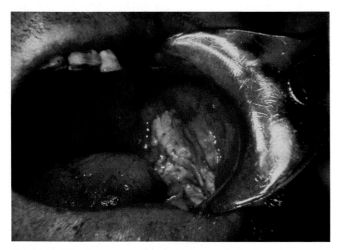

Figure 9–35. Squamous cell carcinoma of the buccal mucosa presenting as an exophytic, tan-white indurated mass.

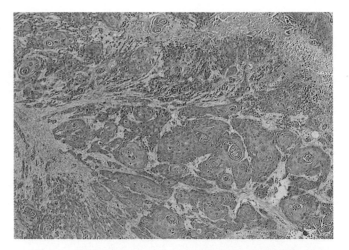

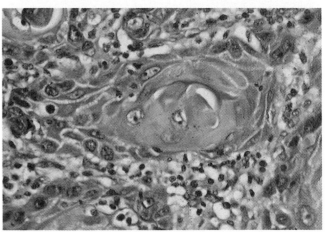

Figure 9–36. *(Top)* Infiltrating keratinizing well-differentiated squamous cell carcinoma of the tongue. *(Bottom)* Designation as a well-differentiated neoplasm is based on attempts of the invasive neoplasm to recapitulate the appearance of the surface epithelium with keratinization and the presence of intercellular bridges (thin parallel lines lying within the clear spaces between cells); mild cellular pleomorphism is seen.

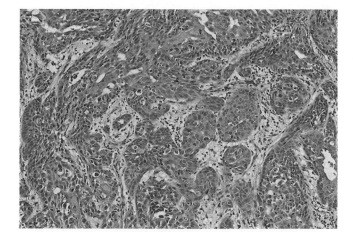

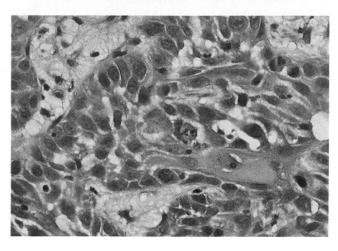

Figure 9-37. *(Top)* Infiltrating, moderately differentiated squamous cell carcinoma of the tongue in contrast to the well-differentiated neoplasm demonstrates only some features of the surface from which it derives; with focal keratinization and with a greater degree of cellular pleomorphism and increased mitotic activity. *(Bottom)* Individual cell keratinization and intercellular bridges represent remnants of squamous epithelial cell derivation in this moderately differentiated squamous cell carcinoma, which is characterized by enlarged nuclei with prominent nucleoli and mitoses.

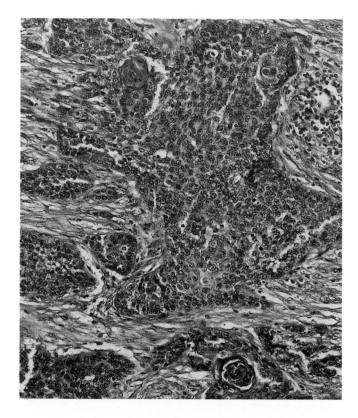

Figure 9-38. Infiltrating, poorly differentiated squamous cell carcinoma of the tongue. In comparison with its better differentiated counterparts, this tumor demonstrates the least similarities to the epithelium from which it derives, as seen by limited foci of keratinization and absence of intercellular bridges; this cohesive cellular infiltrate is characterized by cellular pleomorphism, enlarged nuclei, indistinct cytoplasm, and numerous mitotic figures.

2. Nasopharyngeal Carcinoma (Table 9–2)

Definition: Squamous cell carcinoma arising from the surface epithelium and subtyped according to the World Health Organization (WHO) into three histologic variants: keratinizing, nonkeratinizing, and undifferentiated carcinoma.

Synonyms: Rigaud and Schmincke types of lympho-epithelioma; lymphoepithelioma; transitional carcinoma.

Clinical

- Overall, nasopharyngeal carcinoma is an uncommon neoplasm in the United States, accounting for approximately 0.25% of all cancers; in China, it accounts for 18% of all cancers.
- Affects men more than women; occurs over a wide age range, but is most common in the sixth decade of life.
- Irrespective of the histologic type, the clinical presentation is similar and includes neck mass, hearing loss, nasal obstruction, nasal discharge, epistaxis, pain, otalgia, and headache.
- The signs and symptoms are often subtle and nonspecific, leading to delay in diagnosis and eventual presentation with advanced disease.
- The lateral wall of the nasopharynx (fossa of Rosenmüller) is the most common site of occurrence.
- Suggested etiologic factors include:
  Genetic and geographic: increased incidence in China, especially in southern (Kwantung province) and northern provinces and Taiwan; although the incidence among Chinese people decreases after emigration to low-incidence areas, it still remains higher than in non-Chinese populations; HLA-A2 histocompatibility locus has been suggested as the marker for genetic susceptibility to nasopharyngeal carcinoma.
  Epstein-Barr virus (EBV): elevated titers of anti-EBV antibodies are associated with nasopharyngeal carcinoma (undifferentiated and non-keratinizing types); however, no clear cause and effect has been established between the presence of EBV and the developement of nasopharyngeal carcinoma.
  Other suggested implicating factors are diet, poor hygiene, and environmental.

Radiology

- Plain film radiograph findings are variable and nonspecific, including a soft tissue mass, bone destruction, and sinus opacity.
- CT may demonstrate bone invasion, including invasion of the base of skull and expansion of sinuses, with progression of disease.

Pathology

Gross

- The appearance of nasopharyngeal carcinoma varies from:
  A mucosal bulge with an overlying intact epithelium.
  Clearly demonstrable mass with extensive involvement of the surface epithelium.
  Totally unidentifiable lesion fortuitously sampled and identified by microscopic evaluation.

Histology

Three histologic types are identified, based on the predominant appearance:

1. Keratinizing:
   - Represents approximately 25% of all cases.
   - Conventional squamous carcinoma with keratinization and intercellular bridges; graded as well, moderately or poorly differentiated.
   - Invasion results in a desmoplastic response.
2. Nonkeratinizing:
   - Least common, representing less than 15% of cases.
   - Little to absent keratinization; growth pattern is

Table 9–2
NASOPHARYNGEAL CARCINOMA

	Keratinizing	Nonkeratinizing	Undifferentiated
Percent of cases	Approximately 25%	Least common <15%	Most common >60%
Sex/age	♂ > ♀; >6th decade	♂ > ♀; >6th decade	♂ > ♀; >6th decade
Histology	Keratinization, intercellular bridges; conventional squamous carcinoma graded as well, moderately or poorly differentiated; desmoplastic response to invasion	Little to absent keratinization, growth pattern similar to transitional carcinoma of the bladder; typically, absence of desmoplastic response to invasion	Absence of keratinization, syncytial growth, cohesive or noncohesive cells with round nuclei, prominent eosinophilic nucleoli, scant cytoplasm and mitoses; prominent non-neoplastic lymphoid component; typically, absence of desmoplastic response to invasion
Presence of EBV	Weak association	Strong association	Strong association
Treatment	Radioresponsiveness is not good	Variably radioresponsive	Radiosensitive
Prognosis	10%–20% 5-year survival	35%–50% 5-year survival	60% 5-year survival

similar to transitional carcinoma of the bladder, with stratification of the epithelium composed of cylindrical and spindle-shaped cells.
- Typically, invasion does not create a desmoplastic response.
- Immunohistochemistry: cytokeratin positive; leukocyte common antigen (LCA) negative.

3. Undifferentiated:
- Most common type, accounting for more than 60% of cases.
- Absence of keratinization.
- Noted for the syncytial growth pattern composed of cohesive or noncohesive cells with oval or round vesicular nuclei, prominent eosinophilic nucleoli, scant cytoplasm, indistinct cell margins, and increased mitoses.
- A prominent non-neoplastic lymphoid component is seen, leading to the misnomer lymphoepithelioma.
- Absent desmoplastic response to invasion.
- Immunohistochemistry: cytokeratin positive; LCA negative.

Differential Diagnosis

- Non-Hodgkin's malignant lymphoma (large cell or immunoblastic) (Chapter 9B, #4).
- Rhabdomyosarcoma (Chapter 9B, #5).

Treatment and Prognosis

- As a result of the anatomic constraints imposed by the nasopharynx and the tendency of these neoplasms to present in an advanced stage, supervoltage radiotherapy (6500 to 7000 rads or more) is considered the treatment of choice.
- Responsiveness to radiation varies per histologic type and thereby impacts on prognosis:
  1. Keratinizing:
     Not radioresponsive.
     These tumors have a tendency to remain localized without (nodal) dissemination.
     5-year survival rate is in the range of 10% to 20%.
  2. Nonkeratinizing:
     Variably radioresponsive.
     These tumors have a tendency to metastasize to regional lymph nodes.
     5-year survival rate is in the range of 35% to 50%.
  3. Undifferentiated:
     Radiosensitive.
     These tumors have a tendency to metastasize to regional lymph nodes.
     5-year survival rate of approximately 60%.
- Factors that may affect prognosis include:
  Clinical stage.
  Patient's age (the younger the age, the better the prognosis).
  Lymph node metastasis (positive nodes decrease survival by approximately 10% to 20%).

Additional Facts

- Nasopharyngeal carcinoma, by definition, takes origin from the surface and crypt epithelium; therefore, the use of this term is to the exclusion of all other malignant tumors that may arise in this region (minor salivary gland tumors, sarcomas, lymphomas).
- Nasopharyngeal carcinoma occurring in younger patients is predominantly of the undifferentiated type.
- The sole utility for chemotherapy is for widespread disease.
- The Rigaud and Schmincke types of nasopharyngeal carcinoma refer to those neoplasms with syncytial versus individual cell invasive growth patterns, respectively; these designations and their correlated growth have no bearing on the biology of the disease.
- An in situ component is rarely seen.

References

Batsakis JG, Solomon AR, Rice DH: The pathology of head and neck tumors: carcinoma of the nasopharynx, part II. Head Neck Surg 3:511–524, 1981.

Carbone A, Micheau C: Pitfalls in microscopic diagnosis of undifferentiated carcinoma of nasopharyngeal type (lymphoepithelioma). Cancer 50:1344–1351, 1982.

Gaffey MJ, Weiss LM: Viral oncogenesis: Epstein-Barr virus. Am J Otolaryngol 11:375–381, 1990.

Hyams VJ, Batsakis JG, Michaels L: Squamous cell carcinoma of the nasopharynx mucosa. In: Hyams VJ, Batsakis JG, Michaels L, eds. Tumors of the upper respiratory tract and ear. Fascicle 25, second series. Washington, D.C.: Armed Forces Institute of Pathology, 1986; pp 62–66.

Madri JA, Barwick KW: An immunohistochemical study of nasopharngeal neoplasms using keratin antibodies: epithelial versus nonepithelial neoplasms. Am J Surg Pathol 6:143–149, 1982.

Shanmugaratnam K, Chan SH, de-The G, Goh JEH, Khor TH, Simons MJ, Tye CY: Histopathology of nasopharyngeal carcinoma: correlations with epidemiology, survival rates, and other biological characteristics. Cancer 44:1029–1044, 1979.

Skinner DW, Van Hasselt CA, Tsao SY: Nasopharyngeal carcinoma: modes of presentation. Ann Otol Rhinol Laryngol 100:544–551, 1991.

Weiland LH: Nasopharyngeal carcinoma. In: Barnes L, ed. Surgical pathology of the head and neck. New York: Marcel Dekker, 1985; pp 453–466.

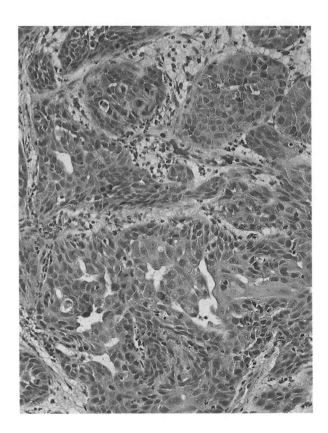

Figure 9–39. Nasopharyngeal keratinization moderately well differentiated squamous carcinoma; invasion by this type of nasopharyngeal carcinoma results in a desmoplastic stromal response.

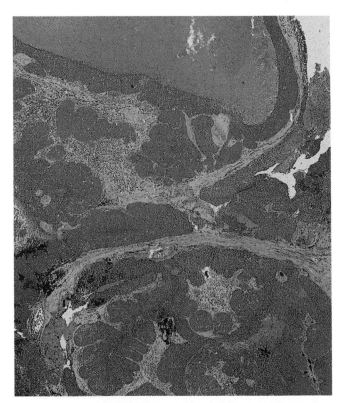

Figure 9–40. Nasopharyngeal, nonkeratinizing squamous carcinoma with little to absent keratinization and cystic degeneration filled with necrotic material. This pattern may be seen in a cervical lymph node, representing metastatic foci from a nasopharyngeal primary neoplasm.

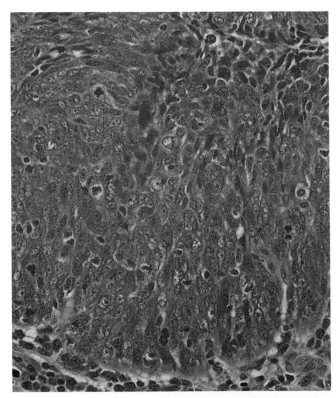

Figure 9–41. The growth pattern in the nonkeratinizing squamous carcinoma is similar to transitional carcinoma of the bladder, with stratification of the epithelium composed of cylindrical and spindle-shaped cells, pleomorphism, loss of cell polarity, and many mitoses.

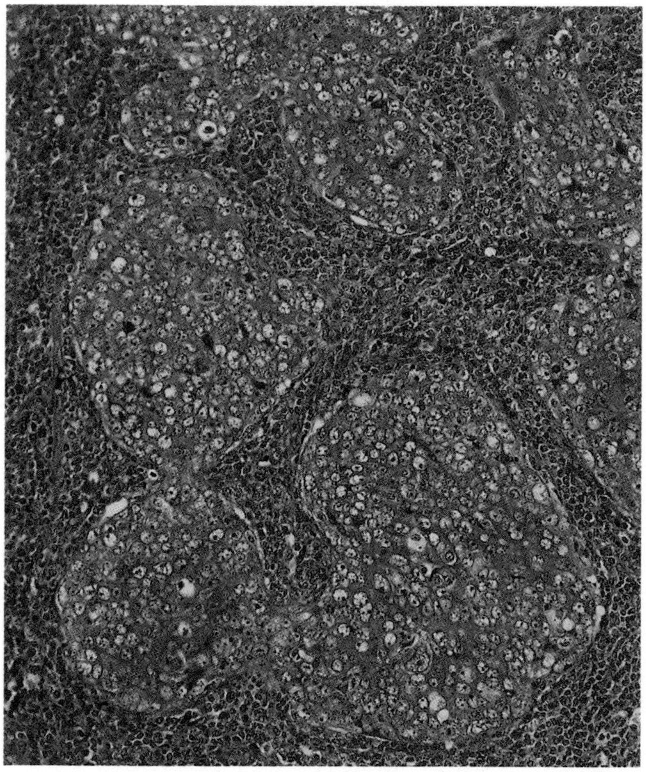

Figure 9–42. Undifferentiated nasopharyngeal carcinoma with a nested growth composed of cells with oval or round vesicular nuclei, prominent eosinophilic nucleoli, scant cytoplasm, indistinct cell margins, and increased mitoses; a prominent non-neoplastic lymphoid component is seen.

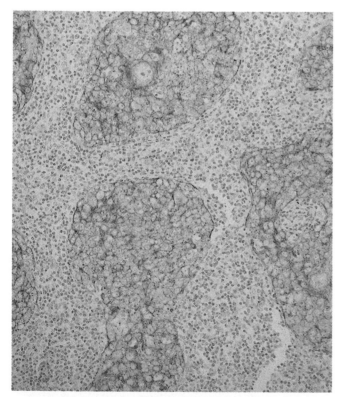

Figure 9–43. Nasopharyngeal undifferentiated carcinoma cells are cytokeratin positive by immunohistochemistry evaluation.

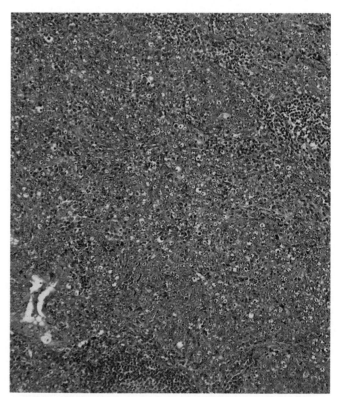

Figure 9–44. Another pattern of the undifferentiated nasopharyngeal carcinoma includes a diffuse, noncohesive cellular proliferation.

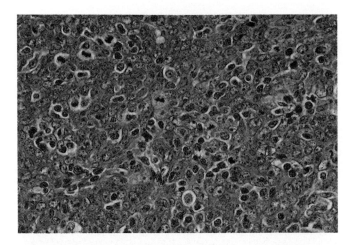

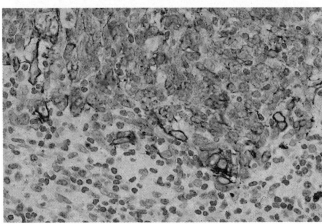

Figure 9–45. *(Top)* Cytologic appearance in this diffuse pattern is similar to that previously described (Fig. 9–42). *(Bottom)* Cytokeratin immunoreactivity confirms the diagnosis of carcinoma and differentiates it from some non-Hodgkin's malignant lymphomas, representing the major differential diagnosis, which share both the diffuse pattern of growth and cytologic appearance seen in nasopharyngeal undifferentiated carcinoma.

3. Low-grade Nasopharyngeal Papillary Adenocarcinoma

Definition: Surface epithelial-derived malignant tumor with adenocarcinomatous differentiation and an indolent biologic behavior.

Clinical

- Uncommon tumor of the nasopharynx.
- No sex predilection; occurs over a wide age range, from the second to seventh decades of life (median, 37 years).
- May occur anywhere in the nasopharynx (posterior wall is often involved).
- The most common symptom is nasal obstruction; other symptoms include otitis media with or without associated hearing deficits and postnasal drip.
- Not associated with any definitive etiologic factors.

Pathology

Gross

- Exophytic, soft to gritty mass, with a papillary, nodular, and cauliflower-like appearance, varying in size from a few millimeters to 3.0 cm.

Histology

- Surface epithelial derivation is identified by transition areas from normal nasopharyngeal surface epithelium to neoplastic proliferation.
- The tumor is unencapsulated, infiltrates the stroma, and is composed of papillary and glandular growth pattern.
- Papillary structures are complex, with arborization and hyalinized fibrovascular cores.
- Complex glandular pattern, characterized by back-to-back and cribriform growth.
- Cells vary in appearance from pseudostratified columnar to cuboidal.
- Nuclei are round to oval with vesicular/optically clear-appearing chromatin pattern; cytoplasm is eosinophilic.
- Nuclear pleomorphism and loss of basal polarity are seen; mitoses and prominent nucleoli are not commonly identified.
- Psammoma bodies and necrosis can be identified.
- Histochemical stains: epithelial mucin is identified —diastase-resistant, PAS-positive (intracytoplasmic), and mucicarmine (intracytoplasmic and luminal).
- Immunohistochemistry: diffusely positive reactivity

with cytokeratin and epithelial membrane antigen (EMA); focal reactivity with carcinoembryonic antigen (CEA); no immunoreactivity with S-100 protein, glial fibrillary acidic protein (GFAP), or thyroglobulin.

Differential Diagnosis

■ Papilloma (surface epithelial or minor salivary gland origin) (Chapter 9, #1; Chapter 19A, #3).
■ Minor salivary gland neoplasms: mucoepidermoid carcinoma (Chapter 19B, #1), acinic cell carcinoma (Chapter 19B, #2), polymorphous low-grade adenocarcinoma (Chapter 19B, #6).
■ Papillary carcinoma of thyroid gland origin.

Treatment and Prognosis

■ Complete surgical excision via a transpalatal approach is the treatment of choice and is curative.
■ Radiotherapy (pre- and postoperative) does not appear to be warranted.
■ Slow-growing tumor with the potential to recur if incompletely excised; metastatic disease does not occur.

Additional Facts

■ Both the light microscopic findings and the immunohistochemical profile support derivation of this neoplasm from the surface epithelium, rather than from the subjacent minor salivary glands.
■ Because of the histologic similarities, thyroglobulin immunohistochemistry must be performed in order to differentiate the nasopharyngeal papillary adenocarcinoma from metastatic papillary carcinoma of the thyroid.

References

Wenig BM, Hyams VJ, Heffner DH: Nasopharyngeal papillary adenocarcinoma: a clinicopathologic study of a low-grade carcinoma. Am J Surg Pathol 12:946–953, 1988.

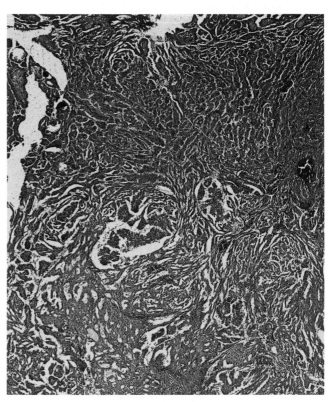

Figure 9–46. Low-grade nasopharyngeal papillary adenocarcinoma (LGNPPA) showing an infiltrating tumor with complex glandular and papillary growth; psammoma bodies can be seen toward the left upper portion of the illustration.

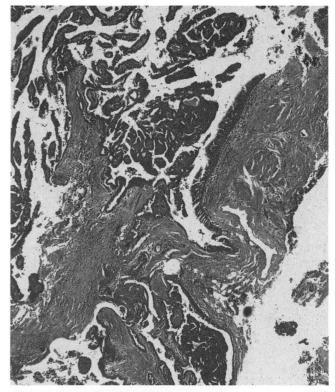

Figure 9–47. LGNPPA arises from the nasopharyngeal surface epithelium, as seen by the transition from normal nasopharyngeal surface epithelium to the neoplastic proliferation.

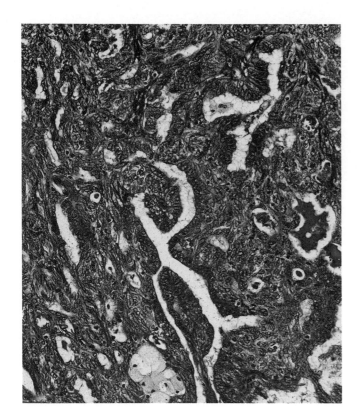

Figure 9–48. The tumor is composed of a complex papillary and glandular growth pattern that consists of pseudostratified columnar to cuboidal cells with round to oval, focally overlapping nuclei with vesicular to optically clear-appearing chromatin pattern and an eosinophilic cytoplasm. The growth pattern, overlapping nuclei, and chromatin pattern are similar to papillary carcinoma of the thyroid, from which LGNPPA must be differentiated. This is accomplished by staining for thyroglobulin, which is not identified in LGNPPA.

4. Malignant Lymphoproliferative Neoplasms

Definition: Primary malignant neoplasms of the lymphoreticular or the immune system.

Nomenclature

■ Malignant lymphomas are generally divided into two major categories: non-Hodgkin's and Hodgkin's lymphomas.

■ Within each category, individual neoplasms are classified according to their morphology, including the pattern of growth and the predominant cytologic appearance; the non-Hodgkin's lymphomas are categorized into low-, intermediate, and high-grades, based on growth and cell type (Table 9–3).

■ The vast array of clinical and pathologic features of the malignant lymphoproliferative diseases are beyond the scope of this text; the approach is to describe the malignant lymphomas of specific extranodal anatomic sites in the head and neck, with examples of specific individual types of lymphoma.

■ The mucosa-associated lymphoid tissue (MALT) has been implicated as giving rise to a variety of extranodal malignant lymphomas; included in this category are head and neck sites (nasopharyngeal, tonsil, salivary glands, and others).

Table 9–3

CLASSIFICTION OF NON-HODGKIN'S MALIGNANT LYMPHOMAS AND HODGKIN'S LYMPHOMAS (Working Formulation)

Non-Hodgkin's lymphomas

Low-grade
Malignant lymphoma, small lymphocytic
Malignant lymphoma, follicular, predominantly small cleaved cell
Malignant lymphoma, follicular, mixed small cleaved and large cell

Intermediate-grade
Malignant lymphoma, follicular, predominantly large cell
Malignant lymphoma, diffuse, small cleaved cell
Malignant lymphoma, diffuse, mixed small cleaved and large cell
Malignant lymphoma, diffuse, large cell

High-grade
Malignant lymphoma, large cell, immunoblastic
Malignant lymphoma, lymphoblastic
Malignant lymphoma, small noncleaved cell (Burkitt's and non-Burkitt's)

Others
Including extramedullary plasmacytoma

Hodgkin's lymphomas
1. Nodular sclerosing
2. Lymphocyte predominant
3. Lymphocyte depleted
4. Mixed cellularity

- MALT lymphomas share clinical, histologic, and immunohistochemical features, including:
  The tendency to remain localized, evolve slowly, and be of B-cell phenotype.
  Salivary gland malignant lymphomas are rare and predominantly arise de novo, but rarely may arise from benign lymphoepithelial lesions.
- AIDS patients may develop malignant lymphomas originating in head and neck sites or involving this region as part of a systemic process.
- Extranodal primary Hodgkin's disease occurring in the head and neck is exceedingly rare and will not be discussed; in general, involvement of head and neck by Hodgkin's disease is predominantly in association with nodal-based disease.

a. Non-Hodgkin's Malignant Lymphoma of Waldeyer's Tonsillar Ring (Nasopharynx, Tonsils, and Base of Tongue)

- Accounts for approximately 50% of all extranodal lymphomas in the head and neck.
- Affects men more than women; can occur at any age, but is most common in the fifth to seventh decades.
- The most common sites of occurrence, in order of frequency, are: tonsils > nasopharynx > base of tongue.
- The most common symptoms include nasal obstruction, otalgia, decreased hearing, pain, and sore throat.
- A large submucosal mass with or without surface ulceration may be seen; in the majority of cases, involvement is unilateral.
- Although any pattern and cell type can be seen, the most common histologic pattern is diffuse with large cell or immunoblastic cytologic features.
- The large cell and immunoblastic lymphomas can be difficult to differentiate from a nasopharyngeal (undifferentiated) carcinoma, and diagnosis depends on immunohistochemical analysis:
  Lymphoma: LCA positive and cytokeratin negative.

Undifferentiated carcinoma: LCA negative and cytokeratin positive.
- Waldeyer's ring lymphomas are predominantly but not exclusively follicular center cell-derived, expressed by positive reactivity with B-cell markers (L-26) and negative reactivity with T-cell markers (UCHL).
- Treatment and prognosis are based on the clinical stage (Table 9–4).

b. Burkitt's Lymphoma

Definition: High-grade non-Hodgkin's malignant lymphoma with distinct clinical, pathologic, and epidemiologic features; according to the Working Formulation, this lymphoma is classified as malignant lymphoma, diffuse, small noncleaved cell, Burkitt's type, high-grade.

Clinical

Two forms are recognized:

I. ENDEMIC OR AFRICAN TYPE

- Affects males more than females; most common in the first decade of life.
- Presents most frequently with extranodal tumor in the jaw, kidneys, ovaries, retroperitoneum, orbit, and meninges.
- Associated with Epstein-Barr virus (approximately 90% of cases have elevated EBV titers and EBV DNA genome).

II. NONENDEMIC OR AMERICAN TYPE

- Affects males more than females; most common in the second decade of life.
- Presents most frequently with intraabdominal tumors in GIT-associated lymphoid tissue; other sites of involvement include the ovary, nasopharynx, retroperitoneum, kidney, peripheral lymph nodes, and bone marrow.
- Evidence of EBV infection is seen in less than 30% of cases.

Table 9–4
CLINICAL STAGING, TREATMENT AND PROGNOSIS OF MALIGNANT LYMPHOMA

Stage	Definition	Treatment	Prognosis (5-year survival)
I	Single lymph node region or single extralymphatic organ or site	Radiotherapy (4500–5000 rads)	50%
II	Two or more lymph node regions or involvement of an extralymphatic site and > one lymph node region on the same side of the diaphragm	Radiotherapy (4500–5000 rads)	25%
III	Lymph node involvement on both sides of the diaphragm with or without splenic and extralymphatic organ involvement	Total lymphoid radiation; chemotherapy if the spleen is involved	17%
IV	Diffuse or disseminated involvement of one or more extralymphatic organs with or without lymph node involvement	Chemotherapy	Poor

Pathology

Gross

■ Homogeneous appearing yellow to tan-white, rubbery to firm mass.

Histology (the histologic features of endemic and nonendemic Burkitt's lymphoma are the same):

■ Diffuse growth pattern characterized by the presence of many macrophages containing phagocytized and cellular debris admixed with a small cell infiltrate and termed "starry-sky" appearance.
■ Neoplastic cells are uniform and small (equal in size to the macrophages) with noncleaved round nuclei, 2 to 5 prominent nucleoli, and a small amount of amphophilic cytoplasm.
■ Cytoplasmic pyroninophilia is seen with methyl green-pyronine stain.
■ Immunohistochemistry: LCA positive with B-cell lymphocyte markers.

Differential Diagnosis

■ Lymphoblastic lymphoma and other lymphomas.
■ Extramedullary plasmacytoma (see below).
■ Rhabdomyosarcoma (Chapter 9B, #5).
■ Neuroblastoma (Chapter 4B, #5).

Treatment and Prognosis (essentially the same for endemic and nonendemic types).

■ Chemotherapy is the treatment of choice and often results in rapid response with marked decrease in the tumor size.
■ Complete response rate can be seen in more than 95% of cases.
■ Relapse rates occur in approximately 60% of cases.
■ 2-year survival is approximately 50%.
■ Burkitt's lymphoma is a rapidly proliferating tumor, requiring immediate diagnosis and treatment.
■ Two clinical staging classifications are used (Table 9–5).
■ Prognosis correlates with the clinical stage, age of the patient, and association with titers for EBV viral capsid antigen, such that better prognosis is seen with:
Lower stage tumors associated with less tumor burden.
Younger patients.
High titers to EBV viral capsid antigen in patients with nonendemic Burkitt's lymphoma (more than 1:160).
■ Distinctive chromosomal translocations involving 14,22,2 (immunoglobulin loci) and 8(c-myc locus).
■ Extramedullary plasmacytoma:
80% occur in the head and neck, primarily in the upper aerodigestive tract (nasal cavity, nasopharynx, paranasal sinuses, and oral cavity).
Affects men more than women; occurs over a wide

Table 9–5
CLINICAL STAGING OF BURKITT'S LYMPHOMA

Stage	Levine et al (I–IV)	Ziegler et al (A–D)
I vs A	Single tumor mass IA = extraabdominal IB = abdominal	Single extraabdominal site
II vs B	Two separate tumor masses above or below the diaphragm	Multiple extraabdominal sites
III vs C	>Two separate masses or diseases above and below the diaphragm	Intraabdominal tumor; AR = Stage C with over 90% of the tumor surgically resected
IV vs D	CNS or bone marrow involvement, pleural effusion or ascites	Intraabdominal tumor with multiple extraabdominal sites

age range, but the vast majority of patients are over 40 years of age.
Histopathology characterized by the presence of sheets of plasma cells, varying from mature to immature; a paranuclear clear area or halo ("hof") representing the Golgi apparatus is a characteristic finding but may not be seen in less well-differentiated tumors.
Cells are methyl green-pyronine positive and monoclonal immunoglobulins are identified by immunohistochemistry; amyloid can be seen in a small percentage of cases.
80% are primary (solitary), without neoplastic foci elsewhere; 20% are part of the generalized picture, associated with multiple myeloma.
Treatment depends on the extent of disease and may include radiotherapy alone or, for large tumors, local resection followed by radiotherapy.
5-year survival ranges from 30% to 75%; up to 50% eventually disseminate into multiple myeloma, usually within 2 years; median survival after dissemination is less than 2 years.

References

Malignant Lymphomas of Waldeyer's Tonsillar Ring

Isaacson PG, Spencer J: Malignant lymphoma of mucosa-associated lymphoid tissue. Histopathology 11:445–462, 1987.
Kapadia SB: Malignant lymphoma of Waldeyer's ring. In: Barnes L, ed. Surgical pathology of the head and neck. New York: Marcel Dekker, 1985; pp 1090–1093.
Kaplan LD, McGrath MS: AIDS-associated non-Hodgkin's lymphoma. AIDS Update 4:1–11, 1991.
Rosenberg SA, Berard CW, Brown BW, et al: National cancer institute sponsored study of classifications of non-Hodgkin's lymphomas: summary and description of a working formulation for clinical usage. Cancer 49:2112–2135, 1982.
Saul SH, Kapadia SB: Primary lymphoma of Waldeyer's ring: clinicopathologic study of 68 cases. Cancer 56:157–166, 1985.
Sciubba JJ, Auclair PL, Ellis GL: Malignant lymphomas. In: Ellis GL, Auclair PL, Gnepp DR, eds. Surgical pathology of salivary glands. Philadelphia: W.B. Saunders Co., 1991; pp 528–543.

Burkitt's Lymphoma

Gaffey MJ, Weiss LM: Viral oncogenesis: Epstein-Barr virus. Am J Otolaryngol 11:375–381, 1990.

Haluska FG, Finger LR, Kagan J, Croce CM: Molecular genetics of chromosomal translocations in B- and T-lymphoid malignancies. *In:* Cossman J, ed. Molecular genetics in cancer diagnosis. New York: Elsevier, 1990; pp 143–162.

Kapadia SB: Extramedullary plasmacytoma. *In:* Barnes L, ed. Surgical pathology of the head and neck. New York: Marcel Dekker, 1985; pp 1140–1149.

Levine AM, Kamaraju LS, Connelly RR, Berard CW, Dorfman RF, Magrath I, Easton JM: The American Burkitt's lymphoma registry: eight years' experience. Cancer 49:1016–1022, 1982.

Levine AM, Pavlova Z, Pockros AW, Teitelbaum AH, Paganini-Hill A, Powars DR, Lukes RJ, Feinstein DI: Small cell non-cleaved follicular center cell (FCC) lymphoma: Burkitt and non-Burkitt variants in the United States. Cancer 52:1073–1079, 1983.

Patton LL, McMillian CW, Webster WP: American Burkitt's lymphoma: a 10-year review and case study. Oral Surg Oral Med Oral Pathol 69:307–316, 1990.

Ziegler JL: Burkitt's lymphoma. N Engl J Med 297:735–745, 1981.

Figure 9–50. Tonsillar biopsy specimen, showing a diffuse cellular infiltrate with areas of necrosis.

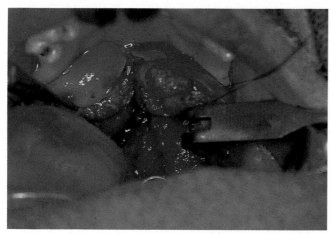

Figure 9–49. Non-Hodgkin's malignant lymphoma of the palate and tonsils, appearing as a diffuse, bilateral, fleshy-appearing tumor mass.

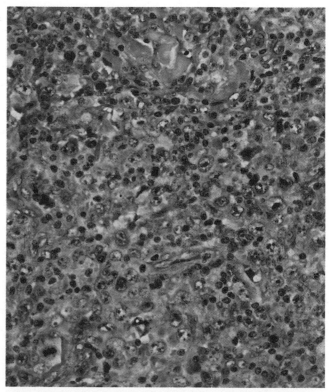

Figure 9–51. Higher power shows the features of an immunoblastic lymphoma composed of a discohesive population of large cells with one or more prominent eosinophilic nucleoli and multiple mitotic figures.

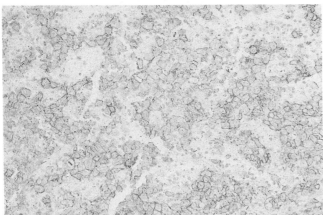

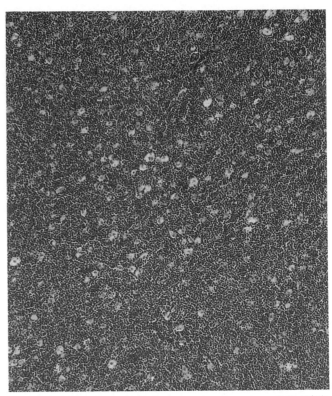

Figure 9–54. Characteristic low-power appearance of Burkitt's lymphoma, showing a "starry-sky" appearance that consists of a diffuse growth pattern characterized by the presence of many macrophages containing phagocytized and cellular debris admixed with a small cell infiltrate.

Figure 9–52. The cytologic features of this lymphoma are similar to those of undifferentiated carcinoma; therefore, immunohistochemical studies are indicated in order to differentiate these neoplasms. *(Top)* Confirmation of lymphoid origin is seen by the presence of diffuse immunoreactivity with leukocyte common antigen (LCA). *(Bottom)* Waldeyer's ring lymphomas are predominantly but not exclusively follicular center cell-derived, expressed by the positive reactivity with B-cell markers (L-26).

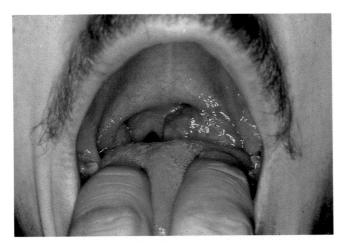

Figure 9–53. Burkitt's lymphoma, presenting as a yellow to tan-white enlarged left tonsillar mass.

Figure 9–55. The neoplastic cells are uniform and small (equal in size to the macrophages), with noncleaved round nuclei, two to five prominent nucleoli, and a small amount of amphophilic cytoplasm.

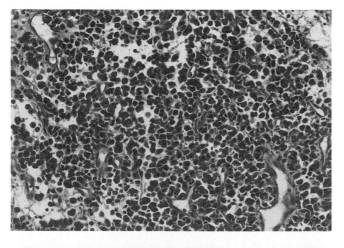

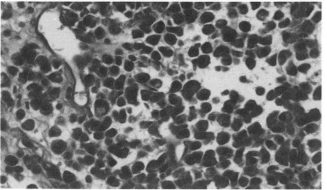

Figure 9–56. Extramedullary plasmacytoma. *(Top)* Diffuse or sheet-like proliferation of plasma cells varying in maturity, distinguished by *(bottom)* eccentrically located, round to oval nuclei with dispersed ("clock-face") nuclear chromatin pattern and a paranuclear clear area or halo ("hof") representative of the Golgi apparatus.

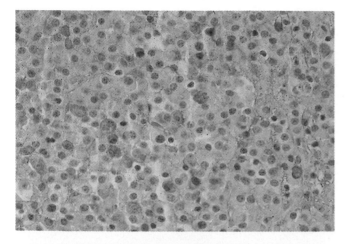

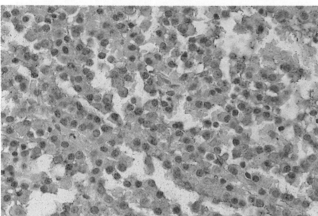

Figure 9-57. Immunohistochemistry of this extramedullary plasmacytoma demonstrates *(top)* reactivity only for IgG and *(bottom)* lambda light chain restriction.

5. Rhabdomyosarcoma

Definition: Malignant tumor of skeletal muscle cells (rhabdomyoblasts) in varying stages of differentiation.

Clinical

- Compose approximately 19% of all sarcomas.
- The most common soft tissue sarcoma in the pediatric, adolescent, and young adult population.
- The most common sarcoma occurring in the head and neck; up to 45% of rhabdomyosarcomas occur in the head and neck region.
- In the pediatric population, 50% of all rhabdomyosarcomas arise in the head and neck, and rhabdomyosarcoma represents the most common aural malignant neoplasm in this population.
- No sex predilection; most common in the first and second decades of life and rarely identified beyond the fifth decade.
- Excluding the orbit, the most common sites in the head and neck are the nasopharynx > ear (middle ear and mastoid) > sinonasal cavity.
- Symptoms vary according to site and include nasal obstruction, epistaxis, pain, refractory otitis media, otorrhea, temporofacial swelling or deformity and neurologic deficits.
- No known associated etiologic factors.

Pathology

Gross

- Nasopharyngeal rhabdomyosarcomas tend to be fairly well circumscribed, polypoid or multinodular, tan-white, glistening or gelatinous, and capable of attaining large sizes.
- Aural rhabdomyosarcomas most commonly present as an otic (external or middle ear) polyp.
- Sinonasal rhabdomyosarcomas tend to be small and appear as a nasal polyp.
- **Note:** approximately 25% of nasopharyngeal and sinonasal cavity rhabdomyosarcomas assume a sarcoma botryoides appearance, with a "grape-like," multinodular, or polypoid configuration.

Histology

Four histologic variants of rhabdomyosarcoma are identified:

1. Embryonal:
   - Most common histologic variant seen in head and neck rhabdomyosarcoma.
   - Typically, there is a variation in the cellularity of these tumors, with alternating hyper- and hypocellular areas; the latter often is associated with a myxoid stroma.
   - The cellular components consist of both round and spindle cells:
     Round cells resemble lymphocytes, and are round to oval with hyperchromatic nuclei and cytoplasm that varies from distinct and eosinophilic to indistinct.
     Spindle cells are elongated, with central hyperchromatic nuclei and eosinophilic cytoplasm.
   - Mitoses and necrosis are commonly seen.
2. Alveolar:
   - Ill-defined collections of noncohesive tumor cells, the central portions of which appear empty or markedly hypocellular, giving the appearance of forming spaces or alveoli.
   - Portions of the tumor do not take on the alveolar appearance but rather are composed of solid aggregates of tumor cells arranged in a trabecular pattern.
   - The cellular portions of the tumor are separated by dense fibrous connective tissue, forming septa and associated with prominent vascular spaces.
   - Tumor cells are round to oval with hyperchromatic nuclei and cytoplasm that varies from scanty and indistinct to distinct and eosinophilic.
   - Multinucleated giant cells with peripherally placed nuclei are a prominent feature.
   - Mitoses are commonly seen.
3. Pleomorphic:
   - Least common histologic variant.
   - Predominantly occurs in adult neoplasms.
   - Composed of pleomorphic-appearing cells composed of spindle-shaped cells admixed with large, pleomorphic cells.
   - The pleomorphic cells have deeply eosinophilic or granular cytoplasm and range from round cells with multiple nuclei to elongated, ribbonlike or strap-shaped cells with multiple nuclei.
4. Mixed
   - Composed of two or more histologic types.

General histologic considerations:

- Rhabdomyoblasts, the cell of origin for this sarcoma, take on numerous appearances, including small round cells to ribbon- or strap-shaped to large and pleomorphic; rhabdomyoblasts with cross-striations are not always identified, and their absence does not exclude the diagnosis of rhabdomyosarcoma.
- An associated benign inflammatory infiltrate may predominate, overrunning and masking the presence of the neoplastic cells.
- In the presence of a poorly differentiated neoplasm lacking evidence of cross-striations, special stains are invaluable in confirming the diagnosis of rhabdomyosarcoma and include:
  Histochemistry: cells contain glycogen as demonstrated by periodic acid-Schiff (PAS) positivity cleared by diastase digestion; intracellular myofibrils can be seen by Masson trichrome and phosphotungstic acid hematoxylin (PTAH) stains.
  Immunohistochemistry: desmin and myoglobin immunoreactivity.

Differential Diagnosis

- Nasal polyps with stromal atypia (Chapter 3, #1).
- Aural polyps (Chapter 24B, #2).
- Small, round cell neoplasms: (olfactory) neuroblastoma (Chapter 4B, #5), Ewing's sarcoma, malignant melanoma (Chapter 4B, #3), malignant lymphoma (Chapters 4B, #5; Chapter 9B, #4).
- Undifferentiated or poorly differentiated carcinoma (Chapter 9B, #2).
- Synovial sarcoma (Chapter 14B, #8).
- Alveolar soft part sarcoma (Chapter 9A, #4).

Treatment and Prognosis

- Multimodality therapy, including nonradical surgery, radiotherapy plus multiagent chemotherapy (vincristine sulfate, dactinomycin, cyclophosphamide, and Adriamycin) is the treatment of choice.
- Prognosis has improved tremendously in a disease that was once considered to be uniformly fatal; the prognostic improvement is based on the multimodality therapeutic regimens and the development of clinical staging, by the Intergroup Rhabdomyosarcoma Study (IRS), which includes:
  1. Stage I: localized disease, with tumor completely resected.
  2. Stage II: grossly resected tumor with:
     Microscopic residual disease and negative regional lymph nodes.
     Microscopic residual disease and positive regional lymph nodes.
     Regional lymph nodes involved or extension of tumor into adjacent viscera without microscopic residual disease.
  3. Stage III: incomplete resection or biopsy of primary tumor with gross residual disease.
  4. Stage IV: metastatic disease present at the time of diagnosis.
- Prognosis (overall 5-year survival) for the clinical stage includes: stage I, 83%; stage II, 70%; stage III, 52%; stage IV, 20%.
- Other factors related to prognosis include:
  Site and extent of disease: orbital tumors have a

more favorable prognosis than nonorbital head and neck rhabdomyosarcomas.

Histologic type: alveolar variant carries a less favorable prognosis than the embryonal variant.

Length of disease-free periods.

■ Rhabdomyosarcomas have a tendency to invade bone and, in the head and neck, this tendency may result in extensive meningeal involvement.

■ Inadequately treated tumors result in recurrence and metastases, most frequently involving the lungs, bone, and lymph nodes.

Additional Facts

■ Both the embryonal and alveolar variants are considered to parallel the embryologic development of striated muscle as it appears in the second and third months (seventh to twelfth weeks) of gestation; given the fact that cross-striations do not appear embryologically until after the twelfth week (generally around the fourteenth week), the presence of cross-striations would not be needed to make the diagnosis.

■ Failure to identify the presence of rhabdomyosarcoma, especially in the innocuous clinical setting of a aural or nasal polyp, results in delay in diagnosis, a higher clinical stage tumor, and a worse prognosis.

■ Sarcoma botryoides is a macroscopic identification and is not considered a separate histologic variant.

■ A mixed histologic type of rhabdomyosarcoma can be seen, but is not necessarily considered an independent histologic variant; rather, it is classified by the predominant growth.

References

Barnes L: Rhabdomyosarcoma. *In*: Barnes L, ed. Surgical pathology of the head and neck. New York: Marcel Dekker, 1985; pp 787–797.

Enzinger FW, Weiss SW: Rhabdomyosarcoma. *In*: Enzinger FW, Weiss SW, eds. Soft tissue tumors; 2nd ed. St. Louis: C.V. Mosby, 1988; pp 448–488.

Dohar JE, Marentette LJ, Adams GL: Rhabdomyosarcoma of the infratemporal fossa: diagnostic dilemmas and surgical management. Am J Otolaryngol 12:146–149, 1991.

Eusebi V, Ceccarelli C, Gorza L, Schiaffino S, Bussolati G: Immunocytochemistry of rhabdomyosarcoma: the use of four different markers. Am J Surg Pathol 10:293–299, 1986.

Feldman BA: Rhabdomyosarcoma of the head and neck. Laryngoscope 92:424–440, 1982.

Healy EB, Upton J, Black PM, Ferraro N: The role of surgery in rhabdomyosarcoma of the head and neck in children. Arch Otolaryngol Head Neck Surg 117:1185–1188, 1991.

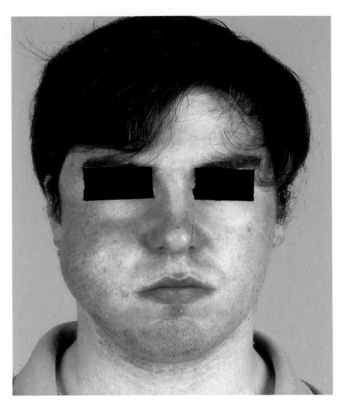

Figure 9–58. Rhabdomyosarcoma presenting with a rapidly enlarging soft tissue mass of the right face.

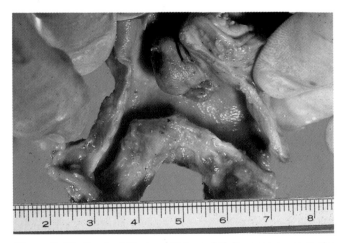

Figure 9–59. Tracheal "botryoid"-type rhabdomyosarcoma at the carina, appearing as a polypoid, well-delineated mass.

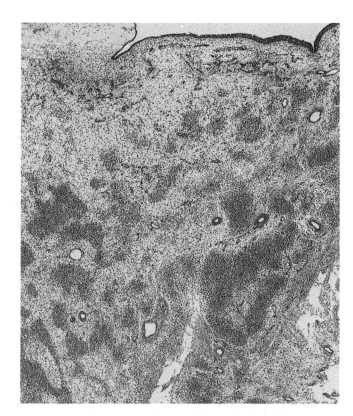

Figure 9–60. Embryonal rhabdomyosarcoma with hyper- and hypocellular areas associated with a myxoid stroma.

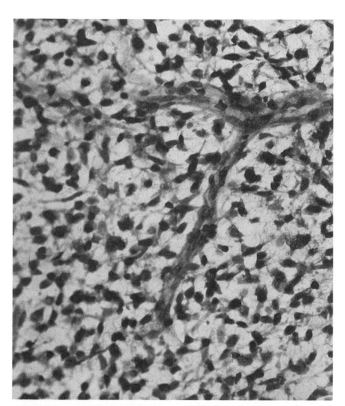

Figure 9–61. Embryonal rhabdomyosarcoma cellular components consist of both round and spindle cells. The round cells resemble lymphocytes, and are round to oval with hyperchromatic nuclei and a cytoplasm that varies from distinct and eosinophilic to indistinct; spindle cells are elongated, with central hyperchromatic nuclei and eosinophilic cytoplasm.

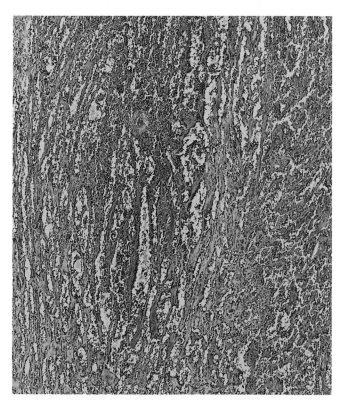

Figure 9–62. Alveolar rhabdomyosarcoma composed of cellular aggregates characterized by poorly differentiated, noncohesive tumor cells, the central portions of which appear empty or markedly hypocellular, giving the appearance of forming spaces or alveoli; this variant may also demonstrate solid cell aggregates (not depicted) in association with the characteristic alveolar pattern or exclusive of an alveolar growth.

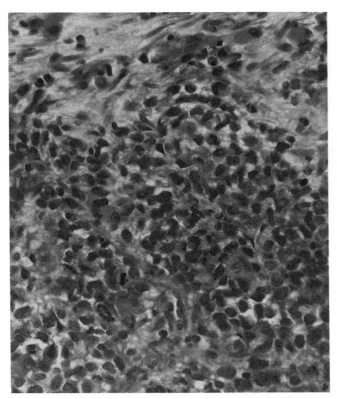

Figure 9–63. Alveolar rhabdomyosarcoma, composed of solid area of tumor cells that are round to oval with hyperchromatic nuclei and cytoplasm that varies from scanty and indistinct to distinct and eosinophilic. Scattered inflammatory cells and a mitotic figure are seen.

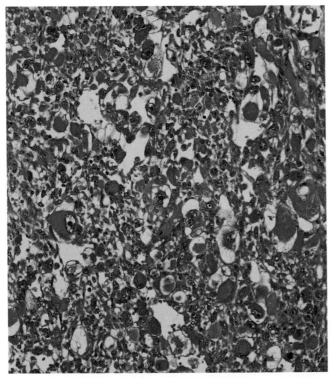

Figure 9–64. Pleomorphic rhabdomyosarcoma, composed of large, pleomorphic-appearing cells with prominent nucleoli and eosinophilic or granular cytoplasm; mitotic figures are seen.

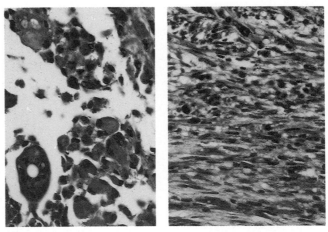

Figure 9–65. Rhabdomyoblasts, the cell of origin for this sarcoma, appear as *(left)* large, pleomorphic cells with hyperchromatic nuclei and abundant eosinophilic cytoplasm, and *(right)* spindle- or strap-shaped.

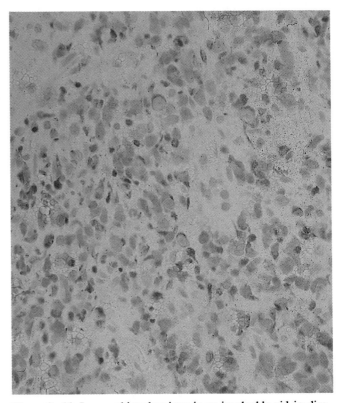

Figure 9–66. Immunohistochemistry is an invaluable aid in diagnosing rhabdomyosarcomas, as depicted here by the immunoreactivity with desmin.

6. Malignant Peripheral Nerve Sheath Tumors (Malignant Schwannoma)

Definition: Malignant tumor of peripheral nerves.
Synonyms: Neurogenic sarcoma; neurofibrosarcoma.

Clinical

- Accounts for approximately 10% of all soft tissue sarcomas; most commonly occurs in the lower extremity.
- Up to 14% of malignant schwannomas occur in the head and neck.
- Malignant schwannomas can occur in two settings, with different epidemiologic findings:
  1. Sporadic occurrence of unknown etiology.
     Affects females more than males; wide age range, but most frequently occurs in the fifth decade.
  2. Associated with von Recklinghausen's disease (VRD).
     Affects males more than females; wide age range, but tends to occur in a younger age group, primarily seen in the third and fourth decades.
- Estimated risk of patients with VRD to develop a malignant schwannoma varies, with figures ranging from 4% to 50%; when malignant schwannoma complicates VRD, it typically occurs after a latent period of 10 to 20 years.
- The most common site of involvement in the head and neck region is the neck; all areas may be involved, including the sinonasal cavity and nasopharynx.
- Symptoms include a neck mass with associated pain, paresthesia, and weakness.

Pathology

Gross

- Fusiform-shaped mass with a fleshy, tan-white appearance and usually measuring more than 5 cm in diameter.

Histology

- Unencapsulated and infiltrating tumor composed of spindle-shaped cells arranged in fascicles.
- Nuclei are irregular in contour and are wavy or buckled in appearance; the cytoplasm is indistinct.
- Hypocellular areas with a myxoid stroma can be seen alternating with areas of greater cellularity.
- Increased cellularity, cellular pleomorphism, and increased mitotic activity are invariably seen; low- versus high-grade malignant schwannomas are based on the degree of these findings.
- Nuclear palisading, cyst formation, and hemorrhage may be seen.
- Heterologous elements can be identified, including bone and cartilage; other cell components include:
  Epithelioid cells (malignant epithelioid schwannoma).

Glands (glandular malignant schwannoma).
Skeletal muscle (malignant Triton tumor).
- Immunohistochemistry: S-100 protein reactivity, which, in contrast to neurilemmomas and neurofibromas, is focal and less intensely positive in low-grade tumors to focal with even less immunoreactivity or no immunoreactivity in high-grade tumors.

Differential Diagnosis

- Fibrosarcoma (Chapter 4B, #7).
- Leiomyosarcoma (Chapter 4B, #8).
- Synovial sarcoma, monophasic variant (Chapter 14B, #8).
- Malignant melanoma (Chapter 4B, #3).

Treatment and Prognosis

- Complete surgical excision is the treatment of choice.
- Radiotherapy may be used in conjunction with surgery or in cases with recurrent disease.
- Survival rates differ for malignant schwannomas arising de novo as compared to those associated with VRD:
  Sporadic malignant schwannomas have a reported 5-year survival rate of approximately 50%.
  In association with VRD, 5-year survival rates are 15% to 30%.
- Poorer survival rates in malignant schwannomas associated with VRD relate to:
  Larger tumors, which tend to be of higher grade.
  Multiple separate malignant schwannomas.
- Local recurrence is common and metastases occur to the lung, liver, bone, and infrequently to lymph nodes.

Additional Facts

- In the sinonasal cavity, malignant schwannomas can occur in the clinical setting of a sinonasal polyp; the malignant schwannoma is often low-grade and appears as a nondescript spindle-cell proliferation in and around a benign glandular proliferation; S-100 protein is invaluable in confirming the diagnosis.

References

Ducatman BS, Sheithauer BW, Piepgras DG, Reiman HL, Ilstrup DM: Malignant peripheral nerve sheath tumors: a clinicopathologic study of 120 cases. Cancer 57:2006–2021, 1986.

Weiss SW, Langloss JM, Enzinger FW: The role of S-100 protein in the diagnosis of soft tissue tumors with particular reference to benign and malignant schwann cell tumors. Lab Invest 49:299–308, 1983.

Enzinger FW, Weiss SW: Malignant tumors of peripheral nerves. *In*: Enzinger FW, Weiss SW, eds. Soft tissue tumors; 2nd ed. St. Louis: C.V. Mosby, 1988; pp 781–815.

Younis RT, Gross CW, Lazar RH: Schwannomas of the paranasal sinuses: case report and clinicopathologic analysis. Arch Otolaryngol Head Neck Surg 117:677–680, 1991.

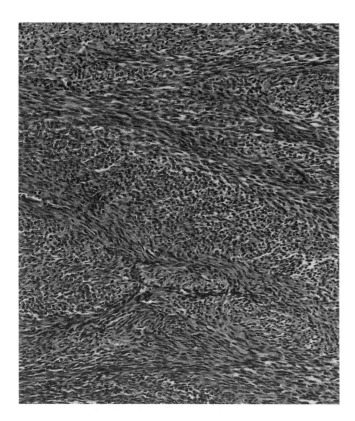

Figure 9–67. Low-grade malignant schwannoma, consisting of an infiltrating cellular tumor composed of spindle-shaped cells that are arranged in fascicles with nuclei having an irregular contour with a wavy or buckled appearance and an indistinct cytoplasm; scattered mitoses were seen. This neoplasm was unencapsulated and had areas of distinct nuclear palisading.

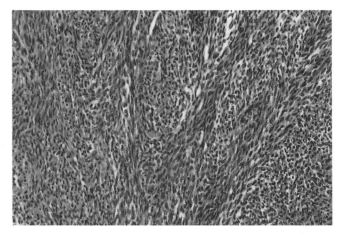

Figure 9–68. Low-grade malignant schwannoma. *(Top)* Fasciculated, cellular neoplasm composed of spindle-shaped cells with mild to moderate pleomorphism. *(Bottom)* S-100 protein is diffusely positive. The cellularity, pleomorphism, and mitotic activity help to rule out the presence of a cellular benign schwannoma, which would have similar diffuse S-100 protein immunoreactivity.

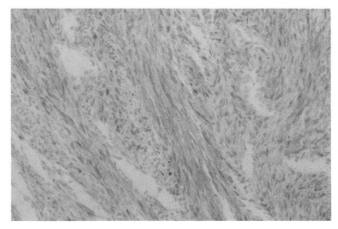

Figure 9–69. High-grade malignant schwannoma: in contrast to the low-grade neoplasm, the high-grade malignant schwannoma shows a spindle and pleomorphic cellular infiltrate with a less conspicuous fasciculated growth, increased cellularity, cellular pleomorphism, hemorrhage, and necrosis.

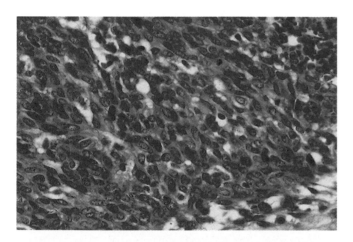

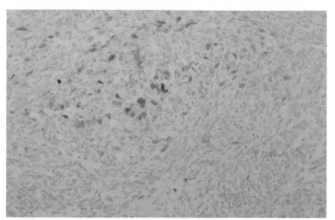

Figure 9–70. *(Top)* High-grade malignant schwannoma, showing a densely cellular, pleomorphic cell infiltrate with increased mitotic activity. *(Bottom)* S-100 protein immunoreactivity, in contrast to low-grade malignant schwannomas, is absent or only focally positive.

7. Chordoma

Definition: Malignant neoplasm arising from the embryonic remnants of the notochord.

Clinical

- Represents approximately 1% of all malignant bone tumors.
- Notochord and chordoma development:
  The notochord functions as a primitive axial skeleton in humans.
  From the time of its development in the third to fourth week of gestation, the notochord extends from the sphenoid bone at the junction of the occipital bone, exits its bony confines to run in close apposition to the primitive pharynx, reenters the bone in the basiocciput, and then courses via the apical odontoid ligament through the center of the vertebral bodies to end at the coccyx.
  In the vertebral column, the notochord is divided into segments and disappears by the seventh week of gestation.
  Persistence of notochordal tissue is seen within the nucleus pulposus of the intervertebral disks.
  Chordomas do not arise from the intervertebral body remnants, but rather from incomplete regression of notochordal tissue along the notochordal tract during development; therefore, chordomas are identified in the sacrococcygeal region, bones of the skull, and the vertebra (cervical > lumbar > thoracic).
- Affects males more than females; can occur at any age, but is generally not common below the fourth decade of life.
- Craniocervical chordomas are identified most frequently in the dorsum sella, clivus, and nasopharyngeal regions.
- Symptoms vary according to the site of occurrence and extension of tumor and include diplopia, visual field defects, headaches, pain, nasal obstruction, epistaxis, nasal discharge, soft tissue mass, and endocrinopathies (secondary to destruction of the sella turcica).

Radiology

- Expansile and destructive osteolytic lesions often associated with a soft tissue mass.
- Nodular or cystic deposits of calcification are often seen.
- Destruction of the sella turcica may be seen.
- Nasopharyngeal chordomas appear as a soft tissue density.

Pathology

Gross

- Well-demarcated or encapsulated, soft, mucoid, or gelatinous mass with a pink to gray color and a variegated appearance with solid and cystic areas.

Histology

- Pseudoencapsulated tumor separated into a lobular growth by fibrous connective tissue.
- The cells are epithelioid with vesicular nuclei and abundant, granular to vacuolated-appearing cytoplasm.
- Vacuolization represents glycogen or mucus and, when extensive, can appear with a "soap bubble" appearance, compressing the nucleus and creating the characteristic physaliferous cells seen in chordomas.
- The cells are associated with a copious extracellular mucinous matrix and are arranged in cords, pseudoacini, or in clusters.
- Cellular pleomorphism and mitoses are not common features; necrosis and calcification can be identified.
- Histochemistry: periodic acid–Schiff and mucin positive.
- Immunohistochemistry: cytokeratin, epithelial membrane antigen, and S-100 protein positive.
- A variant of the chordoma, called *chondroid chordoma,* is identified and is noted for:
  More common occurrence in women and younger patients than nonchondroid chordoma.
  Virtual exclusive occurrence at the base of skull.
  The presence of a cartilaginous component (either benign or malignant).
  S-100 protein immunoreactivity, but absence of cytokeratin immunoreactivity.
  Better prognosis than typical chordomas.
- Dedifferentiation of chordomas may occur and includes transformation to fibrosarcoma, malignant fibrous histiocytoma, osteosarcoma, and chondrosarcoma.

Differential Diagnosis

- Chondrosarcoma (Chapter 14B, #7).
- Liposarcoma (Chapter 9B, #8).
- Mucinous adenocarcinoma (Chapter 4B, #2).

Treatment and Prognosis

- Complete surgical excision is the treatment of choice.
- For advanced disease where complete resection is impossible, high-dose radiotherapy is used.
- Chemotherapy has no proven efficacy.
- Despite its slow growth, chordomas are relentless neoplasms, usually presenting with extensive local infiltration and destruction of adjacent, often vital, structures.
- Prognosis is poor, with less than 20% 5-year survival.
- Metastases are generally a late complication and involve the lungs, bone, liver, and lymph nodes.
- Average survival rate for the chondroid chordoma is reported to be 15.8 years, as compared to 4.1 years for the nonchondroid chordoma.

Additional Facts

■ The calcifications seen in association with chordomas occur as a result of bone sequestration after its destruction or as dystrophic calcification.

■ The mean survival rates for sacrococcygeal chordomas are slightly better than for cervicofacial chordomas.

References

Heffelfinger MJ, Dahlin DC, MacCarty CS, Beabout JW: Chordomas and cartilaginous tumors at the skull base. Cancer 32:410–420, 1973.

Hyams VJ, Batsakis JG, Michaels L: Chordoma. *In:* Hyams VJ, Batsakis JG, Michaels L, eds. Tumors of the upper respiratory tract and ear. Fascicle 25, second series. Washington, D.C.: Armed Forces Institute of Pathology, 1988; pp 192–196.

Miettinen M: Chordoma: antibodies to epithelial membrane antigen and carcinoembryonic antigen in differential diagnosis. Arch Pathol Lab Med 108:891–892, 1984.

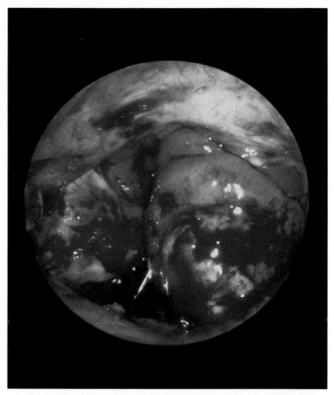

Figure 9–72. Endoscopic appearance of a nasopharyngeal chordoma, appearing as large tan-pink to fleshy, mucoid, or gelatinous mass.

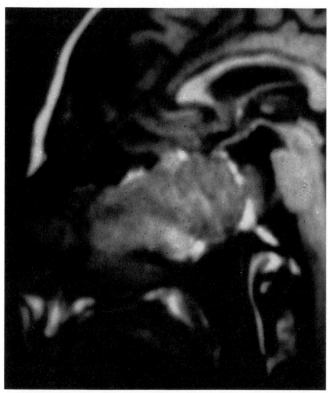

Figure 9–71. Nasopharyngeal chordoma. MR, sagittal view: large nasopharyngeal soft tissue density eroding into and destroying the bone at the base of the skull.

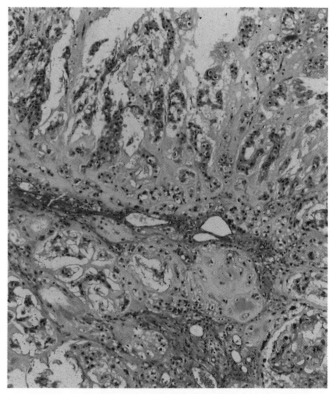

Figure 9–73. Characteristic histologic appearance of nasopharyngeal chordoma, consisting of a lobular neoplastic growth associated with a copious extracellular mucinous matrix.

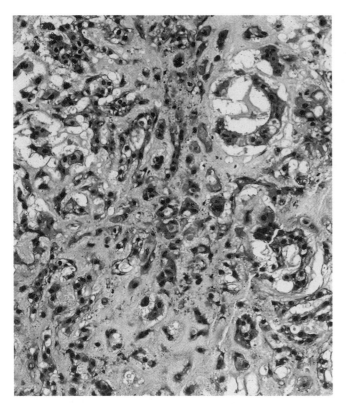

Figure 9–74. The neoplastic growth pattern includes cords, pseudoacini, or cell clusters and trabeculae.

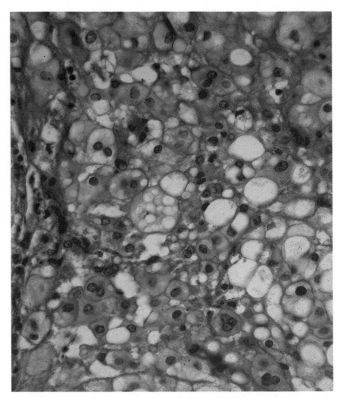

Figure 9–75. Chordoma cells are epithelioid with vesicular to hyperchromatic nuclei and abundant granular to vacuolated-appearing cytoplasm; the vacuolization represents glycogen or mucus, and when extensive can appear with a "soap bubble" appearance, compressing the nucleus and creating the characteristic physaliferous cells.

8. Liposarcoma

Definition: Malignant neoplasm of adipose tissue.

Clinical

■ Second to malignant fibrous histiocytoma, this is the most common soft tissue sarcoma of adult life, representing approximately 16% to 18% of all soft tissue sarcomas; the most common sites of occurrence are the extremities and the retroperitoneum.
■ Head and neck liposarcomas are uncommon, representing approximately 3% to 6% of all cases.
■ Affects males more than females; can occur in all age groups, but is most common in the fifth to seventh decades of life.
■ In the head and neck, the most common site of occurrence is by far the neck region; virtually every other head and neck site can be involved.
■ Symptoms vary according to site, but the most common symptom is an enlarging painless neck mass.
■ Liposarcomas arise from primitive mesenchymal cells rather than mature adipose tissue, accounting

for its presence in areas relatively devoid of fat (i.e., the head and neck).
■ No known associated etiologic factors.

Pathology

Gross

■ Circumscribed or encapsulated, lobulated mass varying in appearance from yellow to tan-white in color and with a myxoid or gelatinous appearance.
■ Although liposarcomas can attain very large sizes, those identified in the head and neck rarely exceed 10 cm and are generally under 5 cm in diameter.
■ **Note:** the variability in the gross appearance is dependent on the histologic type.

Histology

Four histologic variants are identified:
1. Myxoid:
   ■ Most common type, accounting for approximately 40% to 50% of all cases.

- Characterized by:
  Lobular growth.
  Myxoid stroma (rich in glycosaminoglycans or hyaluronidase-sensitive acid mucopolysaccharides).
  Proliferating lipoblasts in all developmental stages.
  Plexiform vascular (capillary) pattern.
2. Round cell:
   - Represents the poorly differentiated form of the myxoid type.
   - Densely cellular, consisting of a proliferation of small round cells with uniform, vesicular nuclei; may have granular to vacuolated-appearing cytoplasm.
   - Vascular pattern is present, but generally is compressed by the cellular proliferation.
   - Intercellular myxoid or mucoid stroma may be seen.
3. Well-differentiated:
   - Synonyms include lipoma-like and sclerosing.
   - Resembles a lipoma, except for:
     The presence of scattered lipoblasts.
     Greater variation in the size and shape of the lipocytes.
   - Sclerosing liposarcomas are composed of broad, dense fibrous bands containing atypical cells with hyperchromatic nuclei and lipoblasts alternating with areas of lipomatous proliferation.
   - May contain a prominent lymphocytic and plasma cell infiltrate ("inflammatory" liposarcoma).
4. Pleomorphic:
   - Composed of a proliferation of large giant cells containing one or more hyperchromatic nuclei.
   - Cytoplasm may contain lipid droplets or eosinophilic hyaline globules, or may be deeply acidophilic.

General histologic considerations:

- Lipoblasts:
  Range in appearance from primitive-appearing cells demonstrating little if any detectable lipid to signet-ring cells with the cytoplasm filled with lipid displacing the nucleus peripherally.
  Classic-appearing lipoblasts have sharply defined lipid droplets, causing scalloping or distortion of the nucleus, which is either centrally or peripherally located in the cell; nuclei are large and hyperchromatic.
  Often require diligence and ample sections for detection.
  Must be distinguished from vacuolated cells closely simulating the appearance of lipoblasts and identified in other soft tissue sarcomas.
- Mitoses, necrosis, and hemorrhage can be identified in all histologic variants and generally correlate to the amount of cellular pleomorphism (mitoses are particularly prominent in the pleomorphic variant).

- Special stains are of little if any assistance in diagnosis.
- Note: adipocytes and lipoblasts have variable S-100 protein immunoreactivity.

Differential Diagnosis

- Lipoma (Chapter 9A, #5).
- Myxoma (intramuscular; nerve sheath) (Chapter 3A, #9).
- Other sarcomas: rhabdomyosarcoma (Chapter 9B, #5), malignant fibrous histiocytoma (Chapter 4B, #6), myxoid chondrosarcoma, Ewing's sarcoma.
- Chordoma (Chapter 9B, #7).
- Signet-ring cell carcinoma or lymphoma.
- Malignant melanoma (Chapter 4B, #3).

Treatment and Prognosis

- Wide local surgical excision is the treatment of choice for well-differentiated liposarcoma; more aggressive surgical procedures may be indicated for the other histologic variants.
- Although controversial, evidence supports the use of postoperative radiotherapy as an adjunct to surgery in order to retard growth and possibly shrink the tumor, allowing for surgical removal.
- Recurrence is common and:
  Generally occurs within 3 years after the initial treatment.
  Usually is of the same histology as the primary tumor, but may be "dedifferentiated" with a histologic appearance less differentiated and with a more aggressive biology than the primary tumor.
- Survival rates correlate to liposarcomas occurring in non-head and neck sites and are influenced by histologic type:
  Well-differentiated: 85% to 100% 5-year survival.
  Myxoid: 71% to 96% 5-year survival.
  Round cell: 12.5% to 55% 5-year survival.
  Pleomorphic: 0% to 45% 5-year survival.
- Other factors important in prognosis include size and location of the tumor.
- Metastases may occur and are more common with the higher grade histologic variants; metastases occur to the lungs, bone, and liver and only infrequently to regional lymph nodes.

Additional Facts

- The term atypical lipoma or atypical lipomatous tumor has been used for superficial (cutaneous or subcutaneous) lipogenic tumors with histologic appearance of well-differentiated liposarcomas and which have a tendency to recur; the use of this term should be viewed with caution in those well-differentiated liposarcomas occurring in more vital areas (deep neck, nasopharynx, sinonasal cavity, larynx, and hypopharynx), where inadequate excision and subsequent recurrence may result in increased morbidity and mortality.

■ The use of the nomenclature well-differentiated liposarcoma rather than atypical lipoma should convey to the surgeon that the neoplasm requires aggressive but not mutilating surgery and not just simple excision.

■ Controversy exists as to the issue of multicentrically occurring liposarcomas versus metastatic liposarcoma.

References

Enzinger FW, Weiss SW: Liposarcoma. *In*: Enzinger FW, Weiss SW, eds. Soft tissue tumors; 2nd ed. St. Louis: C.V. Mosby; 1988; pp 346–382.

Evans HL: Liposarcoma; a study of 55 cases with a reassessment of its classification. Am J Surg Pathol 3:507–523, 1979.

Evans HL, Soule EH, Winkelmann RK: Atypical lipoma, atypical intramuscular lipoma, and well differentiated retroperitoneal liposarcoma: a reappraisal of 30 cases formerly classified as well differentiated liposarcoma. Cancer 43:574–584, 1979.

Fu YS, Perzin KH: Non-epithelial tumors of the nasal cavity, paranasal sinuses, and nasopharynx: a clinical study. VIII. Adipose tissue tumors (lipoma and liposarcoma). Cancer 40:1314–1317, 1977.

Saunders JR, Jacques DA, Casterline PF, Percarpio B, Goodloe S: Liposarcoma of the head and neck: a review of the literature and addition of four cases. Cancer 43:162–168, 1979.

Wenig BM, Weiss SW, Gnepp DR: Laryngeal and hypopharyngeal liposarcoma: a clinicaopathologic study of 10 cases with a comparison to soft-tissue counterparts. Am J Surg Pathol 14:134–141, 1990.

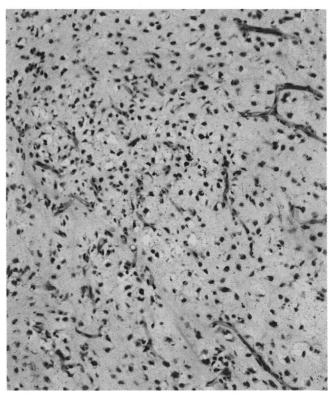

Figure 9–77. Myxoid liposarcoma, showing lipoblasts in varying stages of development, including signet-ring appearance.

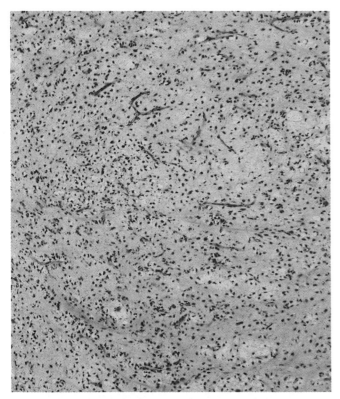

Figure 9–76. Myxoid liposarcoma with scattered lipoblasts and a typical myxoid stroma and plexiform capillary pattern.

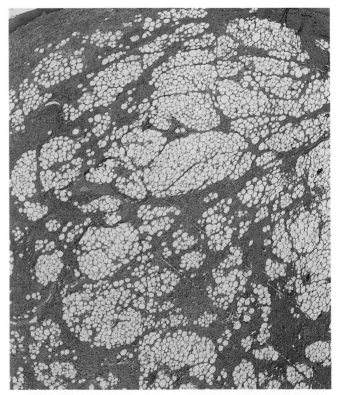

Figure 9–78. Well-differentiated liposarcoma of the larynx, composed of nests of fat cells varying in size and shape, with the cell nests separated by fibrous septa.

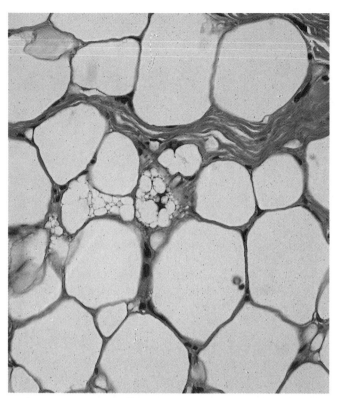

Figure 9-79. Well-differentiated liposarcoma of the larynx with variation in size and shape of fat cells, some of which have hyperchromatic nuclei as well as the presence of a multivacuolar lipoblast.

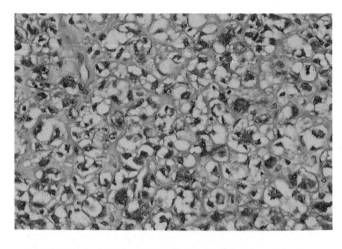

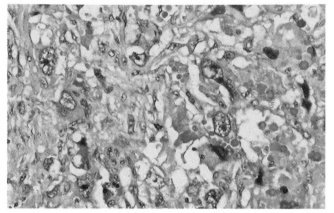

Figure 9-81. Pleomorphic liposarcoma. *(Top)* Tumor cells with intracytoplasmic lipid droplets. *(Bottom)* Eosinophilic hyaline globules within the cytoplasm of the lipoblasts are a frequent finding.

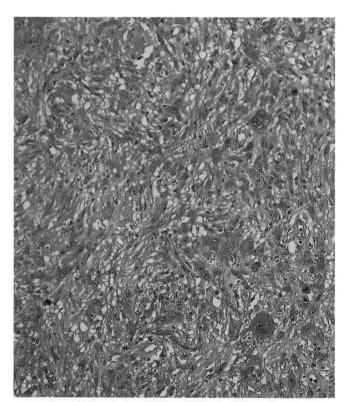

Figure 9-80. Pleomorphic liposarcoma, composed of a proliferation of large, pleomorphic cells containing one or more hyperchromatic nuclei, prominent nucleoli, and increased mitotic activity.

9. Kaposi's Sarcoma

Definition: Angioproliferative neoplastic disorder.

Clinical

- Three forms of Kaposi's sarcoma are identified: classic versus epidemic versus transplantation-associated.

"CLASSIC" KAPOSI'S SARCOMA

- Considered a rare tumor accounting for less than 0.5% of all malignancies.
- Affects men more than women; most common in the sixth and seventh decades of life, affecting people of Jewish or Mediterranean descent.
- Predominantly a cutaneous-related tumor, occurring on the lower extremity > upper extremity; visceral involvement is unusual in the absence of cutaneous disease.
- Initial presentation in the head and neck is decidedly uncommon; however, with progression of disease, mucosal sites in the head and neck can be affected, including oral cavity (palate, tongue, gums, lips, buccal mucosa), tonsils, pharynx, and larynx.
- Association with a second malignant neoplasm (leukemia, lymphoma, myeloma) or autoimmune disease (autoimmune hemolytic anemia) can be seen.
- Not associated with human immunodeficiency virus (HIV) or with the development of AIDS.

"EPIDEMIC" OR AIDS-RELATED KAPOSI'S SARCOMA

- May be seen in all AIDS-related risk groups but appears to be more common among male homosexuals; occurs at a much younger age as compared to the classic type and is most frequently seen in the fourth decade of life.
- Typically, multiple lesions are commonly seen, with involvement of cutaneous sites of the upper extremity, head, and neck, as well as mucosal sites in the oral cavity and the oropharynx; in addition, generalized lymphadenopathy and visceral involvement are frequently seen.
- Identification of Kaposi's sarcoma often is the initial manifestation of AIDS, leading to its diagnosis.

TRANSPLANTATION-ASSOCIATED KAPOSI'S SARCOMA

- Occurs in less than 0.5% of renal transplant patients.
- Probably results as a consequence of immunosuppressive therapy; however, genetic and geographic origin also may be contributing factors because this association occurs in a large percentage of people who are of Jewish or Mediterranean descent.
- In this setting, neoplasm occurs months to years after transplantation and may occur in cutaneous or visceral sites.

Pathology

Gross

- Early lesions in the AIDS group appear as flat, red to pink areas and tend to be small.
- More advanced AIDS-related and "classic" type of Kaposi's sarcoma appear as raised, blue-red or violaceous papules or nodules of varying sizes that with time may coalesce to form plaques.

Histology: (irrespective of the clinical setting, the histology of the more advanced lesions are essentially the same):

- Unencapsulated and infiltrative lesion composed of spindle cells in a fascicular growth.
- Spindle cells are elongated and rather uniform, with scant cytoplasm and indistinct cell borders; scattered mitotic figures can be identified.
- Separating the spindle cell proliferation, slit-like spaces are seen containing erythrocytes that commonly extravasate into the spindle cell component.
- Intra- and extracellular diastase-resistant, PAS-positive hyaline globules can be seen.
- Associated chronic inflammatory cell infiltrates composed of lymphocytes and plasma cells as well as hemosiderin-laden macrophages are seen.
- Cellular pleomorphism, anaplastic changes, and increased mitoses are infrequently seen but may occur; these findings are indicative of more aggressive tumors.
- Immunohistochemistry: variable reactivity with factor VIII-related antigen, *Ulex europaeus,* and CD-34; nonreactivity does not exclude the diagnosis.

Differential Diagnosis

- Lobular capillary hemangioma (Chapter 4A, #2).
- Angiosarcoma (Chapter 4B, #9).
- Spindle cell carcinoma (Chapter 14B, #2).
- Fibrosarcoma (Chapter 4B, #8).

Treatment and Prognosis

- Radiation and chemotherapy are the treatments of choice.
- Other than for diagnostic purposes, surgery is not used in treatment.
- Treatment modalities relate to staging:
  Stage I: cutaneous, locally indolent — radiotherapy.
  Stage II: cutaneous, locally aggressive with or without regional lymph node involvement — radiotherapy.
  Stage III: generalized lymph node or mucocutaneous involvement — chemotherapy.
  Stage IV: visceral involvement — chemotherapy.
- "Classic" form of Kaposi's sarcoma is considered an indolent neoplasm with a prolonged clinical course and low mortality rates.
- AIDS patients with Kaposi's sarcoma have a much more aggressive disease course, with increased

mortality rates as a result of the constellation of problems in this group, including opportunistic infections and visceral Kaposi's sarcoma.

■ Kaposi's sarcoma developing in transplant patients follows a more aggressive course than in the "classic" form, with higher mortality rates due to pulmonary and gastrointestinal involvement.

Additional Facts

■ Jewish population affected are primarily of Eastern European (Ashkenazi) descent.

■ Mediterranean population affected are primarily from European countries.

References

Enzinger FW, Weiss SW: Kaposi's sarcoma. *In*: Enzinger FW, Weiss SW, eds. Soft tissue tumors; 2nd ed. St. Louis: C.V. Mosby, 1988; pp 561–575.

Murphy GF, Elder DE: Kaposi's sarcoma. *In:* Murphy GF, Elder DE, eds. Non-melanocytic tumors of skin. Fascicle I, third series. Washington, D.C.: Armed Forces Institute of Pathology, 1991; pp 214–219.

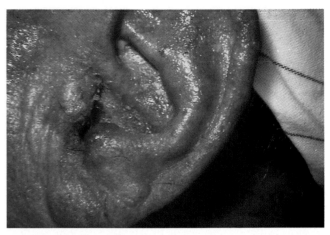

Figure 9–83. KS presenting in a non-AIDS patient as a raised, reddish-appearing nodule immediately outside the external auditory canal.

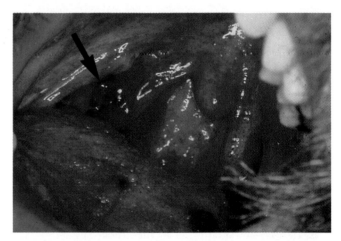

Figure 9–84. KS of the tonsil in an AIDS patient, appearing as an ill-defined deep red mass (*arrow*).

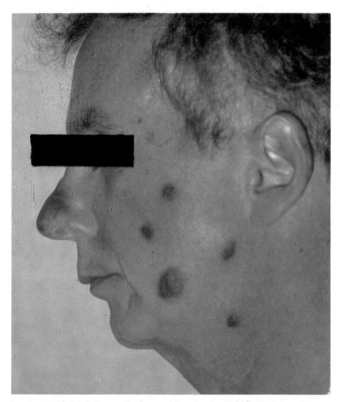

Figure 9–82. Cutaneous Kaposi's sarcoma (KS) in an AIDS patient, represented by multiple, discrete, oval, raised, blue-red or violaceous papules or nodules of varying sizes.

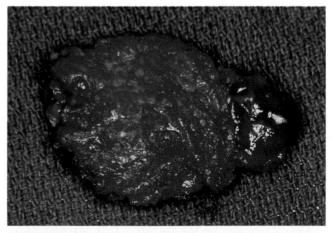

Figure 9–85. KS of the parotid gland in an AIDS patient, appearing as a well-delineated, bright red mass.

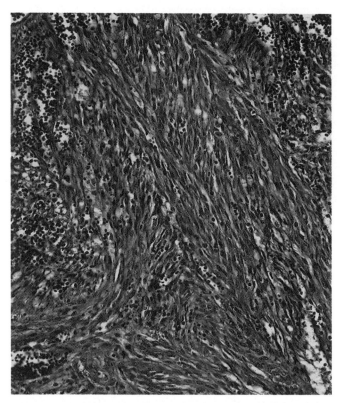

Figure 9–86. Characteristic histologic appearance of KS, consisting of an unencapsulated and infiltrative spindle cell tumor with a fascicular growth. Proliferation of slit-like spaces are seen, containing erythrocytes that extravasate into the spindle cell component.

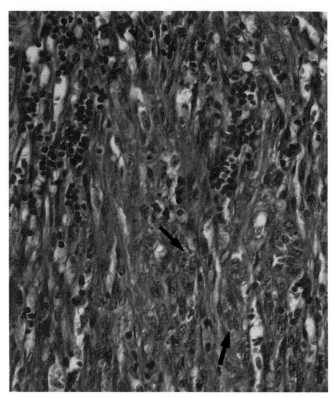

Figure 9–87. The spindle cells of KS are elongated, fairly uniform, with scant cytoplasm and indistinct cell borders; scattered mitotic figures can be identified, as well as intra- and extracellularly hyaline globules (*arrows*).

10. Metastatic Neoplasms to the Neck Region from an Occult Primary Neoplasm

Definition: Overt neck mass harboring a histologically proven metastatic neoplasm in the absence of signs and symptoms of a primary neoplasm or of a clinically detectable mass.

Clinical

■ The most common clinical manifestation of a metastatic tumor to the neck from an occult primary neoplasm is that of a unilateral, fixed mass.

■ Affects men more than women; most frequently seen in the fifth to seventh decades of life.

■ The majority of metastatic tumors to the cervical lymph nodes take origin from a head and neck primary tumor and, therefore, the most common histologic appearance is that of a squamous cell carcinoma.

■ Etiologic factors relate to the development of squamous carcinoma of the head and neck and, as such, are linked to tobacco and alcohol use.

■ Metastatic tumors to the neck are not limited to origin from a head and neck neoplasm, but may represent primary occult neoplasms from organ systems in the thorax, abdomen, and pelvis.

■ The lymphatic drainage to the cervical lymph nodes is predictable and the anatomic location of the metastatic focus assists in the search for the primary focus (Table 9–6).

■ The diagnostic work-up for a patient with a metastatic tumor in the neck of occult primary origin includes:

Panendoscopic evaluation of the upper respiratory tract, including direct laryngoscopy, bronchoscopy, and esophagoscopy.

Any mucosal abnormality should be biopsied and, if no abnormalities are grossly seen, random biopsies especially of Waldeyer's tonsillar ring (nasopharynx, tonsil, and base of tongue) are indicated.

Radiographic studies (head and neck, chest, abdomen).

■ By far, the nasopharynx, tonsils, and base of the tongue, collectively referred to as *Waldeyer's tonsillar ring,* are the areas harboring the occult primary tumor in the majority of squamous carcinomas metastatic to the neck; other common but less

Table 9-6
CERVICAL NODE REGION AND
POSSIBLE ORIGIN OF AN OCCULT
PRIMARY NEOPLASM

Lymph Node(s)	Region Drainage and Potential Source of the Metastatic Neoplasm
Preauricular	Skin of upper face and temple
Submental	Lip, anterior floor of mouth
Submaxillary	Skin of lateral face, floor of mouth and tongue (anterior)
Upper jugular	Tongue (lateral and posterior), palate and tonsil
Middle jugular	Pharynx, larynx
Low jugular	Thyroid, espophagus (cervical segment)
Posterior cervical	Nasopharynx, thyroid
Supraclavicular	Below the clavicle

frequent sites of the occult tumor include thyroid, hypopharynx, and larynx (supraglottic region).
■ The frequency and cystic appearance of tumors originating in Waldeyer's tonsillar ring merit special consideration:

METASTATIC CYSTIC SQUAMOUS CELL CARCINOMA

■ Metastatic deposits from Waldeyer's tonsillar ring often appear as cystic squamous cell carcinomas in cervical lymph nodes.
■ Confusion and controversy exist between the diagnosis of metastatic cystic squamous cell carcinoma versus carcinoma arising in a branchial cleft cyst (branchiogenic carcinoma).
■ Criteria for the diagnosis of a branchiogenic carcinoma include:
The metastatic tumor occurs along the line extending from a point anterior to the tragus along the anterior border of the sternocleidomastoid muscle to the clavicle.
Histology supports origin from a branchial cleft-derived structure.
Histology supports carcinoma arising in the wall of an epithelial-lined cyst.
A minimum of 5-year follow-up demonstrates no evidence of a primary source for this neoplasm.
■ Despite the fulfillment of these criteria, it is highly unlikely that carcinoma arises in a branchial cleft cyst; rather, all these cystic squamous cell carcinomas take origin from a primary tumor in Waldeyer's tonsillar ring; the neoplasm may be so small as to defy clinical detection, but nevertheless is capable of metastasizing.

Pathology

Histology

■ Lymph node is partially or entirely replaced by an epithelial-lined structure with central cystic change.
■ The epithelium varies from areas that are bland, composed of uniform cells lacking pleomorphism, crowding, or loss of polarity, to overtly malignant-appearing epithelium composed of pleomorphic cells with increased cellularity, mitoses, and a loss of polarity.

Differential Diagnosis

■ Metastatic carcinoma from another primary source.

Treatment and Prognosis

■ Treatment modalities are not fixed and are dependent on the clinical stage, location of the lymph node involved, and histologic appearance of the tumor:
Single mobile lymph node in submaxillary, subdigastric, or midjugular regions—neck dissection preferred over radiotherapy due to exposure and complications of radiation to the oral cavity, pharyngeal, and laryngeal mucosae.
Single mobile lymph node in the posterior cervical region—radiotherapy with fields including the nasopharynx, tonsillar fossa, and base of tongue.
Multiple mobile ipsilateral or bilateral lymph nodes—radiotherapy.
Large fixed lymph nodes—neck dissection or radiotherapy to the entire neck.
■ The single most important factor in prognosis is the clinical stage.
■ Other factors that correlate with prognosis include:
Location of the lymph node: supraclavicular nodal involvement has a poor prognosis.
Histologic appearance: metastatic adenocarcinomas have worse survival rates.

Additional Facts

■ It is extremely uncommon for a primary salivary gland neoplasm to manifest as a metastatic tumor in a cervical neck lymph node without a clinically apparent mass at the site of origin.
■ In the head and neck, difficulty in histologically classifying a given tumor or the presence of an unusual histologic appearance should alert the pathologist to the possibility that the neoplasm represents a metastasis from a distant site.
■ Along with the metastatic cystic squamous cell carcinoma, the other metastatic tumor with a histologic appearance virtually identifying the tissue of origin is the undifferentiated carcinoma of the nasopharynx.
■ The most common primary site for a metastatic tumor originating from below the clavicle is the lungs; virtually every other organ may be the primary focus of a metastasis to the head and neck.

References

Luna MA: The occult primary and metastatic tumors to and from the head and neck. *In*: Barnes L, ed. Surgical pathology of the head and neck. Marcel Dekker, New York; 1985; pp 1211–1232.

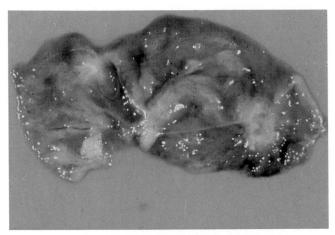

Figure 9–88. Metastatic cystic squamous cell carcinoma, appearing as multiple, tan-yellow, firm nodules in association with a cystic-appearing tissue specimen.

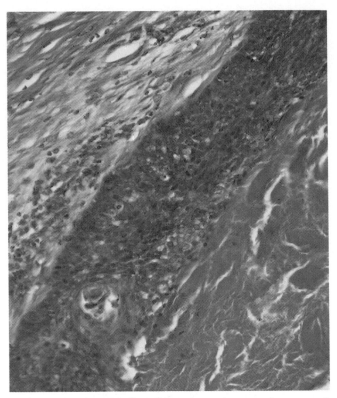

Figure 9–90. The epithelium lining the cystic spaces is composed of a hypercellular and pleomorphic cell population, with loss of polarity and increased mitotic activity.

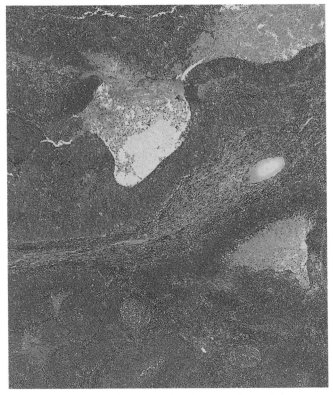

Figure 9–89. Histologic appearance of metastatic cystic squamous cell carcinoma, showing a lymph node that is replaced by epithelial-lined structures with central cystic change.

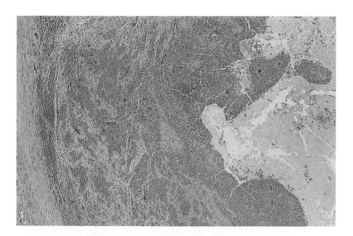

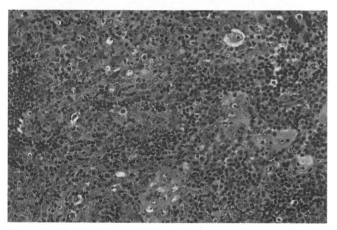

Figure 9–91. *(Top)* Typical histologic picture of metastatic cystic squamous cell carcinoma presenting as an occult neck mass. Endoscopic evaluation failed to detect a primary source for this tumor, and a diagnosis of a carcinoma arising in a branchial cyst (bronchogenic carcinoma) was suggested. *(Bottom)* Three months after removal of the neck mass, biopsy of the nasopharynx revealed an undifferentiated carcinoma, which represented the source of the metastasis.

CHAPTER 10

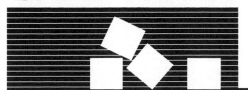

TNM Classification of Oral Cavity, Oropharyngeal, and Nasopharyngeal Tumors

LIP AND ORAL CAVITY
OROPHARYNX

1. T = extent of the primary tumor.
   - Includes both the clinical (T) and pathologic (pT) categories.
   - T designation varies according to the anatomic site involved.

LIP AND ORAL CAVITY

TX — primary tumor cannot be assessed.
T0 — no evidence of primary tumor.
Tis — carcinoma in situ.
T1 — tumor 2 cm or less in greatest dimension.
T2 — tumor more than 2 cm but not more than 4 cm in greatest dimension.
T3 — tumor more than 4 cm in greatest dimension.
T4 — tumor invades adjacent structures (tongue, skin of neck, and through cortical bone).

OROPHARYNX

TX — primary tumor cannot be assessed.
T0 — no evidence of primary tumor.
Tis — carcinoma in situ.
T1 — tumor 2 cm or less in greatest dimension.
T2 — tumor more than 2 cm but not more than 4 cm in greatest dimension.
T3 — tumor more than 4 cm in greatest dimension.
T4 — tumor invades adjacent structures (soft tissues of the neck, deep muscles of the tongue, and through cortical bone).

NASOPHARYNX

TX — primary tumor cannot be assessed.
T0 — no evidence of primary tumor.
Tis — carcinoma in situ.
T1 — tumor limited to one subsite of the nasopharynx.
T2 — tumor invades more than one subsite of the nasopharynx.
T3 — tumor invades nasal cavity or oropharynx.
T4 — tumor invades skull or cranial nerves.

NASOPHARYNX
CLINICAL STAGE

2. N = absence/presence and extent of regional lymph node metastasis; includes both the clinical (N) and pathologic (pN) categories.

NX — regional lymph nodes cannot be assessed.
N0 — no regional lymph node metastasis.
N1 — metastasis in a single ipsilateral lymph node, 3 cm or less in greatest dimension.
N2 — metastasis in a single ipsilateral lymph node, more than 3 cm but not more than 6 cm in greatest dimension *or* metastasis in multiple ipsilateral lymph nodes none more than 6 cm in greatest dimension *or* metastasis in bilateral or contralateral lymph nodes none more than 6 cm in greatest dimension.

- N2a — metastasis in a single ipsilateral lymph node, more than 3 cm but not more than 6 cm in greatest dimension.
- N2b — metastasis in multiple ipsilateral lymph nodes, none more than 6 cm in greatest dimension.
- N2c — metastasis in bilateral or contralateral lymph nodes, none more than 6 cm in greatest dimension.

N3 — metastasis in a lymph node more than 6 cm in greatest dimension.

3. M = absence or presence of distant metastasis; includes both the clinical (M) and pathologic (pM) categories.

MX — not assessed.
M0 — no distant metastasis.
M1 — distant metastasis present.
R — residual tumor.
R0 — no residual tumor.
R1 — microscopic residual tumor.
R2 — macroscopic residual tumor.

CLINICAL STAGE

Stage I   — T1N0M0.
Stage II — T2N0M0.
Stage III — T3N0M0 or T1–T3N1M0.
Stage IV — T4N0M0 or T4N1M0.
         — Any T, N2 or N3, M0.
         — Any T, any N, M1.

References

Spiessl B, Beahrs OH, Hermanek P, Hutter RVP, Scheibe O, Sobin LH, Wagner G (eds): TNM atlas: illustrated guide to the TNM/PTNM-classification of malignant tumours, 3rd ed. Berlin, Springer-Verlag; 1989.

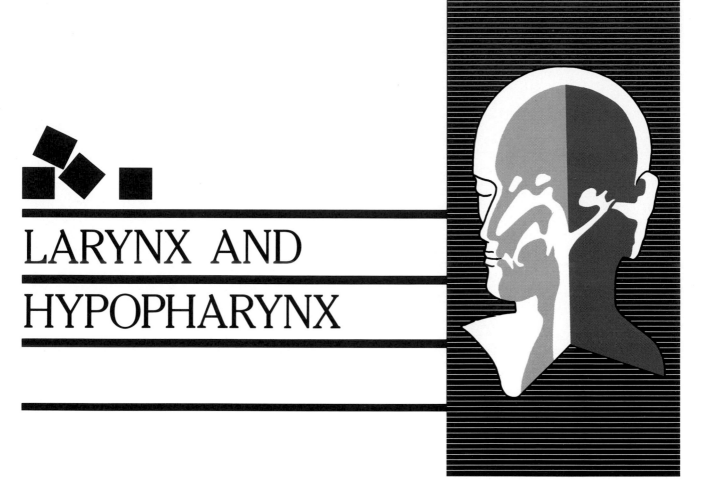

LARYNX AND HYPOPHARYNX

CHAPTER 11

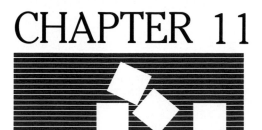

Anatomy and Histology

LARYNX

Anatomic Borders

- Superior: tip of epiglottis.
- Inferior: inferior rim of the cricoid cartilage.
- Anterior: lingual surface of epiglottis (vallecula), thyrohyoid membrane, anterior commissure, thyroid cartilage, cricothyroid membrane, and the anterior arch of the cricoid.
- Posterior: posterior commissure, arytenoid and interarytenoid space, and the mucoperichondrium overlying the cricoid cartilage.
- Lateral: aryepiglottic folds.

Anatomic Compartments

- Supraglottis: extends from the tip of the epiglottis to a horizontal line passing through the apex of the ventricle; structures included in this compartment are the epiglottis (lingual and laryngeal aspects), aryepiglottic folds, arytenoids, false vocal cords, and the ventricle.
   Supraglottic larynx arises from the third and fourth branchial arches.
- Glottis: extends from the ventricle to approximately 0.5 to 1.0 cm below the free level of the true vocal cord and includes the anterior and posterior commissures and the true vocal cord.
- Subglottis: extends from approximately 0.5 to 1.0 cm below the level of the true vocal cord to the inferior rim of the cricoid cartilage.
   Glottis and subglottic larynx arise from the sixth branchial arch.

Histology

- A nonkeratinizing, stratified squamous epithelium lines the epiglottis and true vocal cord.

- A pseudostratified, ciliated respiratory epithelium lines the false vocal cord, ventricle, subglottis.
- Seromucous glands are found in the lower two thirds of the epiglottis and in the ventricular submucosa.
- Thyroid, cricoid, and arytenoid cartilages are hyaline-type cartilage.
- Epiglottis, cuneiform, and corniculate cartilages are elastic-type cartilage.

Facts Regarding the Normal and Aged Larynx

A "transitional"-type epithelium is present between the ventricular epithelium and the true vocal cord epithelium; this transitional epithelium may be misdiagnosed as a dysplasia.

Deep to the true vocal cord lies the vocal cord ligament; biopsy specimens taken in this anatomic location may include the vocal cord ligament, which, if unrecognized, may be misdiagnosed as a myxoma or peripheral nerve sheath neoplasm.

The articulations between the various laryngeal joints are synovial in type and may be involved by an arthritic process.

The hyaline cartilage components of the larynx may calcify or ossify with age; this is a normal aging process in the larynx and, if traumatized, may result in a fractured larynx.

HYPOPHARYNX

- The pharynx is divided into three parts: nasopharynx, oropharynx, and hypopharynx; in this section, only the hypopharynx is discussed.

Anatomic Borders

- Superior: just above the level of the hyoid bone.
- Inferior: lower border of the cricoid cartilage.

205

- Anterior: mucosa on the medial surface of the thyroid cartilage.
- Posterior and lateral: no markings—lateral walls attach to the hyoid bone and thyroid cartilage.
- Medial: larynx and its appendages.
- Pyriform sinus: part of the hypopharynx that expands bilaterally and forward around the sides of the larynx and lies between the larynx and the thyroid cartilage.

Histology

- The epithelium of the hypopharynx is a nonkeratinizing, stratified squamous epithelium.
- Seromucous glands are seen throughout the submucosa.

References

Fawcett DW: The larynx. *In:* Fawcett DW, ed. Bloom and Fawcett: a textbook of histology, 11th ed. Philadelphia: W.B. Saunders Co., 1986; pp 734–735.

Hollinshead WH: The pharynx and larynx. *In:* Hollinshead WH, ed. Anatomy for surgeons, vol. 1, 3rd ed. Philadelphia: Harper & Row, 1982; pp 389–441.

Moore KL: The branchial apparatus and the head and neck. *In:* Moore ML, ed. The developing human: clinically oriented embryology, 4th ed. Philadelphia: W.B. Saunders Co., 1988; pp 170–206.

Moore KL: The respiratory system. *In:* Moore ML, ed. The developing human: clinically oriented embryology, 4th ed. Philadelphia: W.B. Saunders Co., 1988; pp 207–216.

Warwick R, Williams PL: Respiratory system and larynx. *In:* Warwick R, Williams PL, eds. Gray's anatomy, 35th British ed. Philadelphia: W.B. Saunders Co., 1973; pp 1172–1183.

CHAPTER 12

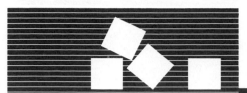

Classification of Non-neoplastic Lesions and Neoplasms of the Larynx and Hypopharynx

NON-NEOPLASTIC LESIONS

Table 12–1
CLASSIFICATION OF LARYNGEAL/
HYPOPHARYNGEAL NON-NEOPLASTIC LESIONS

Congenital and developmental abnormalities
Vocal cord nodules
Laryngocele
Amyloidosis
Contact ulcer
Subglottic stenosis
Epithelial cysts
Reactive epithelial hyperplasia
Dysplastic epithelial changes
Infectious diseases
Others

Table 12–2
CLASSIFICATION OF LARYNGEAL/
HYPOPHARYNGEAL NEOPLASMS

I. Benign
  A. Epithelial
     Squamous papilloma (papillomatosis)
     Minor salivary gland tumors:
        Adenoma (benign mixed tumor)
        Oncocytoma
  B. Mesenchymal/neuroectodermal
     Granular cell tumor
     Chondroma
     Rhabdomyoma
     Hemangioma
     Neurilemmoma/neurofibroma
     Leiomyoma
     Fibrous histiocytoma
     Lipoma
     Paraganglioma

NEOPLASMS

Table 12–2
Continued

II. Malignant
  A. Epithelial
     Squamous cell carcinoma, including:
        "Conventional-type" (in situ; invasive)
        Spindle cell or sarcomatoid
        Exophytic/papillary
     Verrucous carcinoma
     Basaloid squamous cell carcinoma
     Adenosquamous carcinoma
     Minor salivary gland tumors
        Adenoid cystic carcinoma
        Mucoepidermoid carcinoma
  B. Neuroectodermal
     Neuroendocrine carcinoma including:
        Well-differentiated (carcinoid)
        Moderately differentiated (atypical carcinoid)
        Poorly differentiated (small cell carcinoma)
     Malignant melanoma
  C. Mesenchymal
     Chondrosarcoma
     Synovial sarcoma
     Fibrosarcoma/malignant fibrous histiocytoma
     Malignant schwannoma
     Liposarcoma
     Rhabdomyosarcoma
     Angiosarcoma/Kaposi's sarcoma
     Leiomyosarcoma
     Lymphoproliferative (non-Hodgkin's and Hodgkin's lymphomas; extramedullary plasmacytoma)
  D. Metastatic neoplasms to the larynx
     Renal cell carcinoma
     Malignant melanoma
     Others

CHAPTER 13

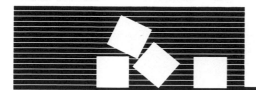

Non-neoplastic Lesions of the Larynx

1. VOCAL CORD NODULES AND POLYPS

Definition: Non-neoplastic stromal reactive process related to inflammation or trauma.

Synonyms: Screamer's, singer's, or preacher's nodules; corditis nodosa.

Clinical

A. Nodules

■ No sex predilection; may be seen in all age groups, but commonly occurs in children and young adults.
■ Usually bilateral, involving the anterior or middle third of the true vocal cord.
■ Follows chronic voice abuse.

B. Polyps

■ No sex predilection; occurs in any age group.
■ Single lesion arising from the true vocal cords, but may take origin from the adjacent ventricular area.
■ Follows voice abuse, infection (laryngitis), alcohol, smoking, or endocrine dysfunction (hypothyroidism).
■ Irrespective of terminology, the symptoms related to both vocal cord polyps and nodules are similar and include hoarseness or voice changes ("breaking" of the voice).
■ The point of maximal vibratory impact in the vocal cord is in the middle third of the true vocal cord (membraneous cord), which represents the most common site for polyps or nodules to occur.

Pathology

Gross

■ Fusiform swelling, sessile or a pedunculated lesion(s) with a soft, rubbery or firm consistency and a white to red to glistening appearance, measuring from a few millimeters to several centimeters.

Histology

■ Four histologic subtypes:
  1. Edematous-myxoid—submucosal accumulation of pale blue to pink material admixed with a sparsely cellular and variably vascularized stroma.
  2. Fibrous—moderately cellular submucosa consisting of uniform oval to spindle-shaped cells associated with a varying amount of fibrous tissue deposition.
  3. Vascular—submucosa is marked by prominent, dilated vascular spaces with or without associated hemorrhage.
  4. Hyaline—dense eosinophilic submucosal deposition of fibrin material, often closely apposed to vascular spaces.
■ The overlying epithelium may be atrophic, hyperplastic, keratotic, and, rarely, dysplastic or malignant.
■ Histochemistry: negative staining for amyloid, which may include Congo red, crystal violet, or Thioflavin T.

Differential Diagnosis

■ Myxoma (Chapter 4A, #9).
■ Amyloidosis (Chapter 13, #4).

Treatment

■ Voice therapy (nodule).
■ Surgery (polyp).

Additional Facts

■ The pathologic process occurs in Reinke's space, the area lying deep to the true vocal cord that is essentially devoid of blood vessels, and in response to injury has a tendency to accumulate fluid.
■ The histologic changes represent different tissue reactions to the initiating event and do not represent progressive (sequential) changes.
■ True myxomas are rarely encountered in the larynx.
■ The hyaline-type vocal cord nodule may be misinterpreted as amyloid deposition; however, staining for amyloid differentiates between these entities.
■ Infrequently, hypothyroidism may cause vocal cord edema, which may progress to formation of a myxoid polyp.

References

Ash JE, Schwartz L: The laryngeal (vocal cord) node. Trans Am Acad Opthalmol Otolaryngol 48:323–332, 1944.

Epstein SS, Winston P, Friedmann I, Ormerod FC: The vocal cord polyp. J Laryngol Otol 71:673–688, 1957.

Kambic V, Radsel Z, Zargi M, Acko M: Vocal cord polyps: incidence, histology and pathogenesis. J Laryngol Otol 95:609–618, 1981.

Kleinsasser O: Pathogenesis of vocal cord polyps. Ann Otol Rhinol Laryngol 91:378–381, 1982.

Rubin HJ, Lehroff I: Pathogenesis and treatment of vocal nodules. J Speech Hear Disord 27:150–161, 1962.

Sena T, Brady S, Huvos AG, Spiro RH: Laryngeal myxoma. Arch Otolaryngol Head Neck Surg 117:430–432, 1991.

Strong MS, Vaughn CW: Vocal cord nodules and polyps—the role of surgical treatment. Laryngoscope 81:911–923, 1971.

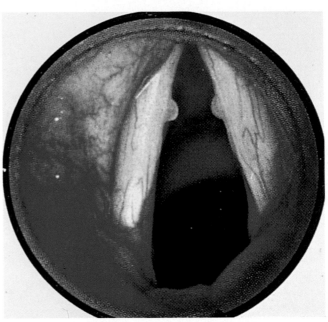

Figure 13–1. Vocal cord nodules, as represented by virtually identical bilateral masses along the true vocal cords.

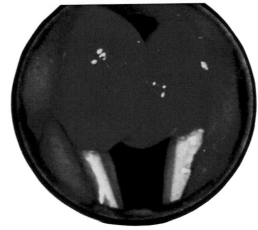

Figure 13–2. Large, beefy-red, bilateral vocal cord polyps of the hemorrhagic type.

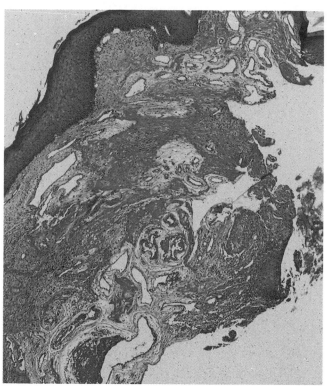

Figure 13–3. Vascular-hyaline vocal cord polyp, characterized by submucosal dilated vascular spaces and deposition of dense eosinophilic fibrin material closely apposed to vascular spaces. The hyaline subtype may be mistaken for amyloid deposition but does not stain for amyloid.

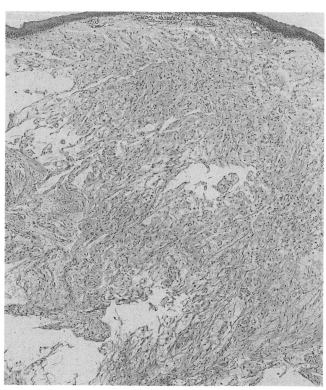

Figure 13–5. The histologic appearance of the edematous-myxoid type of vocal cord polyp appears as submucosal accumulation of pale blue to pink material admixed with a variably cellular and a vascularized stroma.

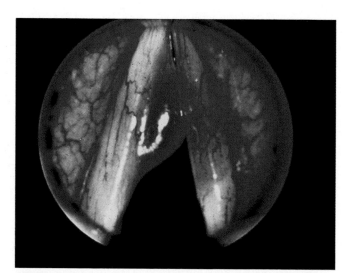

Figure 13–4. Unilateral, glistening, edematous-myxoid type of vocal cord polyp.

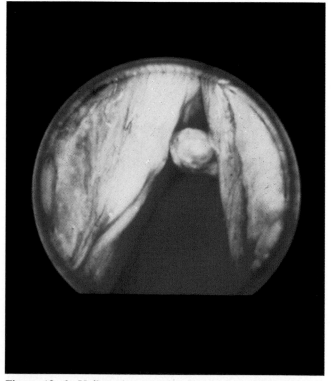

Figure 13–6. Unilateral, tan-white fibrous type of vocal cord polyp.

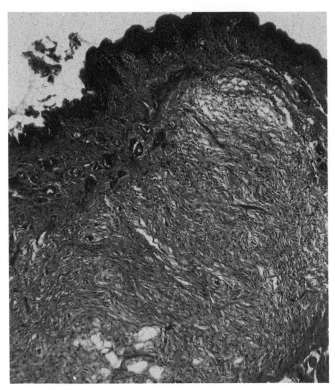

Figure 13–7. The histologic appearance of the fibrous type of vocal cord polyp appears as a moderately cellular submucosal proliferation of uniform, spindle-shaped cells associated with fibrous tissue deposition.

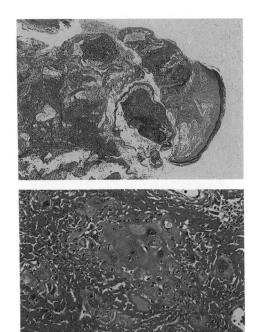

Figure 13–8. (*Top*), Example of a vascular-hyaline vocal cord polyp that was associated with an infiltrating squamous cell carcinoma. (*Bottom*) Nests of infiltrating squamous cell carcinoma were seen within the hyalinized stroma.

2. LARYNGOCELE

Definition: Abnormal dilatation of the saccule (appendix of the ventricle) containing air and maintaining an open communication with the laryngeal lumen.

Clinical

■ Affects men more than women; most common in the fifth to eighth decades of life.

■ The majority of cases are unilateral, but may be bilateral in up to 25% of patients.

■ Symptoms include hoarseness, coughing, a lateral neck mass that fluctuates with changes in intralaryngeal pressure and is compressible, dyspnea, or dysphagia.

■ Infected laryngoceles (laryngopyolocele) are associated with pain and tenderness.

■ The diagnosis of laryngocele is a clinical one.

■ Three types of laryngoceles are identified:
  1. Internal laryngocele—dilatation confined to the intrinsic larynx.
  2. External laryngocele—dilated sac projects upward between the false vocal cord and the thyroid cartilage and laterally through the thyrohyoid ligament.
  3. Both internal and external.

■ Etiology: congenital or acquired; acquired laryngoceles are related to occupation and include those professions in which there is a tendency to excessively increase intralaryngeal pressures, which may result in the development of a laryngocele (glassblowers, musicians, and weight lifters).

■ 15% of patients with a laryngocele may have a coexistent squamous cell carcinoma.

Pathology

Gross

■ Not as impressive as the clinical presentation; resected specimen is a smooth-surfaced, sac-like structure that may be devoid of fluid or, if infected, may contain pus.

Histology

■ Respiratory epithelial-lined (ciliated, columnar) cyst with a fibrous wall.
■ Squamous metaplasia may be seen focally or, if infected, may completely replace the respiratory epithelium; in the latter, a chronic inflammatory cell infiltrate may be seen in the wall of the cyst.
■ Oncocytic metaplasia of the lining epithelium or minor salivary glands may be seen.

Differential Diagnosis

■ Branchial cleft cyst (Chapter 8, #1).
■ Oncocytic papillary cystadenoma (Chapter 19A, #2a).
■ Laryngeal cysts: ductal cysts and saccular cysts.

Treatment

■ Asymptomatic cases require no treatment; however, surgery may be necessary in those cases that become large and symptomatic.
■ Complications associated with laryngoceles include airway obstruction and infection (laryngopyolocele); in the latter, initial treatment is by incision and drainage, followed by antibiotic therapy and then surgical excision after the infection has been controlled.
■ Rare complications include vocal cord paralysis and death due to asphyxia.

Additional Facts

■ Despite clinical assurance of a diagnosis of a laryngocele, prudent therapy would include laryngoscopic examination in order to rule out the presence of a neoplasm.

References

Canalis RF, Maxwell DS, Hemenway CW: Laryngocele—an updated review. J Otolaryngol 6:191–199, 1977.

Celin SE, Johnson J, Curtin H, Barnes L: The association of laryngoceles with squamous cell carcinoma of the larynx. Laryngoscope 101:529–536, 1991.

DeSanto LW: Laryngocele, laryngeal mucocele, large saccules and large saccular cysts: a developmental spectrum. Laryngoscope 84:1291–1296, 1974.

Micheau C, Luboinski B, Lanchi P, Cachin Y: Relationship between laryngoceles and laryngeal carcinomas. Laryngoscope 88:680–688, 1978.

Tucker HM: Degenerative disorders of the larynx. In: Tucker HM, ed. The larynx. New York: Thieme, 1987; pp 209–220.

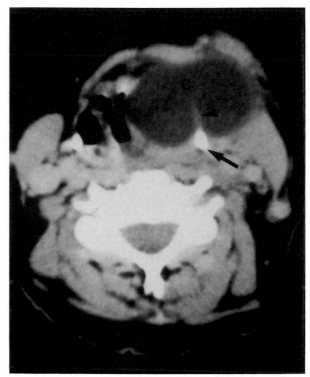

Figure 13-9. Axial CT, enhanced, mixed internal and external laryngocele: large, fluid-filled cyst (c) straddling the thyrohyoid ligament (*arrowhead*) and thyroid cartilage (*arrow*). The wall does not enhance after the administration of intravenous contrast. (Courtesy of Philip Trotta, M.D., Barnes Hospital, St. Peters, MO.)

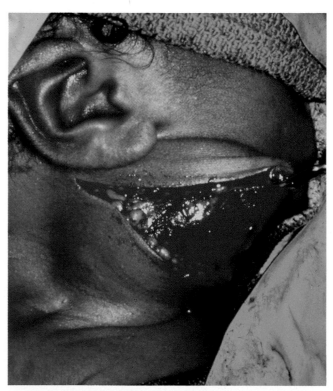

Figure 13-10. Laryngocele that has resulted in a large neck mass, seen as a subcutaneous bulging mass at surgery.

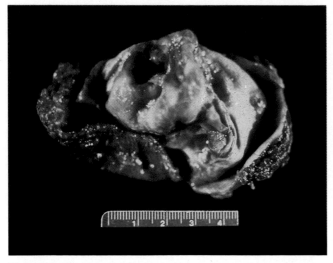

Figure 13-11. Resected laryngocele—smooth-walled cystic structure that contained clear fluid before its puncture.

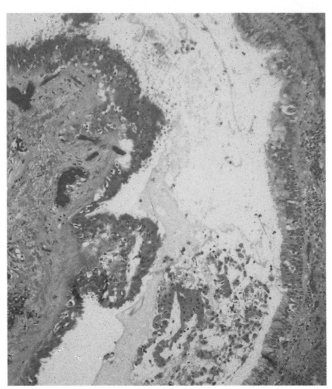

Figure 13-12. The histologic picture of a laryngocele is less dramatic than its clinical presentation and is characterized by a ciliated respiratory epithelial-lined cyst filled with clear to pink-appearing fluid. Note the oncocytic cytoplasmic changes in the epithelia to the left of midline, representing a metaplastic process.

3. CONTACT ULCERS OF THE LARYNX

Definition: Benign, tumor-like condition, occurring most commonly along the posterior aspect of one or both vocal cords.

Synonyms: Pyogenic granuloma of the larynx.

Clinical

■ Affect men more than women; occur over a wide age range and, although generally seen in the adult population, not restricted to any specific age group.
■ Most common site of occurrence is along the posterior aspect of one or both vocal cords; uncommon sites include the middle third or anterior portions of the true vocal cords.
■ Wide variety of symptoms: hoarseness, dysphagia, sore throat, dysphonia, difficulty breathing, choking, pain.
■ Duration of symptoms may be from weeks to years.
■ Etiologic factors include: 1) vocal abuse (shouting, persistent coughing, or throat clearing), 2) acid regurgitation secondary to hiatal hernia, 3) postintubational trauma.

Pathology

Gross

■ Ulcerated, polypoid, nodular, or fungating mass with a beefy red to tan-white appearance, ranging in size up to 3 cm in diameter.

Histology

■ Most often an ulcerated lesion with associated fibrinoid necrosis, granulation tissue, acute and chronic inflammation.
■ As a result of recurrent (chronic) disease, the lesion may demonstrate a hyperplastic epithelium with no ulcerative component.
■ Additional histologic findings may include giant cells, marked vascular proliferation, and spindle cells (fibroblasts).

Differential Diagnosis

■ Infectious disease(s).
■ Squamous carcinoma (Chapter 14B, #1).
■ Spindle cell carcinoma (Chapter 14B, #2).
■ Vascular neoplasms—lobular capillary heman-

gioma (Chapter 4A,#2), angiosarcoma (Chapter 4B, #9), Kaposi's sarcoma (Chapter 9B, #9).

Treatment

■ Identify and treat (nonsurgically) the underlying cause.

Additional Facts

■ Although the majority of contact ulcers occur along the posterior vocal cords, other vocal cord sites may be affected.
■ Propensity for contact ulcers to occur along the posterior vocal cords include:
　Posterior vocal cord experiences the greatest excursion during opening and closing of the glottis.
　Mucoperichondrium overlying the posterior vocal cord is extremely thin and prone to trauma.
■ Squamous cell carcinoma occurring in the posterior vocal cord area is decidedly uncommon.
■ Postintubational contact ulcers tend to occur more frequently in women as a result of the smaller luminal diameter seen in women.

References

Ward PH, Zwitman D, Hanson D, Berci G: Contact ulcers and granulomas of the larynx: new insights into their etiology as a basis for more rational treatment. Otolaryngol Head Neck Surg 88:262–269, 1980.

Wenig BM, Heffner DK: Contact ulcers of the larynx: a reacquaintance with the pathology of an often underdiagnosed entity. Arch Pathol Lab Med 114:825–828, 1990.

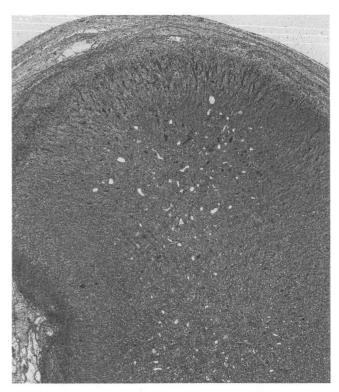

Figure 13–14. Histology of CUL includes a morphologic appearance similar to that of lobular capillary hemangioma, as seen by this polypoid, ulcerated lesion with associated granulation tissue and inflammation.

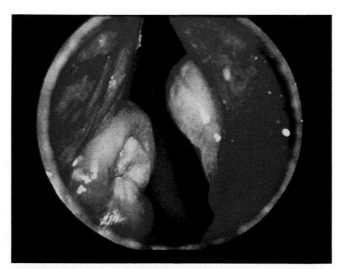

Figure 13–13. Contact ulcers of the larynx (CUL), as depicted by bilateral polypoid and focally ulcerated, tan-white masses along the posterior aspect of the vocal cords.

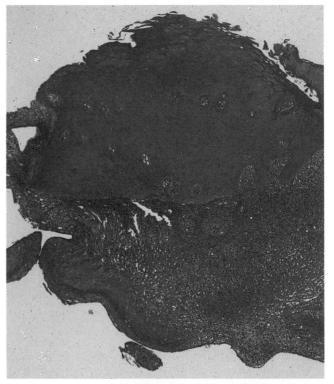

Figure 13–15. As a result of recurrent (chronic) disease, this CUL demonstrates a hyperplastic squamous epithelium, associated with fibrinoid necrosis and a marked inflammatory component.

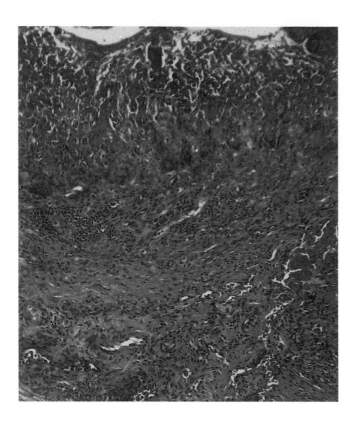

Figure 13–16. Additional histologic findings in CUL may include giant cells, vascular proliferation, or a spindlecell (fibroblasts) component; these findings may be prominent, necessitating differentiation from an infectious process, a vascular neoplasm, or a spindle-cell neoplasm (carcinoma, sarcoma).

4. AMYLOIDOSIS

Definition: Extracellular accumulation of fibrillar proteins identified in association with a variety of clinical settings and occurring in a variety of tissue sites.

Clinical

■ Amyloidosis may manifest in several forms and, in decreasing order of frequency, includes systemic amyloidosis (primary and secondary), multiple myeloma-associated amyloidosis, localized or solitary amyloidosis, and familial amyloidosis.
■ In the head and neck, amyloid generally is localized or solitary in form.
■ Amyloidosis can affect almost every head and neck site, but the most common sites of occurrence are the larynx and tongue.

Laryngeal Amyloidosis

■ Affects men more than women; occurs in the fifth to sixth decades of life.
■ The most common complaint is hoarseness.
■ Can affect any portion of the larynx, but most frequently is seen along the true vocal cord.

Pathology

Gross

■ Mucosal covered, firm, tan-yellow to gray, polypoid mass (glottis and supraglottis) or diffuse swelling (subglottis).

Histology

■ Extracellular eosinophilic, acellular, amorphous material deposited randomly throughout the submucosa; generally does not alter the appearance of the surface epithelium.
■ The deposition is often seen around blood vessels ("angiocentric") or within the walls of vascular spaces without producing vascular compromise.
■ Submucosal deposition of amyloid results in the disappearance of the seromucous glands.
■ An associated chronic inflammatory infiltrate, including plasma cells, lymphocytes, and histiocytes may be seen; often, a foreign body-type giant-cell reaction is identified.
■ Histochemistry: stains for amyloid (Congo red, crystal violet, thioflavin-T) are positive; apple-green birefringence is seen under polarized light with Congo red staining.

- Electronmicroscopy: nonbranching fibrils varying in size from 50 to 150 Å in diameter.

Differential Diagnosis

- Vocal cord nodules/polyps of the hyalinized type (Chapter 13, #1).
- Lipoid proteinosis (see below).

Treatment and Prognosis

- Local endoscopic resection is curative.

Additional Facts

- Although laryngeal amyloidosis is generally a solitary lesion, up to 15% of patients may have amyloid deposition in other head and neck sites (trachea, bronchus, tongue).
- In contrast to laryngeal amyloidosis, lingual amyloidosis is frequently a target organ as part of primary systemic amyloidosis or myeloma-related amyloidosis; in this setting there is marked enlargement of the tongue (macroglossia).
- *Lipoid proteinosis (hyalinosis cutis et mucosae):*
  Familial disorder, possibly associated with autosomal recessive inheritence, characterized by amorphous deposits of lipoprotein, primarily in the skin and mucous membranes.
  Clinical features include skin lesions, beady deposits under the eyelid margins, and intracranial (hippocampal gyrus) calcifications as seen by radiography.
  Localized laryngeal involvement may occur, but more often widespread involvement is seen, including the oral cavity and oropharynx.
  Involvement of the larynx results in hoarseness or an abnormal cry (a common sign in infancy); dysphagia may also occur.
  Multinodular growths may be seen in the laryngeal mucosa, which appear as a diffuse deposition of hyaline-like material in submucosal tissues by light microscopy.
  Neutral and acid mucoploysaccharides can be demonstrated by special stains; amyloid stains are negative.
  Endoscopic removal or tracheostomy may be necessary in cases that attain a large size and cause airway obstruction.

References

Barnes EL, Zafar T: Laryngeal amyloidosis: clinicopatholgic study of seven cases. Ann Otol Rhinol Laryngol 86:856–863, 1977.

Kyle RA, Bayrd ED: Amyloidosis: review of 236 cases. Medicine 54:271–299, 1975.

Michaels L, Hyams VJ: Amyloid in localized deposits and plasmacytomas of the respiratory tract. J Pathol 128:29–38, 1979.

Richards SH, Bull PD: Lipoid proteinosis of the larynx. J Laryngol Otol 87:187–190, 1973.

Ryan RE, Pearson BW, Weiland LH: Laryngeal amyloidosis. Trans Am Acad Ophthalmol Otolaryngol 84:872–877, 1977.

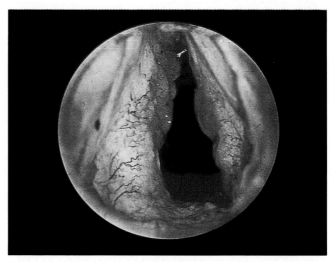

Figure 13–17. Laryngeal amyloidosis, as seen by the presence of mucosal-covered, diffuse swelling in the glottic and subglottic region.

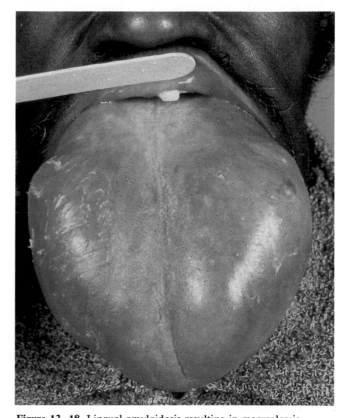

Figure 13–18. Lingual amyloidosis resulting in macroglossia.

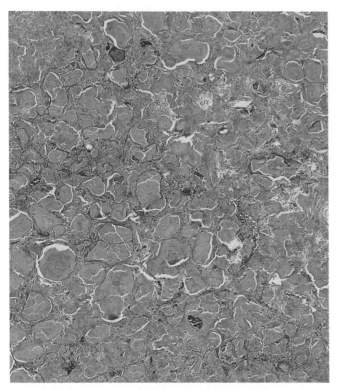

Figure 13–19. Histologic appearance of amyloid deposition, characterized by random deposition of eosinophilic, acellular, amorphous material throughout the submucosa and often around vascular spaces.

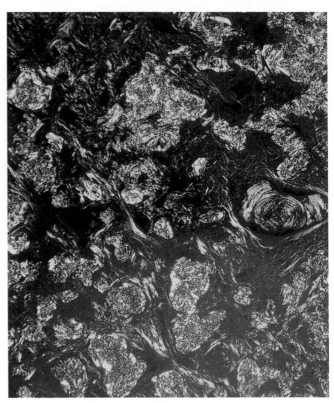

Figure 13–20. Congo red staining for amyloid, showing the characteristic apple-green birefringence.

5. SUBGLOTTIC STENOSIS

Definition: Partial or complete narrowing of the larynx, which may be congenital or acquired.

Clinical

- Relatively rare condition with acquired stenosis, much more common than congenital stenosis.
- No sex predilection; affects all age groups.
- Symptoms relate to airway obstruction with progressive respiratory difficulty, biphasic stridor, dyspnea, and air hunger; other symptoms include hoarseness, abnormal cry, aphonia, dysphagia, and feeding abnormalities.
- In congenital stenosis, symptoms appear at or shortly after birth; in acquired stenosis, usually there is a history of trauma followed by a latent period of 1 month or longer prior to the manifestations of symptoms.
- Etiologies of acquired subglottic stenosis include:
  Trauma: blunt or penetrating trauma, prolonged endotracheal intubation, endotracheal burns, postsurgical, postradiotherapy.
  Neoplasms (carcinoma, sarcomas, others).
  Infectious or autoimmune disease (tuberculosis, syphilis, sarcoidosis, lupus erythematosus, Wegener's granulomatosis, relapsing polychondritis, amyloidosis).
  Idiopathic.
- In both children and adults, trauma is the most common cause of stenosis.
- In cases of subglottic stenosis, complete physical evaluation of the entire upper aerodigestive tract is indicated in order to rule out separate congenital anomalies or other acquired injuries.

Pathology

Gross

- Partial or complete narrowing of the endolaryngeal luminal diameter.
- Depending on the etiologic cause, a mucosal or submucosal mass or submucosal bulging may be seen.

Histology

- The histologic picture is dependent on the cause of the stenosis.
- In idiopathic stenosis, a submucosal fibrous proliferation with associated nonspecific chronic inflammation may be seen; this histologic picture is similar to that of fibromatosis or tumefactive fibroinflammatory lesions identified in the sinonasal tract and may, in fact, represent the same pathologic process.

Differential Diagnosis

- Infectious disease(s).
- Wegener's granulomatosis (Chapter 3, #8).
- Collagen vascular disease(s).
- Neoplasms (clinical).

Treatment and Prognosis

- Treatment is based on the age of the patient, degree of stenosis, and underlying pathology.
- In general, cases of acquired stenosis initially require tracheotomy to establish an airway followed by endoscopic dilatation, laser excision, or external surgical (open excision with reconstruction) management.
- Prognosis is dependent on multiple factors, with the etiologic cause probably the most important:
  Congenital subglottic stenosis is less severe than acquired types, and many patients outgrow their condition, making surgical reconstruction often unnecessary, with management by conservative methods.

Additional Facts

- Congenital stenosis is the third most common laryngeal congenital disorder, preceded by laryngomalacia and vocal cord paralysis.
- Laryngeal Wegener's granulomatosis occurs much more frequently in women and generally affects the larynx (subglottis) only when the disease already affects other, more common sites (sinonasal tract, lungs, genitourinary system).
- A concomitant pseudotumor of the orbit has been seen in association with idiopathic subglottic stenosis; both lesions display identical histologic features.

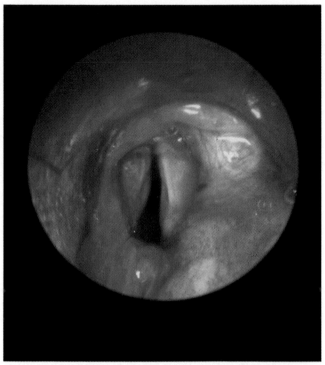

Figure 13–21. Subglottic stenosis, resulting in partial narrowing of the endolaryngeal luminal diameter.

References

Brandenburg JH: Idiopathic subglottic stenosis. Trans Am Acad Ophthalmol Otolaryngol 76:1402–1406, 1972.

Cotton RT, Manuokian JJ: Glottic and subglottic stenosis. *In:* Cummings CW, Frederickson JM, Harker LA, Krause CJ, Schuller DE, eds. Otolaryngology—head and neck surgery. St. Louis: C.V. Mosby Co., 1986; pp 2159–2180.

Hoare TJ, Jayne D, Rhys Evans P, Crofti CB, Howard DJ: Wegener's granulomatosis, subglottic stenosis and anti-neutrophil cytoplasm antibodies. J Laryngol Otol 103:1187–1191, 1989.

Rosenberg HS, Vogler C, Close LG, Warshaw HE: Laryngeal fibromatosis in the neonate. Arch Otolaryngol Head Neck Surg 107:513–517, 1981.

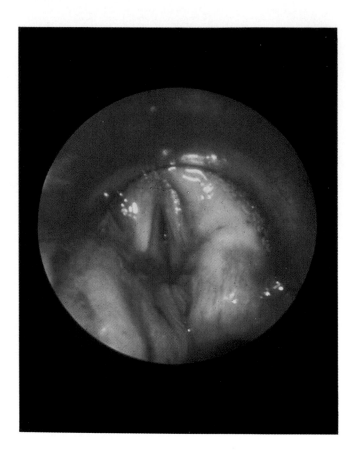

Figure 13–22. Subglottic stenosis, causing complete narrowing of the endolaryngeal lumen.

Figure 13–23. Laryngectomy specimen, showing a tan-white mass bulging into the endolaryngeal lumen at the lower subglottic region (*arrow*).

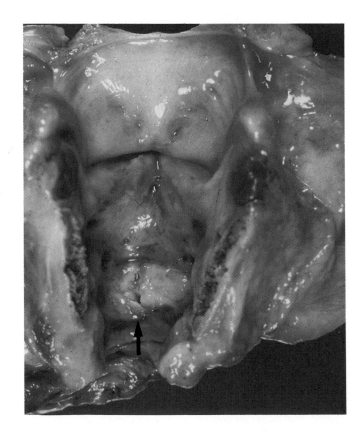

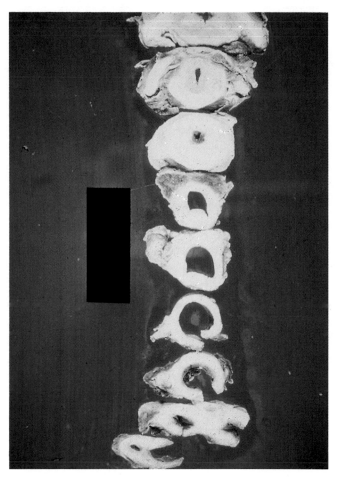

Figure 13–24. Another resected specimen, showing progressive narrowing of the endolaryngeal lumen at the top portion of the photograph; the endotracheal lumen is patent, without compromise of this space.

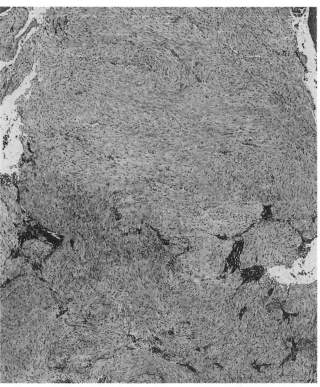

Figure 13–25. Despite the impressive clinical picture, the histology of (idiopathic) subglottic stenosis is remarkably bland, as seen by the presence of a moderately cellular fibroblastic proliferation.

6. LARYNGEAL EPITHELIAL CHANGES

a. Terminology of Epithelial-Associated Changes

■ Leukoplakia — **clinical** term describing any white lesion on a mucous membrane; **not** indicative of underlying malignant tumor.

■ Erythroplakia — **clinical** term describing any red lesion on a mucous membrane; often indicative of an underlying malignant tumor.

■ Hyperplasia — thickening of an epithelial surface as a result of an absolute increase in the number of cells.

■ Pseudoepitheliomatous hyperplasia (PEH) — exuberant reactive or reparative overgrowth of squamous epithelium (hyperplasia) displaying no cytologic evidence of malignancy; frequently associated with granular cell tumor and may be mistaken for an invasive squamous cell carcinoma.

■ Keratosis — presence of keratin on an epithelial suface (**Note:** the use of the term hyperkeratosis is redundant when applied to the larynx, which has a nonkeratinizing epithelium).

■ Parakeratosis — presence of nuclei in the keratin layer.

■ Dyskeratosis — abnormal keratinization of epithelial cells.

■ Ulceration — erosion or loss of the surface epithelium.

■ Metaplasia — change from one histologic tissue type to another; generally occurs as a result of tissue insult or injury.

■ Koilocytosis — descriptive term for cytoplasmic vacuolization of squamous cells; this morphologic

Table 13-1
ABNORMALITIES OF THE SURFACE
EPITHELIUM

Morphologic Change	Pathologic Lesion(s)
Hyperplasia/acanthosis	Benign reactive processes, infections, papillomas, carcinoma
Keratosis/parakeratosis	Benign reactive processes, infections, papillomas, carcinoma
Ulceration or necrosis	Benign reactive processes, infections, polyps, papillomas, carcinoma
Pseudoepitheliomatous hyperplasia	Benign reactive processes, infections, granular cell tumor
Papillary/verrucoid growth	Benign reactive processes, verrucae, papillomas, carcinoma
Koilocytosis	Benign reactive processes, verrucae, papillomas, carcinomas
Dysplasia/atypia	Benign reactive processes, infections/inflammatory conditions, papillomas, carcinoma
Dyskeratosis	Dysplastic lesions; carcinoma
Metaplasia	Benign reactive processes

change is suggestive of viral (Human papillomavirus) infection.
■ Dysplasia or atypia—synonomous terms describing abnormal maturation and cellular aberrations.
■ Carcinoma in situ—full thickness epithelial dysplatic change with an intact basement membrane. (**Note:** as applied to the larynx, carcinoma in situ is not a requirement prior to the developement of an invasive squamous cell carcinoma, which may arise from the basal layer in the absence of overlying dysplastic changes.)
■ Superficially invasive or microscopically invasive squamous cell carcinoma—squamous carcinoma in which there is violation of the basement membrane with invasion into the underlying stroma; the identification of superficial or microinvasive carcinoma is significant, given the presence of vascular spaces high in the lamina propria, so that access to vessels may occur in the face of limited invasion, potentially resulting in metastatic disease.

These morphologic changes may be identified in an array of pathologic lesions and are not necessarily specific for any single disease (Table 13-1).

b. Hyperplastic Epithelial Changes

Definition: Reactive or reparative benign process, reflecting the epithelial response to a stimulus or to injury.

Clinical

■ Affects men more than women; generally limited to the adult population.
■ May occur anywhere in the larynx, but mainly identified along the true vocal cord.
■ The most frequent symptom is hoarseness.
■ Etiologic causes include smoking, alcohol, voice abuse, and chronic inflammation.

Pathology

Gross

■ Array of appearances, including a flat, papillary, or verrucoid lesion with a white (leukoplakic) or red (erythroplakic) appearance.
■ May be localized to a small area of the vocal cord or may be diffuse, involving virtually the entire larynx (pachyderma laryngis).

Histology

The following changes may be an isolated finding; however, multiple changes often occur within a single specimen.

■ Thickening of the surface epithelium by an absolute increase in the number of cells (simple epithelial hyperplasia).
■ Presence of a superficial keratin layer (keratosis) or nuclei in the superficial keratin layer (parakeratosis).
■ Papillary or verrucoid appearance.
■ Presence of keratohyaline granules in the granulosa cell layer.
■ Presence of koilocytosis.
■ Presence of cytologic atypia (see below).
■ Presence of dyskeratosis.

Differential Diagnosis

■ Contact ulcer (Chapter 13, #3).
■ Verruca vulgaris (Chapter 14A, #1).
■ Verrucous carcinoma (Chapter 14B, #3).
■ Well-differentiated ("conventional") squamous cell carcinoma (Chapter 14B, #1).

Treatment

■ Excisional biopsy and close clinical follow-up.
■ If associated etiologic factors are identified, then attempts to control the inciting cause should be attempted.
■ Risk of development of a carcinoma in the face of a hyperplastic process without significant atypia is minimal.

c. Dysplastic Epithelial Changes

Definition: Qualitative alteration in a malignant direction in the appearance of cells.
Synonyms: Atypia.

Clinical

■ Affects males more than females; generally limited to the adult population.
■ Can occur anywhere in the larynx, but majority occur along the anterior portion of the true vocal cord; bilateral involvement seen in approximately 25% of all patients.
■ Hoarseness is the most frequent complaint.

■ Etiologic factors include smoking (single most common cause), alcohol, chronic infections and, less commonly, secondary to voice abuse, environmental/industrial exposure, and vitamin A deficiency.

■ Any degree of dysplasia/atypia short of carcinoma in situ is a potentially reversible process.

Pathology

Gross

■ Localized, circumscribed flat or papillary area with white (leukoplakic), red (erythroplakic), or gray appearance.

Histology

■ Cytologic alterations—increase in the nuclear chromatin (hyperchromasia) with irregularity of distribution, increase in nuclear size relative to the cytoplasm, increased mitoses, and crowding of cells with loss of cellular polarity.

■ Process begins in the basal and parabasal area.

■ Graded as mild, moderate, and severe:

Mild: dysplasia limited to the lower portions or inner third of the epithelium (basal zone dysplasia).

Moderate: dysplasia involves up to two thirds of the thickness of the epithelium.

Severe: dysplasia involves from two thirds to almost complete thickness of the epithelium.

■ Normal maturation of the superficial layers of the epithelium.

■ Intact basement membrane.

■ May be associated with keratosis or dyskeratosis, as well as other hyperplastic epithelial changes.

■ Full-thickness dysplasia (carcinoma in situ) is **not** a prerequisite prior to the development of an invasive squamous cell carcinoma.

Differential Diagnosis

■ Reactive epithelial changes (Chapter 13, #6a).

■ Infectious disease(s).

■ Squamous cell carcinoma (Chapter 14B, #1).

Treatment

■ Excisional biopsy is the treatment of choice.

■ Dysplastic epithelial changes short of carcinoma in situ require no additional treatment; close follow-up of the patient is indicated and, if clinically warranted, rebiopsy may be necessary and should be performed months after any procedure so as to allow adequate healing and less surgical-associated pathologic changes, which may obscure a neoplastic process.

■ Cessation of contributing risk factors should be undertaken.

■ Development of a squamous cell carcinoma from a dysplastic process varies, according to the literature, from 8% to 15% of cases.

■ Statistically, the more severe the dysplasia, the greater the association with the development of carcinoma.

References

Crissman JD: Laryngeal keratosis preceding laryngeal carcinoma: a report of four cases. Arch Otolaryngol 108:445–448, 1982.

Fechner RE: Centennial conference on laryngeal carcinoma. New York: Appleton-Century-Crofts, 1976; pp. 110–115.

Hellquist H, Oloffson J, Grontoft O: Carcinoma in situ and severe dysplasia of the vocal cords: a clinicopathological and photometric investigation. Acta Otolaryngol 92:543–555, 1981.

Hellquist H, Lundgren J, Oloffson J: Hyperplasia, dysplasia and carcinoma in situ of the vocal cords: a follow up study. Clin Otolaryngol 7:11–27, 1982.

McGavran MH, Bauer WC, Ogura JH: Isolated laryngeal keratosis: its relation to carcinoma of the larynx based on a clinicopathologic study of 87 consecutive cases with long-term follow-up. Laryngoscope 70:932–951, 1960.

Sllamniku B, Bauer W, Painter C, Sessions D: The transformation of laryngeal keratosis into invasive cancer. Am J Otolaryngol 10:42–54, 1989.

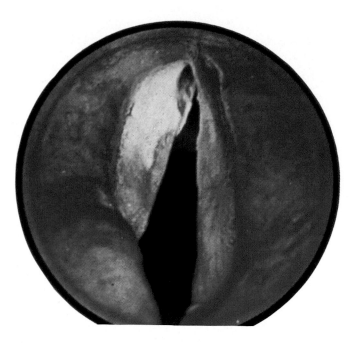

Figure 13-26. Laryngeal leukoplakia, as depicted by the presence of a focal, flat, white lesion along the anterior true vocal cord.

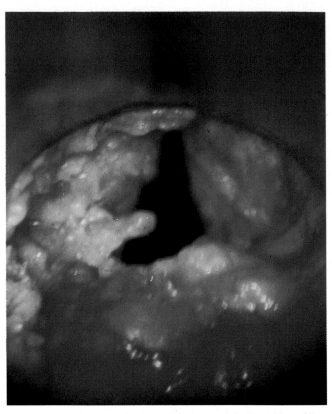

Figure 13-28. Another example of laryngeal leukoplakia, with a papillary or verrucoid appearance.

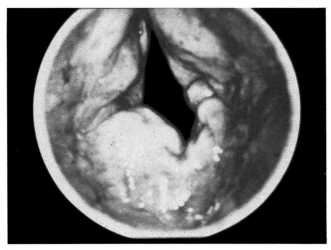

Figure 13-27. Laryngeal leukoplakia; in contrast to the previous example, this lesion is raised and more diffuse in its extent.

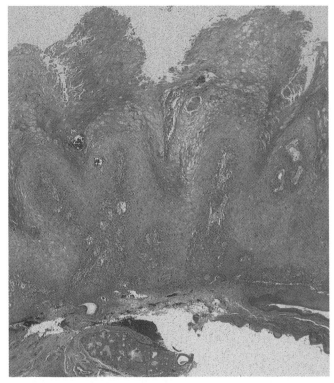

Figure 13-29. Papillary or verrucoid epithelial hyperplasia of the larynx, with marked keratosis without dysplasia.

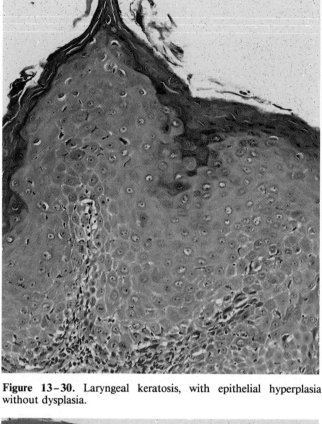

Figure 13-30. Laryngeal keratosis, with epithelial hyperplasia without dysplasia.

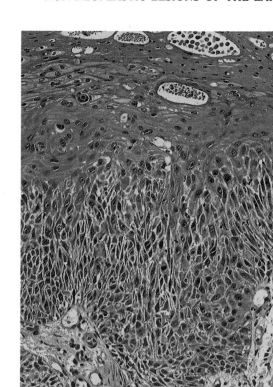

Figure 13-32. Laryngeal biopsy specimen, showing keratosis with moderate dysplasia involving up to two thirds of the thickness of the epithelium; note incidental finding of intraepithelial eosinophilic pooling.

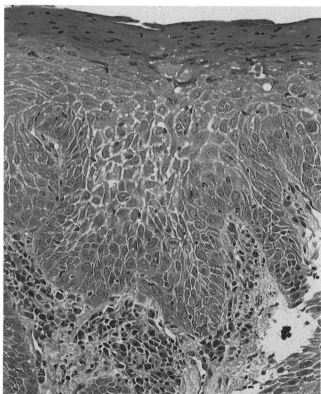

Figure 13-31. Laryngeal biopsy specimen, showing a flat type of keratosis with epithelial hyperplasia and mild dysplasia limited to the basal zone area, characterized by loss of cellular polarity, increase in nuclear size relative to the cytoplasm, and slight increase in the nuclear chromatin.

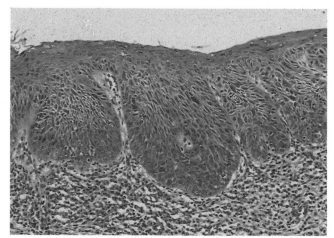

Figure 13-33. Laryngeal biopsy specimen without keratosis, showing severe dysplasia involving greater than two thirds of the thickness of the epithelium (carcinoma in situ). While some degree of maturation is seen at the epithelial surface, the downward growth of the epithelium associated with marked dysplastic changes warrants classification as severe dysplasia even in the absence of dysplastic involvement of the entire epithelium.

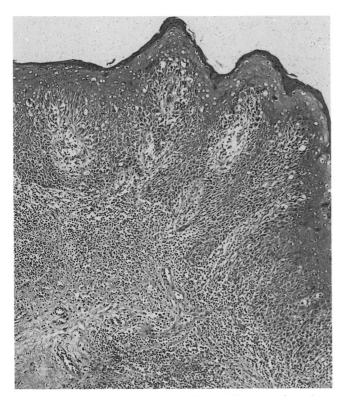

Figure 13-34. Laryngeal biopsy specimen with keratosis and severe dysplasia; although the dysplasia does not involve two thirds or greater of the epithelial surface, this biopsy specimen qualifies as severe dysplasia, given the downward growth of the epithelium, which manifests marked dysplastic changes. This biopsy specimen borders on superficially invasive squamous cell carcinoma.

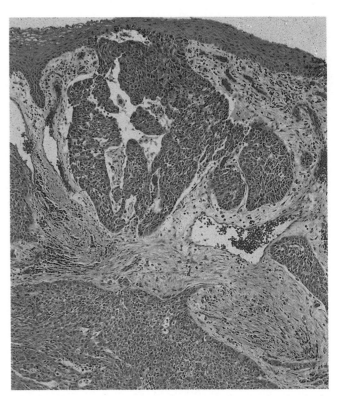

Figure 13-35. Unlike cervical intraepithelial neoplasia, dysplastic changes involving the entire thickness of the epithelium are not a prerequisite prior to the development of an invasive squamous cell carcinoma, as seen in this specimen. An invasive carcinoma arises from the basal zone region of the epithelium without overlying dysplastic epithelial changes.

CHAPTER 14

Neoplasms of the Larynx and Hypopharynx

A. BENIGN NEOPLASMS

1. Laryngeal Papillomatosis

Definition: Benign, exophytic neoplastic growth composed of branching fronds of squamous epithelium with fibrovascular cores.
Synonym: Squamous papilloma.

Clinical

- Most common benign neoplasm occurring in this anatomic region.
- No sex predilection; affects all age groups.
- Single or multiple lesions occurring anywhere in the larynx, but primarily identified along the true and false vocal cords, the anterior commissure, and ventricles.
- Symptoms: changes in phonation, dyspnea, cough, dysphagia, stridor.
- Clinical course correlated to age at onset:
  Juvenile type—often multiple lesions with extensive growth and rapid recurrence; may remit spontaneously or persist into old age.
  Adult type—more often single, recurs less often, and is less likely to spread.

Pathology

Gross

- Exophytic, warty, friable, tan-white to red growth(s).
- A characteristic feature is their ease of bleeding after minor trauma.

Histologic

- Papillary fronds of multilayered benign squamous epithelium containing fibrovascular cores.
- Little or no keratin production.
- Absence of stromal invasion.
- A certain degree of cellular atypia may be seen; however, the presence of severe atypia may be indicative of the development of a squamous carcinoma arising in papillomatosis or may in fact represent an exophytic squamous cell carcinoma.

Differential Diagnosis

- Verruca vulgaris (see below).
- Verrucous carcinoma (Chapter 14B, #3).
- Exophytic squamous cell carcinoma (Chapter 14B, #1).

Treatment and Prognosis

■ Laryngeal papillomatosis is treated by surgical excision, with CO_2 laser surgery the preferred modality; additional modalities used in the treatment of laryngeal papillomatosis, all with essentially equal success rates, include antibiotics, steroids, hormones (estrogen), electrocautery, cryosurgery, radiotherapy, ultrasound, and interferon.

■ Tracheostomy should be avoided if possible and may be complicated by spread of disease into the tracheobronchial tree; however, a tracheostomy may be required in order to maintain a functional airway in as high as 65% of patients.

■ Recurrence of tumor is common, requiring long-term and repeated management.

■ Overall mortality rate is 2% to 14%; extension into the trachea or bronchi occurs in 2% to 15%, and involvement of lower respiratory tract parenchyma is associated with increased mortality rates.

■ In general, treatment should be as conservative as possible; the primary aims of therapy include airway maintanence, voice preservation, and disease eradication.

■ Complications of aggressive management may include laryngoceles, scarring, or stenosis.

■ Radiotherapy is contraindicated because of its associated complications, including laryngeal destruction, scarring and laryngeal stenosis, and risk of inducing malignant transformation.

Additional Facts

■ Overall incidence of developing carcinoma is 2%.

■ Increasing evidence implicates human papillomavirus (HPV) as a major etiologic factor.

■ Only approximately 1% of laryngeal papillomas are associated with tracheal papillomas.

■ *Laryngeal verruca vulgaris:*
  Rare lesion of the larynx; exclusively described in men.
  Histologically similar to verruca vulgaris of the skin and includes a verrucoid appearance, keratosis, prominent granular cell layer, coarse and irregular keratohyaline granules, and thin, pointy rete pegs.

References

Abramson AL, Steinberg BM, Winkler B: Laryngeal papillomatosis: clinical, histologic and molecular studies. Laryngoscope 97:678–685, 1987.

Arends MJ, Wyllie AH, Bird CC: Papillomavirus and human cancer. Hum Pathol 21:686–698, 1990.

Batsakis JG, Raymond AK, Rice DH: The pathology of head and neck tumors: papillomas of the upper respiratory tracts, part 18. Head Neck Surg 5:332–344, 1983.

Braun L, Kashima H, Eggleston J, Shah K: Demonstration of papillomavirus antigen in paraffin sections of laryngeal papillomas. Laryngoscope 92:640–643, 1982.

Fechner RE, Mills SE: Verruca vulgaris of the larynx: a distinctive lesion of probable viral origin confused with verrucous carcinoma. Am J Surg Pathol 6:357–362, 1982.

Gaylis B, Hayden RE: Recurrent respiratory papillomatosis: progression to invasion and malignancy. Am J Otolaryngol 12:104–112, 1991.

Holinger PH, Johnstone KC, Anison GC: Papillomas of the larynx: a review of 109 cases with a preliminary report of aureomycin therapy. Ann Otol Rhinol Laryngol 59:547–564, 1950.

Johnson TL, Plieth DA, Crissman JD, Sarkar FH: HPV detection by polymerase chain reaction (pcr) in verrucous lesions of the upper aerodigestive tract. Mod Pathol 4:461–465, 1991.

Schnadig VJ, Clark WD, Clegg TJ, Yao CS: Invasive papillomatosis and squamous carcinoma complicating juvenile laryngeal papillomatosis. Arch Otolaryngol Head Neck Surg 112:966–971, 1986.

Steinberg B: Human papillomavirus and upper airway oncogenesis. Am J Otolaryngol 11:37–374, 1990.

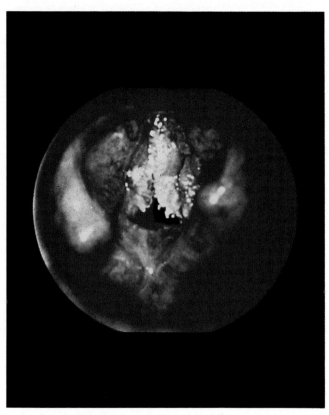

Figure 14–1. Laryngeal papillomatosis, characterized by an exophytic, warty-appearing, tan-white growth.

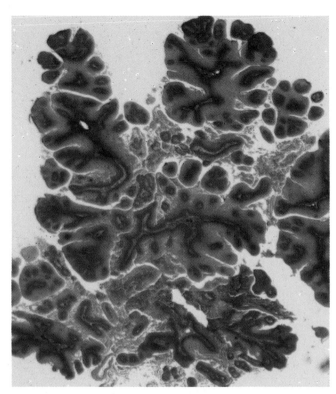

Figure 14–3. Histologic appearance of laryngeal papilloma, characterized by papillary fronds of multilayered benign squamous epithelium that contain fibrovascular cores; no surface keratinization is seen.

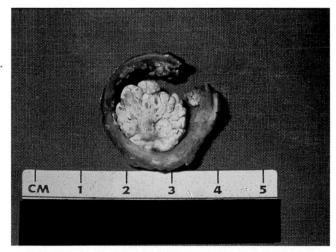

Figure 14–2. Resected portion of larynx, showing the characteristic appearance of a papilloma growing into the lumen and confined to the surface without gross evidence of an endophytic growth phase.

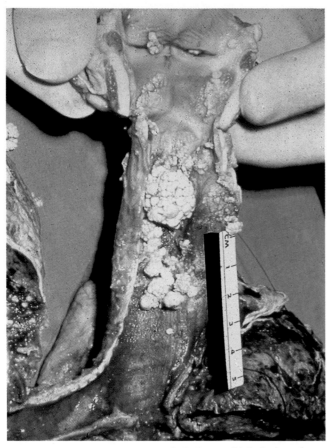

Figure 14–4. Autopsy specimen displaying multiple laryngeal papillomas extending into the trachea; histologic examination identified papillomas in the lower respiratory tract parenchyma that contributed to the demise of this person.

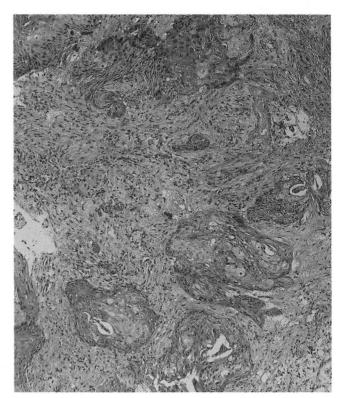

Figure 14–6. Histologic section from the previously depicted laryngectomy specimen, showing an invasive, well-differentiated squamous cell carcinoma; in situ hybridization revealed the presence of human papillomavirus 6/11. The tumor was metastatic to paratracheal and cervical neck lymph nodes.

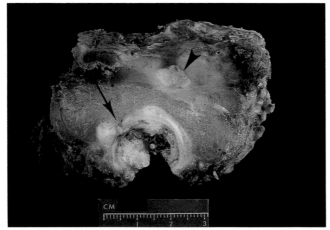

Figure 14–5. Rare example of horizontal section from a laryngectomy specimen from a teenaged girl with multiply recurrent laryngeal papillomas, eventually transforming into an invasive squamous cell carcinoma; the tumor invades through cartilage (arrow) with a separate focus deep within skeletal muscle (arrowhead).

2. Granular Cell Tumor

Definition: Benign tumor of probable neural (Schwann cell) origin, primarily identified in the skin and the mucous membranes of various head and neck sites.

- Two forms of granular cell tumors are seen:
  1. Mucosal granular cell tumor.
  2. Congenital epulis or gingival granular cell tumor.

a. Mucosal Granular Cell Tumor

Clinical

- Females affected more than males; primarily affects young adults in the 30- to 40-year age range.
- Can involve virtually every organ; most frequent sites of occurrence include: skin > tongue > breast > larynx > gastrointestinal tract > bronchus.
- Symptoms vary according to site but, in general, patients complain of a painless mass.

Laryngeal Granular Cell Tumors

- Slightly more common in men than in women.
- Hoarseness is the most common complaint.
- Most frequently identified along the posterior aspect of the true vocal cord, but can also be seen in the supraglottic and subglottic areas.
- No known etiology.

Pathology

Gross

- Solitary, polypoid, sessile, papillary, or cystic lesion measuring from 0.3 to 3.0 cm in diameter.
- Rarely associated with epithelial ulceration.

Histology

- Irrespective of location, the histology of granular cell tumors is the same.
- Unencapsulated or poorly circumscribed subepithelial lesion with a syncytial, trabecular, or nested growth pattern.
- Round to polygonal cells with round to oval vesicular nuclei and coarsely granular cytoplasm; cell borders are poorly defined.
- Cellular pleomorphism varies, and although usually minimal, may be markedly pleomorphic.
- Mitoses and necrosis are not seen.
- Occasionally, within the collagenous tissue and in the proximity of vessels, interstitial cells with large, "needle-shaped" bodies may be seen (angulate bodies).
- Pseudoepitheliomatous hyperplasia (PEH)—an exuberant epithelial hyperplasia that may be mistaken for an invasive squamous cell carcinoma may be seen in association with granular cell tumor; in contrast to squamous cell carcinoma, PEH displays no cytologic evidence of malignancy, and the epithelial proliferation does not extend beyond the limit of the associated granular cell tumor.
- Granular cell tumor cells may involve ("invade") nerves, but this is not an indication of malignancy.
- Histochemistry: cytoplasmic granules are diastase resistant, PAS positive, stain with alcian blue at pH 2.5, stain red with trichrome, and vary in size from being minute to as large as red blood cells; angulate bodies are intensely PAS positive.
- Immunohistochemistry—granular cells are S-100 protein and neuron specific enolase positive; interstitial cells with angulate bodies are myelin protein positive and S-100 protein negative.
- Electronmicroscopy—granular cells consist of membrane-bound autophagic vacuoles containing mitochondria, rough endoplasmic reticulum, myelin figures, and myelinated and nonmyelinated axonlike structures.

Differential Diagnosis

- Rhabdomyoma (Chapter 14A, #4).
- Invasive squamous cell carcinoma (Chapter 14B, #1).
- Alveolar soft part sarcoma (Chapter 9A, #4).

Treatment and Prognosis

- Conservative but complete surgical excision is considered curative.

Additional Facts

- The histogenesis of granular cell tumors is thought to be of neural (Schwann cell) origin and is supported by:
  Granular cells are S-100 protein and neuron specific enolase positive.
  Presence of myelinated and nonmyelinated axonlike structures by ultrastructural analysis.
  Presence of residual axons in many granular cell tumors.
  Development of tumors in multiple, different sites.
- *Malignant granular cell tumors* are rare neoplasms, accounting for approximately 1% of all granular cell tumors, and have the following features:
  Clinically are similar to benign granular cell tumors except that they do not occur in newborns or children, usually measure more than 4.0 cm in diameter, and tend to occur in the extremities.
  Histologically, there is increased cellularity and cellular pleomorphism, necrosis, prominent nucleoli, spindle-shaped cells, and increased mitotic activity (more than 2 mitoses per 10 high-power fields).
  Transition from benign granular cell tumor to malignant granular cell tumor is frequently apparent.
  Differential diagnosis includes alveolar soft part sarcoma and paraganglioma.
  Surgery is the treatment of choice; radio- and chemotherapy are ineffective.

Metastasize via lymphatics and blood vessels (lymph nodes, lung, liver, and bone).

b. Congenital Epulis

Synonym: Gingival granular cell tumor.

Clinical

■ Affects females more than males; occurs exclusively in newborns.
■ Identified on the gum pads in the oral cavity on the crest of the alveolar ridge in the incisor region.
■ Affects the maxilla more often than the mandible, but can occur in both locations simultaneously.

Pathology

Gross

■ Smooth, pink, multilobulated mass, ranging in size from millimeters up to 5 cm.

Histology

■ Similar to granular cell tumor, with the following exceptions:
Greater degree of vascularity.
Absence of associated pseudoepitheliomatous hyperplasia.
Less conspicuous nerve bundles.
Incorporation of odontogenic epithelium may be seen.

Treatment

■ May regress spontanously.
■ Complete surgical excision.

References

Cadotte M: Malignant granular cell myoblastoma. Cancer 33:1417–1422, 1974.

Compagno J, Hyams VJ, Ste-Marie P: Benign granular cell tumors of the larynx: a review of 36 cases with clinicopathologic data. Ann Otol Rhinol Laryngol 84:308–314, 1975.

Fisher ER, Wechsler H: Granular cell myoblastoma—a misnomer: electron microscopic and histochemical evidence concerning its schwann cell derivation and nature (granular cell schwannoma). Cancer 15:936–954, 1962.

Regezi JA, Batsakis JG, Courtney RM: Granular cell tumors of the head and neck. J Oral Surg 37:402–406, 1979.

Regezi JA, Zarbo RJ, Courtney RM, Crissman JD: Immunoreactivity of granular cell lesions of skin, mucosa, and jaw. Cancer 64:1455–1460, 1989.

Tucker MC, Rusnock EJ, Azumi N, Hoy GR, Lack EE: Gingival granular cell tumors of the newborn: an ultrastructural and immunohistochemical study. Arch Pathol Lab Med 114:895–898, 1990.

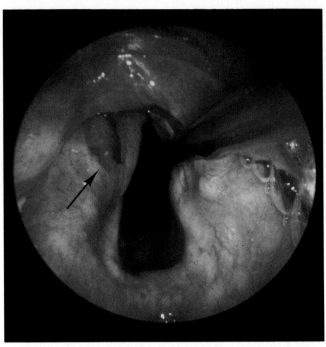

Figure 14–7. Solitary, polypoid, fleshy-appearing, mucosal-covered granular cell tumor is seen in the supraglottic larynx (*arrow*).

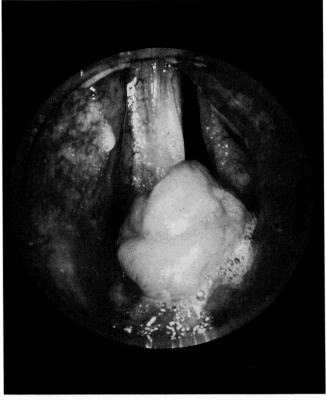

Figure 14–8. Large, solitary tan-yellow appearing granular cell tumor seen along the posterior aspect of the true vocal cord.

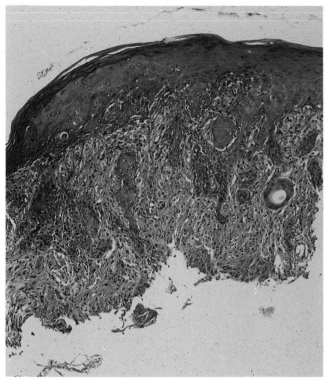

Figure 14-9. Laryngeal granular cell tumor inducing a pseudoepitheliomatous hyperplastic reaction in the overlying epithelium; the tumor cells can be seen between and below the epithelial reactive changes.

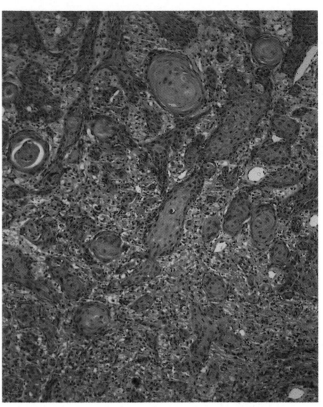

Figure 14-10. This pseudoepitheliomatous hyperplasia is easily misinterpreted as an invasive squamous carcinoma; however, in between the squamous nests, the cells of the associated granular cell tumor are seen.

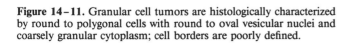

Figure 14-11. Granular cell tumors are histologically characterized by round to polygonal cells with round to oval vesicular nuclei and coarsely granular cytoplasm; cell borders are poorly defined.

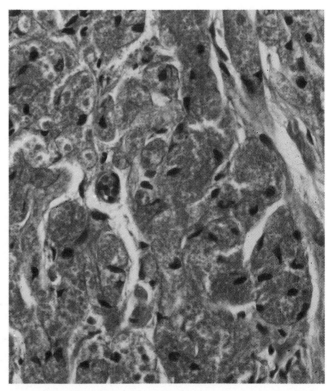

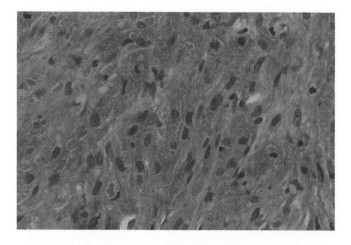

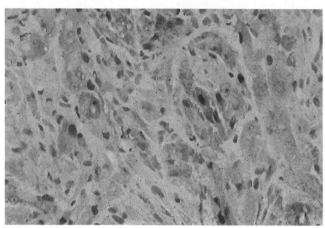

Figure 14-12. (*Top*) Typical histologic picture of a granular cell tumor. (*Bottom*) Granular cells are S-100 protein immunoreactive, aiding in the diagnosis.

2. Chondroma

Definition: Benign tumor of cartilage.

Clinical

■ Cartilaginous neoplasms of the head and neck are uncommon.
■ Affects males more than females; occurs most frequently in the fourth to seventh decades.
■ Most common sites of occurrence of head and neck chondromas include paranasal sinuses (ethmoid > maxillary > sphenoid), nasal cavity and nasal septum, maxilla and mandible, larynx, palate, pharynx and nasopharynx, and ear.
■ Symptoms vary according to the site of origin:
Sinonasal: nasal obstruction, mass lesion, asymptomatic found during routine examinations.
Larynx: dyspnea, stridor, and hoarseness.
■ In the larynx, chondromas may originate from epiglottis, cricoid, arytenoid, or thyroid cartilages; chondromas may arise in the soft tissues of the true vocal cords (Reinke's space).

Radiology

■ Sinonasal: sinus opacification; circumscribed radiolucent lesion.
■ Laryngeal: discrete soft-tissue mass contiguous with its laryngeal cartilaginous origin; coarse calcifications and ossification may be seen.

Pathology

Gross

■ Sinonasal:
Polypoid, firm, smooth-surfaced nodule measuring from 0.5 to 2.0 cm and rarely greater than 3.0 cm.
Overlying epithelium generally intact.

■ Laryngeal:
Lobulated, firm to hard, blue-gray, submucosal mass, seldom measuring more than 1 cm.

Histology

■ Lobulated tumor composed of chondrocytes that recapitulate the normal histology of cartilage.
■ Absence of cellular pleomorphism, binucleate chondrocytes, or mitotic activity.

Differential Diagnosis

■ Cartilaginous hamartoma.
■ Chondrosarcoma (Chapter 14B, #7).

Treatment and Prognosis

■ Conservative but wide surgical excision, including an adequate margin of normal tissue.
■ Following adequate surgery, recurrences are uncommon.

Additional Facts

■ Involvement of Reinke's space most probably represents a metaplastic, rather than a true neoplastic, process with derivation from the vocal cord ligament.
■ Although laryngeal chondromas seldom attain sizes greater than 1 cm, occasionally they may grow to sizes up to 4 cm.
■ In comparison to cartilaginous tumors of the larynx, chondrogenic tumors of the sinonasal and craniofacial bones are more often malignant.

References

Fu YS, Perzin KH: Non-epithelial tumors of the nasal cavity, paranasal sinuses, and nasopharynx: a clinicopathologic study. III: cartilaginous tumors (chondroma, chondrosarcoma). Cancer 34:453–463, 1974.

Hyams VJ, Rabuzzi DD: Cartilaginous tumors of the larynx. Laryngoscope 80:755–767, 1970.

Neel HB, Unni KK: Cartilaginous tumors of the larynx: a series of 33 cases. Otolaryngol Head Neck Surg 90:201–207, 1982.

Singh J, Black MJ, Fried I: Cartilaginous tumors of the larynx: a review of the literature and two case experiences. Laryngoscope 90:1872–1879, 1980.

Zizmor J, Noyek AM, Lewis JS: Radiologic diagnosis of chondromas and chodrosarcomas of the larynx. Arch Otolaryngol Head Neck Surg 101:232–234, 1975.

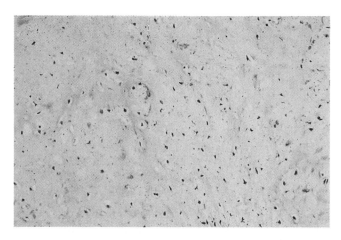

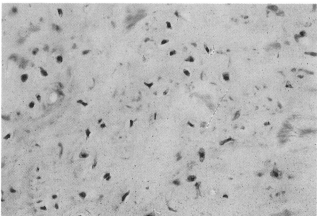

Figure 14–13. Laryngeal chondroma. (*Top*) Portion of a lobulated neoplasm composed of a hypocellular population of chondrocytes. (*Bottom*) Cytologic features seen in chondromas noteworthy for bland-appearing chondrocytes and lacking cellular pleomorphism, binucleate chondrocytes, or mitotic activity.

4. Rhabdomyoma

Definition: Benign tumor of striated muscle.

Two types:
I. Adult-type.
II. Fetal-type.

Clinical

ADULT-TYPE RHABDOMYOMA
- Considerably less common than their malignant counterparts (rhabdomyosarcoma).
- Affects males more than females; occurs in adults over 40 years of age.
- Predilection for the head and neck; the most commonly affected sites are the neck, pharynx, larynx, oral cavity (tongue and floor of mouth), and the soft palate.
- Symptoms vary according to site: painless neck mass, dysphagia, dyspnea, hoarseness.

Pathology

Gross

- Well-delineated, lobulated, red-brown mass ranging in size from 0.5 to 6.0 cm.

Histology

- Large, polygonal to round cells with abundant, deeply eosinophilic, granular cytoplasm and one or two peripherally placed vesicular nuclei.
- Nucleoli may be prominent.
- Cytoplasmic vacuolization may be prominent.
- Cross-striations are usually readily apparent and stain with phosphotungstic acid-hematoxylin (PTAH).
- Mitoses are absent.
- Contain abundant cytoplasmic glycogen (diastase sensitive, PAS positive).
- Immunohistochemistry: desmin and myoglobin positive.

Differential Diagnosis

- Granular cell tumor (Chapter 14A, #2).
- Alveolar soft part sarcoma (Chapter 9A, #4).

Treatment and Prognosis

- Cured by complete surgical excision.
- May recur if incompletely excised.

FETAL-TYPE RHABDOMYOMA

Clinical

- Very rare.

- Primarily affects male children under 3 years of age.
- Most common sites of occurrence are posterior auricular subcutaneous tissue > nasopharynx, parotid gland, neck.
- Symptoms vary according to site; in posterior auricular region, presents as a slow-growing, painless mass.

Pathology

Gross

- Solitary, well to moderately circumscribed nodule, measuring from 1 to 8 cm, with a gray to pink, mucoid appearance.

Histology

- Superficially located.
- Undifferentiated spindle cells and immature muscle fibers within a myxoid stroma.
- Cross-striations rarely discernible; cellular differentiation (mature muscle fibers) can be seen at the periphery of the tumor.
- Mitoses, necrosis, and significant cellular pleomorphism are absent.

Differential Diagnosis

- Rhabdomyosarcoma (Chapter 9B, #5).

Treatment and Prognosis

- Cured by local excision.

Additional Facts

- The separation of adult-type from fetal-type rhabdomyomas is based on histologic appearance rather than on the age of the patient.
- Fetal-type may represent a hamartoma or congenital anomaly, rather than a true neoplasm; in support of the hamartoma is the reported association of fetal-type rhabdomyoma with nevoid basal cell carcinoma syndrome.

References

Dehner LP, Enzinger FM, Font RL: Fetal rhabdomyoma: an analysis of nine cases. Cancer 30:160–166, 1972.
Ferlito A, Frugoni P: Rhabdomyoma purum of the larynx. J Laryngol Otol 89:1131–1141, 1975.
Moran JJ, Enterline HT: Benign rhabdomyoma of the pharynx: a case report, review of the literature, and comparison with cardiac rhabdomyoma. Am J Clin Pathol 42:174–181, 1964.
Modlin B: Rhabdomyoma of the larynx. Laryngoscope 92:580–582, 1982.
Winther LK: Rhabdomyoma of the hypopharynx and larynx. J Laryngol Otol 90:1041–1051, 1976.

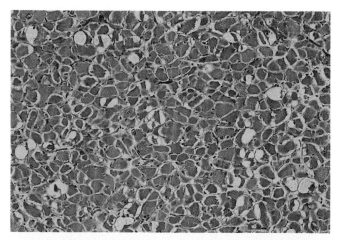

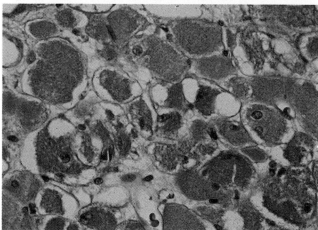

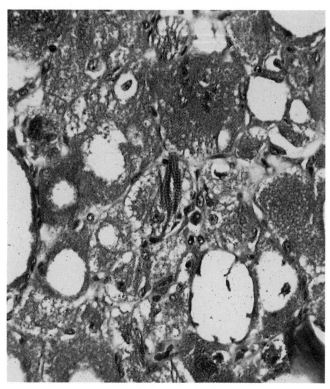

Figure 14–15. Cross striations are usually readily apparent in rhabdomyoma, as depicted in the center of the figure by staining with phosphotungstic acid-hematoxylin (PTAH).

Figure 14–14. Hypopharyngeal adult rhabdomyoma. (*Top*) Variably sized, polygonal cells with eosinophilic cytoplasm and peripherally placed nuclei; scattered vacuolated cells can be seen. (*Bottom*) Large polygonal to round cells with peripheral nuclei, abundant deeply eosinophilic, granular-appearing cytoplasm, and intracellular vacuoles.

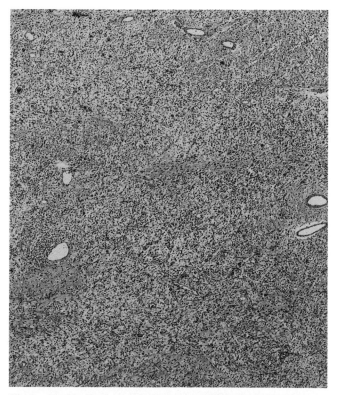

Figure 14–16. Fetal rhabdomyoma: undifferentiated spindle cell proliferation admixed with immature muscle fibers within a myxoid stroma.

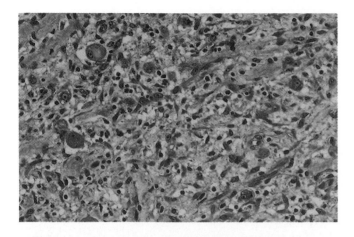

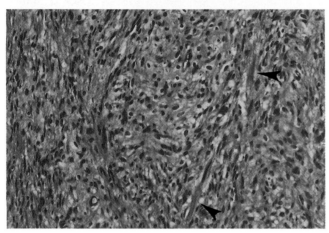

Figure 14–17. Fetal rhabdomyoma. (*Top*) Undifferentiated mesenchymal cells admixed with larger, more mature-appearing (differentiated) cell population within a myxoid matrix. (*Bottom*) Little variation in size or shape of the cells and no mitoses are seen; focally, myofibrils can be seen (arrowheads).

B. MALIGNANT NEOPLASMS

1. Squamous Cell Carcinoma

a. In Situ Squamous Cell Carcinoma (CIS)

Definition: Cellular dysplasia involving the entire thickness of the mucosa without compromise of the basement membrane; the dyplasia may extend into adjacent seromucous glands and is still considered an in situ lesion.

Clinical

- Affects males more than females; most frequently seen in the sixth to seventh decades of life.
- Can occur anywhere in the larynx, but most often involves the anterior portion of one or both true vocal cords.
- May exist as an isolated lesion.
- Hoarseness is the most frequent presenting complaint.

- Frequently associated with an invasive squamous cell carcinoma, lying either adjacent to or remote from one another.
- May exist as an isolated lesion; multifocal areas can occur.

Pathology

Gross

- Circumscribed or diffuse lesion with a white, red, or gray color and a smooth to granular appearance.

Histology

- Dysplastic process involves the entire thickness of the squamous epithelium.
- The squamous epithelium may or may not be thickened.
- Loss of cellular maturation and polarity.
- Increase in the nuclear:cytoplasmic ratio.

- Presence of mitoses (normal and abnormal).
- Keratosis and dyskeratosis may be present.
- Extension into adjacent seromucous glands.

Differential Diagnosis

- Reactive epithelial changes (Chapter 13, #6).

Treatment and Prognosis

- Conservative management is indicated and involves either mucosal stripping or irradiation.
- Either type of management offers a high cure rate, but periodic laryngoscopic examinations should be maintained.
- Treatment failures result from extensive or multifocal disease, associated undetected invasive squamous carcinoma, extension of CIS to subjacent seromucous glands that harbor residual disease after the mucosal stripping.

Additional Facts

- In the face of a diagnosis of CIS, the pathologist should liberally section the biopsy specimen to rule out the presence of an invasive squamous cell carcinoma, particularly for supra- and subglottic CIS.
- Unlike cervical intraepithelial neoplasia, laryngeal CIS is not a requirement prior to the development of an invasive squamous cell carcinoma.

b. Microinvasive or Superficially Invasive Squamous Cell Carcinoma

Definition: Nests of malignant cells that have penetrated the basement membrane and invaded superficially into the submucosa.

Clinical

- Clinical manifestations are similar to those of carcinoma in situ.
- Biologically malignant lesion, capable of metastasizing either via lymphatic or vascular channels.

Pathology

Gross

- Similar to carcinoma in situ.

Histology

- Microinvasive carcinoma can occur in two unrelated phases:
  1. Development from and as a continuum of carcinoma in situ.
  2. Invasion from an epithelium that demonstrates no evidence of carcinoma in situ.

Differential Diagnosis

- Pseudoepitheliomatous hyperplasia (Chapter 13, #6; Chapter 14, #2).

Treatment

- Behavior is similar to that of carcinoma in situ; if the presence of a coexisting invasive squamous cell carcinoma can be ruled out, the therapy is similar to that of carcinoma in situ.
- Treat conservatively with endoscopic removal of the lesion and close clinical follow-up.

c. Invasive Squamous Cell Carcinoma

- Accounts for approximately 2.5% of all cancers in men and approximately 0.5% of all cancers in women.
- Represents greater than 95% of all laryngeal carcinomas.
- Affects men more than women; most commonly occurs in the fifth to seventh decades of life.
- Etiologic factors linked to the development of squamous cell carcinoma and also linked to specific sites in the larynx: alcohol is linked to supraglottic carcinoma, and tobacco is linked to glottic carcinoma; other contributing etiologic factors associated with but not definitively linked as a direct cause of squamous cell carcinoma include environmental/occupational exposure (asbestos, nickel, wood, air pollution, isopropyl alcohol, mustard gas), dietary deficiencies, previous irradiation to the neck.
- Clinicopathology, therapy, staging, and biology differ according to laryngeal compartment involved by carcinoma (supraglottic versus glottic versus subglottic).
- The differential diagnosis of laryngeal invasive squamous cell carcinoma includes:
  Reactive epithelial changes (Chapter 13, #6).
  Pseudoepitheliomatous hyperplasia (Chapter 13, #6; Chapter 14, #2).

SUPRAGLOTTIC SQUAMOUS CELL CARCINOMA

Clinical

- Accounts for 25% to 40% of all laryngeal squamous cell carcinomas.
- Majority arise at the epiglottis (base) and false vocal cords and extend to the base of the tongue or to the pyriform sinus.
- Symptoms vary according to the site of involvement, but generally relate to changes in the quality of voice; other symptomatic manifestations of supraglottic carcinoma include dysphagia, odonophagia, hoarseness, hemoptysis, dyspnea.
- Marginal carcinomas (suprahyoid epiglottis, aryepiglottic folds) tend to remain quiescent for longer periods and present with more advanced disease.

Pathology

Gross

- Vary in size and appearance, ranging from 1 to 4 cm; appearing ulcerated, flat, exophytic or, rarely, papillary.

Histology

- Tend to be nonkeratinizing, moderately to poorly differentiated; but keratinizing, well-differentiated squamous cell carcinomas are also seen.
- An in situ component is common and may be extensive.
- Invasive pattern can be pushing or infiltrative.
- Mitoses and necrosis can be seen, and their presence relates to the grade of the tumor (tend to more common with more poorly differentiated tumors).

Treatment and Prognosis

- Dependent on staging:
  T1 and T2: conservation surgery (supraglottic laryngectomy) or radiotherapy.
  T3 and T4: surgery or combined surgery and radiotherapy.
- Overall 5 year survival rate of 75%.

Additional Facts

- Prognosis is better for the more inferiorly located supraglottic tumors.
- Rarely will supraglottic carcinomas extend to the arytenoids, invade the thyroid cartilage, or invade the glottic region.
- Invasion of the preepiglottic space is associated with increased incidence of cervical lymph node metastasis.
- The supraglottic larynx is rich in lymphatic spaces, increasing the likelihood of cervical lymph node metastasis, even in early stage disease; the incidence of nodal disease ranges from 25% to 35%, and increased rates of cervical lymph node metastasis are correlated to:
  Size: the larger the tumor (>4 cm), the higher the rate of metastasis.
  Location: tumors arising from the marginal supraglottis have a higher rate of metastasis; anterior tumors or tumors that cross the midline may produce bilateral metastases.
- The supraglottic lymphatic drainage is to the upper and middle jugular chains.
- Distant metastasis from laryngeal cancers are uncommon, and when it occurs, it more commonly involves the lung and mediastinal lymph nodes.

GLOTTIC SQUAMOUS CELL CARCINOMA

Clinical

- Constitutes the majority of all laryngeal squamous cell carcinomas, representing from 60% to 75% of all carcinomas.
- Majority arise from the anterior portion of the true vocal cord.
- Posterior portion of true vocal cord is an uncommon site for carcinoma to develop.
- The most common presenting symptom is hoarseness.

- As a result of interference with vocal cord mobility, symptoms develop early in the course of disease; many glottic carcinomas are small, limited in size, tend to be localized, and are amenable to conservative therapy (stripping or radiotherapy).

Pathology

Gross

- Early lesions: irregular area of mucosal thickening of varying size.
- Advanced lesions: exophytic, fungating, endophytic, or ulcerated mass that can attain a large size.

Histology

- More commonly, keratinizing well- to moderately differentiated squamous cell carcinomas, but can be nonkeratinizing, poorly differentiated squamous cell carcinoma.
- An in situ component is commonly seen and may occur without concomitant invasive carcinoma.
- Invasive pattern is predominantly infiltrative, but can be pushing.

Treatment and Prognosis

- Therapy is dependent on staging:
  T1 and T2 with normal cord mobility: conservation surgery, including mucosal stripping or radiotherapy.
  T1, bilateral: radiotherapy.
  T2 with impaired vocal cord mobility: treated as a T3 lesion.
  T3 and T4: surgery (total laryngectomy) or combined surgery and radiotherapy.
- Overall 5-year survival rates:
  T1: >90%.
  T2: 85%.
  T3: 55%.
  T4: 25%.

Additional Facts

- Spread of glottic carcinomas includes:
  Spread across the anterior commissure to involve the opposite vocal cord, or spread posteriorly to involve the posterior commissure (T1).
  Extension to the supraglottis or subglottis (T2).
  Extension into Reinke's space along the vocal cord ligament, with infiltration into the vocalis muscle; this pattern of invasion defines vocal cord fixation (T3).
  Anterior extension with deep invasion and penetration of the thyroid cartilage or invasion into the soft tissues of the neck (T4).
- Involvement of the arytenoid indicates a worse prognosis and may necessitate total laryngectomy.
- The glottic region of the larynx has sparse lymphatic drainage; as such, the overall incidence of lymph node metastasis is less than 10%; the vast majority of cervical lymph node metastasis occur-

ring in glottic carcinomas are seen in T3 and T4 lesions.

■ The glottic lymphatic drainage is to the upper and lower jugular chains.

SUBGLOTTIC SQUAMOUS CELL CARCINOMA

Clinical

■ Considered rare, accounting for less than 5% of all laryngeal squamous cell carcinomas.
■ Tend to remain clinically quiescent, presenting with advanced disease.
■ Most common presenting symptoms relate to airway obstruction (dyspnea, stridor) and to vocal cord fixation (voice changes).

Pathology

Gross

■ Large, exophytic, fungating, ulcerating, or endophytic mass.

Histology

■ Tend to be keratinizing moderately to poorly differentiated squamous cell carcinoma.
■ An in situ component is less common and tends to be seen adjacent to the carcinoma.
■ Invasive pattern is predominantly infiltrative.

Treatment and Prognosis

■ Dependent on staging:
Limited tumors (T1 and T2): radiotherapy alone or conservative surgery.
In general, subglottic tumors present with advanced disease and, because of the proximity to the cricothyroid space and the cricoid cartilage, surgical treatment usually necessitates a total laryngectomy.
■ Overall 5-year survival rate is less than 40%.

Additional Facts

■ Spread of subglottic carcinomas includes:
Into the thyroarytenoid muscle to produce vocal cord fixation.
Anteriorly through the cricothyroid membrane, with thyroid gland involvement.
Superiorly to involve the glottic and supraglottic regions.
Inferiorly into the trachea.
Posteriorly below the cricoid cartilage and into the esophagus.
■ Up to 20% of patients with subglottic squamous cell carcinoma present with cervical lymph node metastases.
■ The subglottic region of the larynx has lymphatic drainage to upper and lower jugular lymph node chains.
■ In addition to the drainage to the jugular chains, the subglottic region has lymphatic drainage ante-

riorly to the prelaryngeal (delphian) lymph node and posterolateral to the paratracheal lymph nodes; the latter are clinically silent and may harbor metastatic tumor from a subglottic primary carcinoma in up to 50% of cases.
■ Stomal recurrent tumor is not uncommon after treatment of a primary subglottic carcinoma.

TRANSGLOTTIC SQUAMOUS CELL CARCINOMA

Definition: Those carcinomas that extend in a vertical direction to involve both glottic and supraglottic structures.

■ Usually represent advanced tumors.
■ High incidence of nodal metastases and extralaryngeal spread.
■ May be understaged as a result of undetectable cartilaginous invasion.
■ Treatment generally requires radical surgery and radiotherapy.
■ In limited patients, conservation techniques may be used.
■ Overall 5-year survival parallels that of subglottic carcinomas and is less than 40%.

Additional Facts Relating to Laryngeal Squamous Cell Carcinoma

■ Factors adversely affecting prognosis:
Tumor location: transglottic tumors have a higher incidence of lymph node metastasis compared with supraglottic and subglottic carcinomas.
Tumor size: the larger the tumor, the greater the chances of metastasis.
Tumor histology: the poorer the differentiation (grade), the more likely dissemination will occur.
Cervical lymph node metastasis: metastatic tumor to cervical lymph nodes decreases survival by 50%; tumor extending beyond the confines of the lymph node (extranodal spread) represents an important finding relating to recurrent disease in the neck and should be specifically commented on in the pathology report.
Multiple malignancies: up to 12% of patients with laryngeal carcinoma will develop a secondary primary malignant tumor, either in the lung, another upper aerodigestive tract site or, less commonly, in a distant, unrelated site.

References

Barnes L: Carcinoma in situ, microinvasive carcinoma and squamous cell carcinoma of the larynx. *In*: Barnes L, ed. Surgical pathology of the head and neck. New York: Marcel Dekker, 1985; pp 159–174.

Barnes EL, Johnson JT: Pathologic and clinical considerations in the evaluation of major head and neck specimens resected for cancer. Pathol Annu 21 (Pt 1):173–250, 1986.

Crissman JD, Gnepp DR, Goodman ML, Hellquist H, Johns ME: Preinvasive lesions of the upper aerodigestive tract: histologic and clinical implications. Pathol Annu 22 (Pt 1):311–352, 1987. ■

DeStefani E, Correa P, Oreggia F, et al: Risk factors for laryngeal cancer. Cancer 60:3087–3091, 1987.

Elman AJ, Goodman M, Wang CC, Pilch B, Busse J: In situ carcinoma of the vocal cords. Cancer 43:2422–2428, 1979.

Gillis TM, Incze MS, Vaughan CW, Simpson GT: Natural history and management of keratosis, atypia, carcinoma in situ and microinvasive cancer of the larynx. Am J Surg 146:512–516, 1983.

Hirabayashi H, Koshii K, Uno K, et al: Extracapsular spread of squamous cell carcinoma in neck lymph nodes: prognostic factor of laryngeal cancer. Laryngoscope 101:502–506, 1991.

McGuirt WF, Browne JD: Management decisions in laryngeal carcinoma in situ. Laryngoscope 101:125–129, 1991.

Miller AH: Carcinoma in situ of the larynx—clinical appearance and treatment. *In:* Alberti PW, Bryce DP, eds. Centennial conference on laryngeal carcinoma. New York: Appleton-Century-Crofts, 1976; pp 161–166.

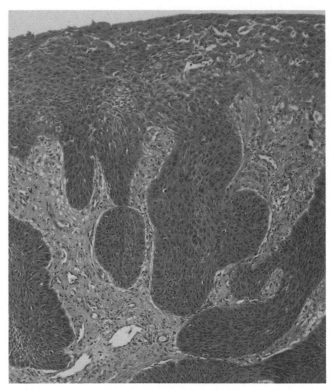

Figure 14–19. Superficially invasive (microinvasive) carcinoma developing from an epithelium without evidence of carcinoma in situ (full-thickness dysplasia).

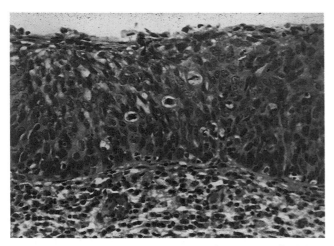

Figure 14–18. Laryngeal carcinoma in situ, characterized by a dysplastic process involving the entire thickness of the squamous epithelium with loss of cellular maturation and polarity, an increase in the nuclear:cytoplasmic ratio, and mitoses scattered throughout all layers of the epithelium; the squamous epithelium is not thickened.

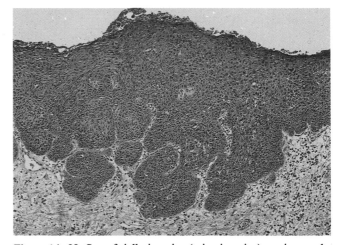

Figure 14–20. Superficially invasive (microinvasive) carcinoma developing as a continuum of carcinoma in situ, seen in the overlying epithelial component.

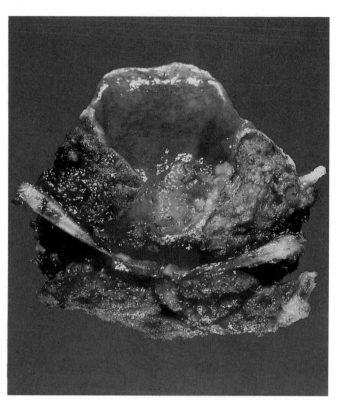

Figure 14-21. Laryngeal squamous cell carcinoma as seen by a large, tan-white neoplasm in the right supraglottis, extending upward toward the epiglottis.

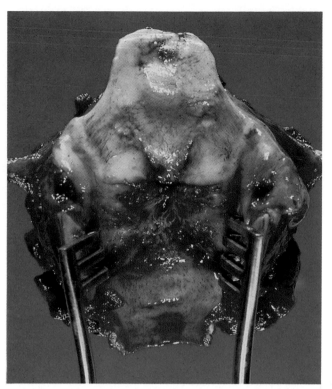

Figure 14-23. Laryngeal (subglottic) squamous cell carcinoma appearing as a flat, indurated lesion diffusely involving the subglottic compartment.

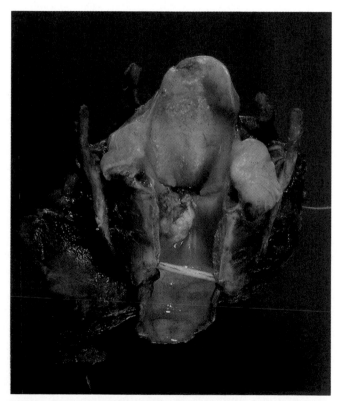

Figure 14-22. Laryngeal squamous cell carcinoma that began in the left glottis and eventually crossed the midline to involve the opposite vocal cord and with subglottic extension.

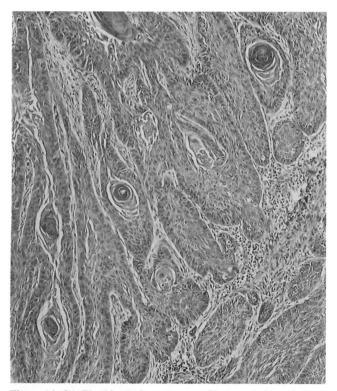

Figure 14-24. The histologic spectrum of laryngeal squamous cell carcinoma is varied, including well, moderately, and poorly differentiated carcinomas; this illustration is that of an invasive moderately well-differentiated squamous cell carcinoma.

2. Spindle Cell (Squamous) Carcinoma (SCSC)

Definition: Foci of conventional squamous cell carcinoma (in situ or invasive carcinoma) associated with a malignant spindle cell stromal component.

Synonyms: Carcinosarcoma, pleomorphic carcinoma, metaplastic carcinoma, collision tumor, pseudosarcoma, Lane tumor.

Clinical

- Majority occur in men (85%); occur most frequently in sixth to eighth decades of life.
- Can occur anywhere in the upper aerodigestive tract; most common sites include larynx (true vocal cords > false vocal cords and supraglottis) > oral cavity (lips, tongue, gingiva, floor of mouth, buccal mucosa) > skin > tonsil and pharynx.
- Symptoms vary according to site: larynx—hoarseness, voice changes, airway obstruction, dysphagia; oral cavity or skin—mass or nonhealing sore with or without pain; sinonasal tract and nasopharynx—airway obstruction, pain, epistaxis, discharge, facial deformity, unilateral otitis media, orbital symptoms.
- No specific correlation with known risk factors (alcohol, tobacco, or environment/occupation); tumors have been reported in areas of prior irradiation.

Pathology

Gross

- Variations in the gross appearance may correlate with the primary site of occurrence: larynx—polypoid or exophytic; sinonasal/nasopharynx—fungating or ulcerative.
- Firm, tan-white, gray, or pink mass, varying in size from 1 to 6 cm.

Histology

- Conventional squamous cell component either in situ or frankly invasive that is typically keratinizing and of varying differentiation (well- to poorly differentiated). **Note:** this component may be limited and may require multiple sectioning for identification.
- Spindle cell component:
  Generally is the dominant cell type.
  Varies from a bland to an overtly pleomorphic-appearing infiltrate.
  Growth pattern varies, including fascicular, storiform, or palisading with associated myxomatous stroma.
  Generally is hypercellular and pleomorphic, with large, hyperchromatic nuclei, prominent nucleoli, many mitoses (typical and atypical), multinucleated giant cells.
  May be a bland, sparsely cellular infiltrate with atypical nuclear features.

- Heterologous elements can be seen, including bone and cartilage, which may in and of itself be malignant.
- Necrosis is not uncommon.
- Immunohistochemistry: spindle cells are keratin positive in the majority of cases; however, the spindle cells may be keratin negative, which does not exclude the diagnosis.

Differential Diagnosis

- Reactive (fibroblastic) proliferation, including fibromatosis (Chapter 4A, #4; Chapter 13, #5).
- Malignant fibrous histiocytoma (Chapter 4B, #6).
- Fibrosarcoma (Chapter 4B, #7).
- Malignant melanoma (Chapter 4B, #3).
- **Note:** Sarcomas, although uncommon in the head and neck region, do occur; in general, these tumors are deeply seated in any given location and do not usually result in a polypoid mass protruding from a mucosal surface.

Treatment and Prognosis

- Surgery is the preferred therapy.
- Radiotherapy may be used as an adjunct to surgery, but neither radiotherapy nor chemotherapy have merit as the sole therapeutic modality.
- Prognosis is dependent on the site of occurrence, as well as the clinical stage:
  Polypoid lesions may behave less aggressively than flat, ulcerative tumors, perhaps correlating with limited (superficial) invasion.
  Vocal cord lesions that manifest symptoms early in the disease course may have a better prognosis than SCSC arising in other sites (supraglottis, hypo- and nasopharynx), where symptoms occur only after the tumor has become large and extensively infiltrative.
- In general, prognosis is poor.
- Metastases primarily occur to cervical lymph nodes and lung.

Additional Facts

- The histogenesis of the spindle cells is controversial, as evidenced by the array of names given to this tumor; epithelial derivation is supported by:
  Intimate association with conventional squamous cell carcinoma.
  Presence of cytokeratin immunoreactivity in the majority of cases and lack of immunoreactivity with other antibodies.
  Despite the presence of heterologous elements, including malignant bone or cartilage, neither of these components have been reported to metastasize and in all probability represent a metaplastic phenomenon.
- Metastasis from a SCSC may include:
  The conventional squamous cell carcinoma alone.
  The spindle cell carcinoma alone.

Both conventional and spindle cell squamous carcinoma.

References

Batsakis JG, Rice DH, Howard DR: The pathology of head and neck tumors: spindle cell lesions (sarcomatoid carcinomas, nodular fasciitis, and fibrosarcoma) of the upper aerodigestive tracts, part 14. Head Neck Surg 4:499–513, 1982.

Ellis GL, Langloss JM, Heffner DK, Hyams VJ: Spindle-cell carcinoma of the aerodigestive tract: an immunohistochemical analysis of 21 cases. Am J Surg Pathol 11:335–342, 1987.

Lasser KH, Naeim F, Higgins J, Cove H, Waisman J: "Pseudosarcoma" pf the larynx. Am J Surg Pathol 3:39–404, 1979.

Leventon GS, Evans HL: Sarcomatoid squamous cell carcinoma of the mucous membranes of the head and neck: a clinicopathologic study of 20 cases. Cancer 48:994–1003, 1981.

Zarbo RJ, Crissman JD, Venkat H, Weiss MA: Spindle-cell carcinoma of the aerodigestive tract mucosa: an immunohistologic and ultrastructural study of 18 biphasic tumors and comparison with seven monophasic spindle-cell tumors. Am J Surg Pathol 10:741–753, 1986.

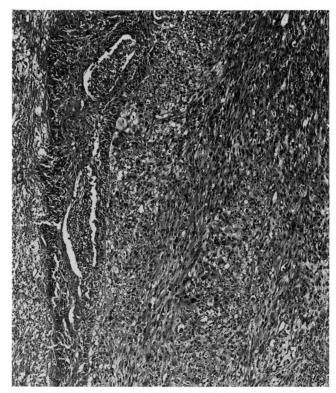

Figure 14–26. Spindle cell carcinoma, showing an invasive squamous carcinoma (along the left side) in association with a malignant spindle cell stroma.

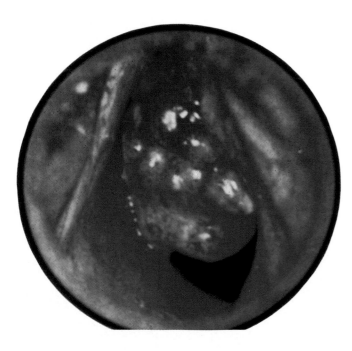

Figure 14–25. Laryngeal spindle cell carcinoma, seen as a polypoid or exophytic mass protruding into the laryngeal lumen.

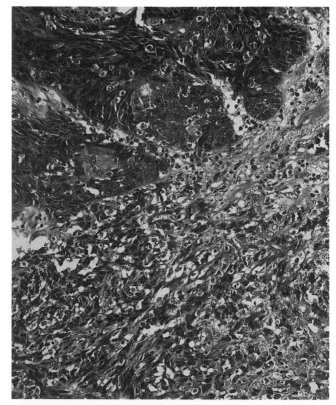

Figure 14–27. Carcinoma in situ, as seen at the top, also is acceptable as the differentiated epithelial component seen in spindle cell carcinoma; a malignant spindle cell component is depicted in the lower aspect of the illustration.

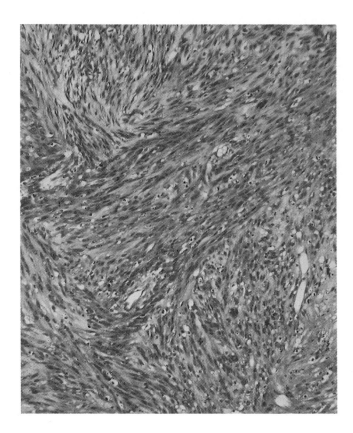

Figure 14–28. The spindle cell component may histologically appear with growth patterns and cytomorphologic features of fibrosarcoma or malignant fibrous histiocytoma, as seen by the presence of a fasciculated or storiform growth in association with spindle cells, histiocytic-like cells, and multinucleated cells; scattered mitotic figures can be seen.

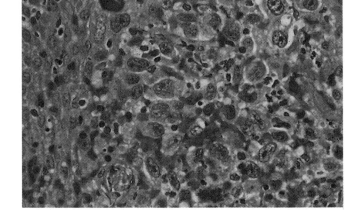

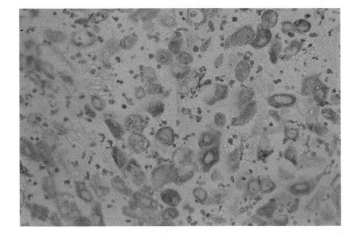

Figure 14–29. (Top) Pleomorphic cellular infiltrate of spindle cell carcinoma. (Bottom) In addition to the superficial location and unequivocal presence of a squamous carcinoma (in situ or invasive), the presence of cytokeratin immunoreactivity assists in confirming the diagnosis of spindle cell carcinoma.

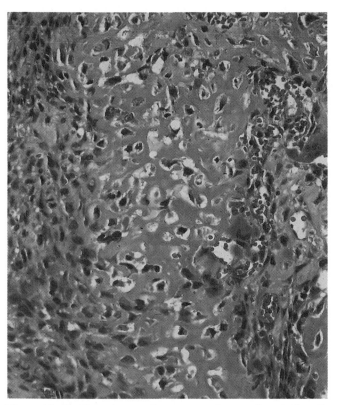

Figure 14-30. Heterologous elements can be seen in spindle cell carcinoma, including this focus of osteosarcoma.

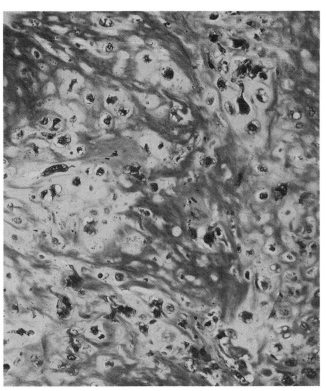

Figure 14-31. Additional heterologous components that may be identified in spindle cell carcinoma include chondrosarcomatous foci.

3. Verrucous Carcinoma

Definition: Highly differentiated variant of squamous cell carcinoma with locally destructive but not metastatic capabilities.

Clinical

■ Verrucous carcinoma represents 1% to 3% of all laryngeal carcinomas.
■ Affects men more than women; generally occurs in the sixth and seventh decades of life.
■ Can occur anywhere in the upper aerodigestive tract; most common sites include oral cavity > larynx > nasal fossa > sinonasal tract, nasopharynx.
■ Symptoms vary according to site: larynx — hoarseness is the most common complaint, less frequent symptoms include airway obstruction, hemoptysis, dysphagia; oral cavity — mass with or without pain; sinonasal tract — airway obstruction; nasopharynx — dysphagia.
■ The most common site of occurrence in the larynx is the glottic area; oral cavity verrucous carcinomas most commonly arise on the buccal mucosa and gingiva.

■ Potential but not definitive etiologic factors include tobacco smoking or chewing and viral-induced.

Pathology

Gross

■ Tan or white, warty, fungating or exophytic, firm to hard mass of varying size, measuring up to 9 to 10 cm in diameter.
■ In general, the tumors are attached by a broad base.

Histology

■ Squamous cell proliferation with the following characteristics:
  Uniform cells without dysplastic features or mitoses.
  Marked surface keratinization ("church-spire" keratosis).
  Broad or bulbous rete pegs with a pushing, **not** infiltrative, margin.
■ A mixed chronic inflammatory cell infiltrate composed of lymphocytes, plasma cells, and histiocytes may be prominent along the adjacent stroma.

Differential Diagnosis

■ Keratotic squamous papilloma (Chapter 9A, #1; Chapter 14A, #1).
■ Reactive keratosis and epithelial hyperplasia (Chapter 13B, #6).
■ Pseudoepitheliomatous hyperplasia (Chapter 13B, #6; Chapter 14A, #2).
■ Verruca vulgaris (Chapter 14A, #1).
■ Keratoacanthoma (when verrucous carcinoma affects cutaneous sites) (Chapter 25A, #1).
■ "Conventional" type of squamous cell carcinoma (Chapter 14B, #1).

Treatment and Prognosis

■ Surgery (conservation or total laryngectomy) is the definitive therapeutic modality.
■ Radiotherapy can be used in patients with advanced disease or in patients who are not good surgical candidates.
■ Metastatic tumor to regional lymph nodes is rare, and distant metastases do not occur.
■ Prognosis is excellent after complete surgical removal.
■ Local recurrence may occur if incompletely excised.
■ Anaplastic transformation may result in distant metastases.

Additional Facts

■ The pathologic diagnosis of verrucous carcinoma may be extremely difficult, requiring multiple biopsies over several years before identification of diagnostic features supporting appropriate interpretation; both clinician and pathologists should be aware of this fact. To this end, adequate biopsy material is critical to interpretation and should include a good epithelial–stromal interface. The pathologist should not overinterpret a verrucoid lesion as a carcinoma without seeing the relationship to the underlying stroma.
■ The differentiation of verrucous carcinoma from a "conventional" type of carcinoma is based on the presence or absence of cytologic abnormalities. Dysplastic features limited in scope and confined to the basal zone areas can be seen in verrucous carcinoma. Any dysplastic features greater than this should exclude a diagnosis of verrucous carcinoma.
■ The literature supports the dogma that radiotherapy is contraindicated in the treatment of verrucous carcinoma because of its purported increased association with anaplastic transformation of the verrucous carcinoma; however, similar transformations can occur after surgery or cryosurgery alone, and even without any treatment. Therefore, radiotherapy is not contraindicated in the treatment of verrucous carcinoma and can be used in selected clinical settings.

■ Cervical adenopathy may be associated with verrucous carcinoma, representing reactive changes and not metastatic disease.

References

Abramson AL, Brandsma JL, Steinberg BM, Winkler B: Verrucous carcinoma of the larynx: possible human papillomavirus etiology. Arch Otolaryngol Head Neck Surg 111:709–715, 1985.

Ackerman LV: Verrucous carcinoma of the oral cavity. Surgery 23:670–678, 1948.

Brandsma JL, Steinberg BM, Abramson AL, Winkler B: Presence of HPV-16 related sequences in verrucous carcinoma of the larynx. Cancer Res 46:2185–2188, 1986.

Crissman JD, Gnepp DR, Goodman ML, Hellquist H, Johns ME: Preinvasive lesions of the upper aerodigestive tract: histologic definitions and clinical implications (a symposium). Pathol Annu 22 (Pt 1):311–352, 1987.

Fechner RE, Mills SE: Verruca vulgaris of the larynx: a distinctive lesion of probable viral origin confused with verrucous carcinoma. Am J Surg Pathol 6:357–362, 1982.

Ferlito A, Recher G: Ackerman's tumor (verrucous carcinoma) of the larynx: a clinicopathologic study of 77 cases. Cancer 46:1617–1630, 1980.

Kraus FT, Perez-Mesa C. Verrucous carcinoma: clinical and pathologic study of 105 cases involving oral cavity, larynx and genitalia. Cancer 19:26–38, 1966.

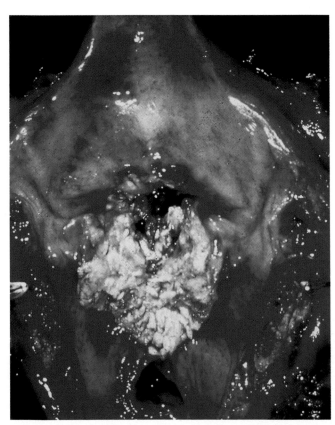

Figure 14–32. Laryngeal verrucous carcinoma, consisting of a large, tan-white, warty or fungating mass.

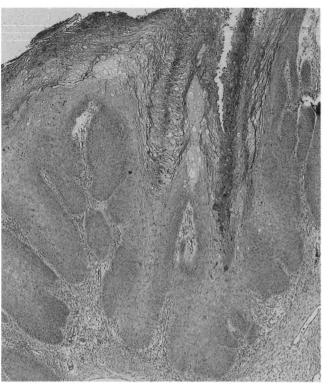

Figure 14–33. Histologic appearance of verrucous carcinoma includes marked surface keratinization ("church-spire" keratosis), bulbous rete pegs "pushing" into the underlying stroma, absence of cellular atypia, and a mixed chronic inflammatory cell infiltrate.

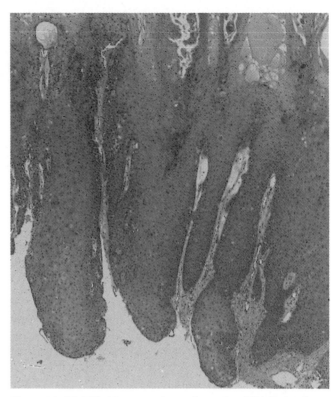

Figure 14–35. This biopsy specimen shows the difficulty confronting the pathologist in the diagnosis of verrucous carcinoma, in that the features of verrucous carcinoma are present; however, the absence of an adequate stromal component without a good epithelial–connective tissue interface precludes a definitive diagnosis of verrucous carcinoma. In this situation, additional (deeper) biopsy specimens would be necessary before definitively diagnosing a verrucous carcinoma.

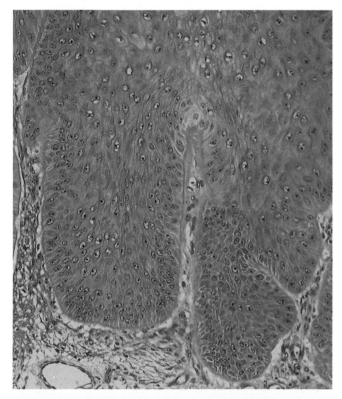

Figure 14–34. Portion of verrucous carcinoma showing a rounded rete peg pushing downward into the stroma, which is composed of epithelial cells with uniform appearance without dysplastic features or mitoses.

4. Basaloid Squamous Cell Carcinoma

Definition: An invasive neoplasm, composed of basaloid cells intimately associated with either a dysplastic squamous epithelium, in situ squamous cell carcinoma, or invasive squamous cell carcinoma.

Clinical

■ Uncommonly occurring variant of squamous cell carcinoma.
■ Affects males more than females; predominantly occurs in the sixth to seventh decades of life.
■ Predilection for the hypopharynx (pyriform sinus), larynx (supraglottis), and tongue.
■ Symptoms depend on the site of occurrence and include hoarseness, dysphagia, pain, and a neck mass.
■ Etiologic factors include excessive alcohol or tobacco use.
■ Cell of origin not definitively identified, but in all probability is a single totipotential cell that is capable of divergent differentiation and is located either in the basal cell layer of the surface epithelium or within seromucous glands.

Pathology

Gross

■ Firm to hard, tan-white mass, often with associated central necrosis, measuring up to 6.0 cm in greatest dimension.
■ Infrequently, these neoplasms may be exophytic in appearance.

Histology

■ Infiltrating tumor arranged in a variety of growth patterns, all of which may be seen within any given tumor and include solid, lobular, cell nests, cribriform, cords, trabeculae, and gland-like or cystic.
■ One of the important cytologic features is the presence of a basaloid cell component, consisting of small, closely apposed cells with hyperchromatic nuclei, scanty cytoplasm, and marked mitotic activity; large cells or pleomorphism may be seen.
■ Frequently, comedonecrosis is seen in the center of the neoplastic lobules.
■ Intercellular deposition of a hyalin or mucohyalin material can be seen.
■ The other important cytologic feature is the intimate association with foci of squamous differentiation, as manifested by squamous carcinoma (in situ squamous cell carcinoma or invasive squamous cell carcinoma), dysplastic squamous epithelium, or focal squamous differentiation; in addition, a neoplastic, spindle cell carcinomatous component may be identified in association with the basaloid–squamous elements.

■ Histochemistry: material within the cystic spaces is periodic acid-Schiff and alcian blue positive.
■ Immunohistochemistry: cytokeratin, EMA, CEA, S-100 protein positive; chromogranin, synaptophysin, muscle-specific actin negative.
■ Electronmicroscopy: basaloid component—desmosomes, rare tonofilaments and loose stellate granules or replicated basal lamina within the cystic spaces.

Differential Diagnosis

■ Adenoid cystic carcinoma (Chapter 19B, #3)
■ Neuroendocrine carcinoma (Chapter 14B, #6).
■ Adenosquamous carcinoma (Chapter 14b, #5).
■ Spindle cell carcinoma (Chapter 14B, #2).

Treatment and Prognosis

■ Radical surgical excision is the treatment of choice and, as a result of both early regional lymph node as well as distant visceral metastases, radical neck dissection and supplemental radio- and chemotherapy may be included in the initial management protocol.
■ This neoplasm is aggressive and high grade, with increased tendency to be multifocal, deeply invasive, and metastatic.
■ Metastases occur via lymphatics and blood vessels, with sites of predilection including regional and distant lymph nodes, lung, bone, skin, and brain.
■ Rapidly fatal neoplasm, associated with high mortality rates within the first year after diagnosis.

Additional Facts

■ Shallow biopsy specimens may belie the depth and extent of invasion and may not be representative of the lesion, thereby leading to erroneous classification.
■ Metastases include both basaloid and squamous cell components.

References

Banks ER, Frierson HF Jr, Mills SE, George E, Zarbo RJ, Swanson PE: Basaloid squamous cell carcinoma of the head and neck: a clinicopathologic and immunohistochemical study of 40 cases. Am J Surg Pathol 16:939–946, 1992.

Batsakis JG, El Naggar A: Basaloid-squamous carcinomas of the upper aerodigestive tracts. Ann Otol Rhinol Laryngol 98:919–920, 1989.

Luna MA, El Naggar A, Parichatikanond P, Weber RS, Batsakis JG: Basaloid squamous cell carcinoma of the upper aerodigestive tract: clinicopathologic and DNA flow cytometric analysis. Cancer 66:537–542, 1990.

McKay MJ, Bilous AM: Basaloid-squamous carcinomas of the hypopharynx. Cancer 63:2528–2531, 1989.

Wain SL, Kier R, Vollmer RT, Bossen EH: Basaloid-squamous carcinoma of the tongue, hypopharynx and larynx. Hum Pathol 17:1158–1166, 1986.

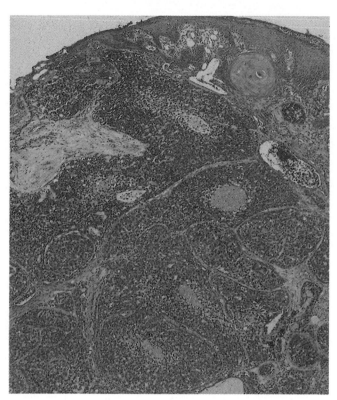

Figure 14–36. Basaloid squamous cell carcinoma, showing an infiltrating tumor originating from the surface epithelium and arranged in a predominantly solid growth pattern, with comedonecrosis seen in the center of several neoplastic lobules.

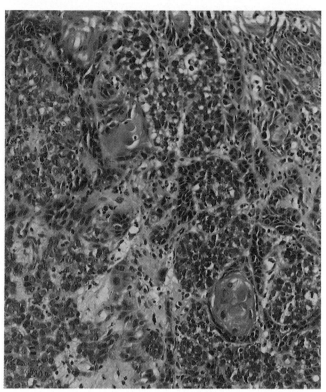

Figure 14–37. Basaloid squamous cell carcinoma is characterized by the presence of a basaloid cell component, which consists of small, closely apposed cells with hyperchromatic nuclei, scanty cytoplasm, and marked mitotic activity intimately associated with cellular foci of squamous differentiation (dysplastic, in situ, or invasive squamous cell carcinoma).

Figure 14–38. Basaloid squamous cell carcinoma may manifest varied growth patterns, including cribriform areas associated with hyalin or mucohyalin material similar to that of adenoid cystic carcinoma; superficial biopsy specimens that include these foci may erroneously be diagnosed as an adenoid cystic carcinoma.

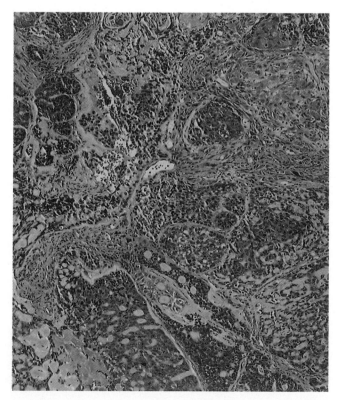

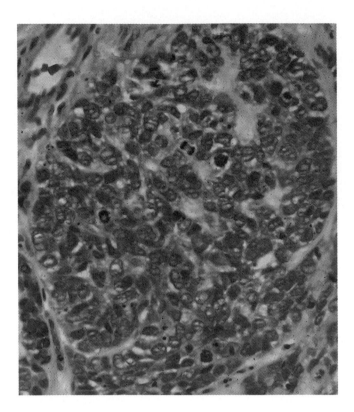

Figure 14–39. In addition to the small basaloid cells typically identified in basaloid squamous-cell carcinoma, a large cell or pleomorphic population may also be seen.

5. Adenosquamous Carcinoma

Definition: Malignant, high-grade, epithelial neoplasm with histologic features of both an adenocarcinoma and a squamous cell carcinoma.

Clinical

■ Uncommon neoplasm.

■ Affects males more than females; occurs over a wide age range, but most frequently seen in the sixth and seventh decades of life.

■ This neoplasm may occur in virtually all upper aerodigestive tract sites, but is most frequently identified in the larynx, hypopharynx, oral cavity (tongue, floor of mouth, tonsil, and palate), and sinonasal cavity.

■ Symptoms vary according to the site of occurrence and include dysphagia, hoarseness, a mass with or without pain, and nasal obstruction.

■ Etiology is not clearly defined and may be related to alcohol or tobacco use.

■ Cell of origin is not definitively identified, but in all probability is a single totipotential cell that is capable of divergent differentiation and is located either in the basal cell layer of the surface epithelium or within seromucous glands; in the latter, the cell arises from excretory or interlobular salivary gland ducts.

Pathology

Gross

■ Exophytic or submucosal, friable, edematous or granular mass with or without surface ulceration, measuring from 0.6 to 5.0 cm.

Histology

■ Infiltrating neoplasm composed of solid and glandular growth.

■ Squamous cell carcinoma component varies from well- to poorly differentiated; often there is an in situ carcinoma of the surface epithelium, extension of the in situ component to the contiguous minor salivary glands, or an invasive carcinoma arising from the surface epithelium.

■ Squamous cell differentiation is evident by the presence of individual cell keratinization, intercellular bridges, keratin pearl formation, or dyskeratosis.

■ Adenocarcinoma is identified in the submucosa and may be easily recognized by its glandular differentiation; mucous cell differentiation may not be seen and is not a prerequisite for diagnosis.

- The squamous cell carcinoma and adenocarcinoma may be admixed, but may also be distinct and separate from one another.
- Cellular pleomorphism, increased mitoses, foci of necrosis, and perineural invasion may be prominent.
- Histochemistry: the intracellular and intraluminal mucicarmine and diastase-resitant, PAS-positive material seen is associated with the glandular component.
- Immunohistochemistry: cytokeratin positive.

Differential Diagnosis

- Mucoepidermoid carcinoma (Chapter 19B, #1).
- Adenoid squamous cell carcinoma (Chapter 25C, #2).

Treatment and Prognosis

- Radical surgical excision is the treatment of choice.
- As a result of the propensity for this neoplasm to demonstrate early regional lymph node metastasis, radical neck dissection may be necessary as part of the initial management; radiotherapy is of questionable benefit.
- Prognosis is poor, because this neoplasm is aggressive and high grade, with increased tendency to be multifocal, deeply invasive, and metastatic.
- Metastases occur via lymphatics and blood vessels, with sites of predilection including regional lymph nodes, lung, and liver.
- 5-year survival rates are approximately 25%.

Additional Facts

- Metastatic disease histologically is similar to the primary neoplasm and includes both malignant histologic components.
- These neoplasms behave very aggressively, irrespective of the size of the neoplasm.

References

Damiani JM, Damiani KK, Hauck K, Hyams VJ: Mucoepidermoid-adenosquamous carcinoma of the larynx and hypopharynx: a report of 21 cases and a review of the literature. Otolaryngol Head Neck Surg 89:235–243, 1981.

Gerughty RM, Henniger GR, Brown RM: Adenosquamous carcinoma of the nasal, oral and laryngeal cavities: a clinicopathologic survey of 10 cases. Cancer 22:1140–1155, 1966.

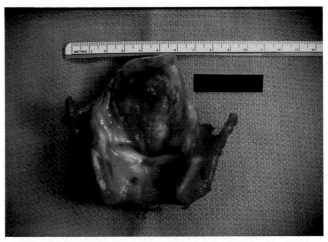

Figure 14–40. Adenosquamous carcinoma appearing as a large supraglottic mass extending down to involve the laryngeal ventricle.

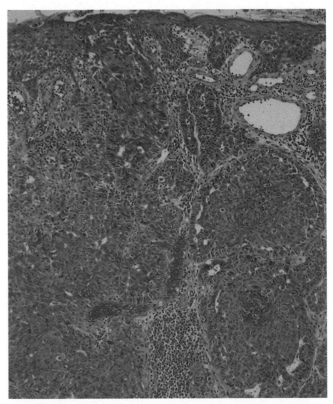

Figure 14–41. Adenosquamous carcinoma characterized by a neoplasm arising from the surface epithelium conisting of an admixture of glandular and squamous differentiation. The squamous component often shows evidence of keratinization (squamous pearls and/or individual cell keratinization).

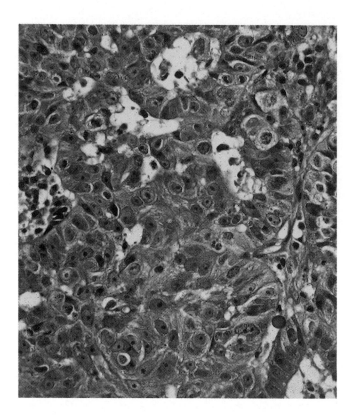

Figure 14–42. Adenosquamous carcinoma is a high-grade neoplasm composed of pleomorphic cells with enlarged round to oval nuclei, prominent eosinophilic nucleoli, and increased mitotic activity.

6. Neuroendocrine Carcinoma

Definition: Malignant neoplasm with divergent differentiation along both epithelial and neuroendocrine cell lines.

Clinical

■ In general, an uncommon class of neoplasms.
■ May be identified in virtually all sites of the head and neck, including larynx, sinonasal cavity, salivary glands, and middle ear.

LARYNGEAL NEUROENDOCRINE CARCINOMA

■ Affects males more than females; generally occurs in the sixth to seventh decades of life.
■ The supraglottic larynx is overwhelmingly the most common site of occurrence; however, both the glottis and subglottis occasionally may be the site of origin.
■ Hoarseness is the most common complaint.
■ Over 60% have a history of cigarette smoking.
■ *Classification of laryngeal neuroendocrine tumors:*
  1. Carcinoid tumor or well-differentiated neuroendocrine carcinoma (WDNEC).
  2. Atypical carcinoid or moderately differentiated neuroendocrine carcinoma (MDNEC).

  3. Small ("oat") cell carcinoma or poorly differentiated neuroendocrine carcinoma (PDNEC).
■ In order of frequency of occurrence: MDNEC > PDNEC > WDNEC.

Pathology

Gross

■ Submucosal nodular or polypoid mass with a tan-white appearance, varying in size from a few millimeters up to 4 cm in diameter.
■ Surface ulceration is generally absent in WDNEC and is often identified in association with MDNEC and PDNEC.

Histology

CARCINOID TUMOR (WDNEC)

■ Submucosal tumor arranged in organoid or trabecular growth pattern, with fibrovascular stroma.
■ Uniform cells with centrally located round nuclei, vesicular chromatin, and eosinophilic cytoplasm.
■ Absence of pleomorphism, mitoses, necrosis.
■ Glands or squamous differentiation can be seen.
■ Low nuclear:cytoplasmic ratio.
■ Surface ulceration uncommon.

- Vascular, lymphatic, and perineural invasion absent.
- Histochemistry: presence of epithelial mucin (diastase resistant, PAS positive), argyrophilia.
- Immunohistochemistry: cytokeratin, chromogranin, synaptophysin, Ber-EP4 and neuron-specific enolase positive.
- Electronmicroscopy: abundant neurosecretory granules (90–230 nm); cellular junctional complexes, inter- and intracellular lumina are present.

ATYPICAL CARCINOID (MDNEC)

Synonyms: Pleomorphic, malignant, or anaplastic carcinoid tumors.

- Submucosal tumor arranged in organoid, trabecular, cribriform, or solid growth with a prominent fibrovascular stroma.
- Mild to marked cellular pleomorphism with round to oval nuclei, vesicular to hyperchromatic chromatin and eosinophilic cytoplasm; nuclei can be centrally or eccentrically located.
- Nucleoli may be prominent.
- Mitoses, although uncommon, can be seen; necrosis may be focally seen.
- Glandular and squamous differentiation can be identified.
- Variable nuclear:cytoplasmic ratio.
- Surface ulceration may be prominent.
- Vascular, lymphatic, and perineural invasion may be present.
- Histochemistry: presence of epithelial mucin (diastase resistant, PAS positive, and occasionally mucicarmine positive), argyrophilia; rarely, argentaffin positive.
- Immunohistochemistry: cytokeratin, chromogranin, synaptophysin, calcitonin, Ber-EP4, S-100 protein- and neuron-specific enolase positive; HMB-45 negative.
- Electronmicroscopy: neurosecretory granules are commonly seen (70–420 nm); cellular junctional complexes, inter- and intracellular lumina are present.

SMALL CELL CARCINOMA (PDNEC)

Synonym: Oat cell carcinoma.

- Submucosal tumor arranged in solid nests, sheets, or ribbons, with absence of a fibrovascular stromal component.
- Marked cellular pleomorphism associated with "crush" artifact, cellular necrosis, hyperchromatic oval to spindle nuclei, abundant mitoses.
- Glands and squamous differentiation rarely seen.
- High nuclear:cytoplasmic ratio.
- Surface ulceration present.
- Vascular, lymphatic, and perineural invasion commonly seen.
- Histochemistry: epithelial mucin may be present; argyrophilia rarely is present.
- Immunohistochemistry: cytokeratin, chromogranin,

synaptophysin, Ber-EP4 and neuron-specific enolase may be present; calcitonin rarely is present.
- Electronmicroscopy: scanty neurosecretory granules (50–200 nm); cellular junctional complexes, inter- and intracellular lumina are usually absent.

Differential Diagnosis

- Poorly differentiated squamous cell carcinoma (Chapter 14B, #1).
- Basaloid squamous cell carcinoma (Chapter 14B, #4).
- Adenosquamous carcinoma (Chapter 14B, #5).
- Paraganglioma (Chapter 9A, #4).
- Extramedullary plasmacytoma (Chapter 9B, #4).
- Medullary carcinoma of the thyroid.
- Primary laryngeal malignant melanoma and metastatic melanoma to the larynx (Chapter 4B, #3).

Treatment and Prognosis

CARCINOID TUMOR (WDNEC)
- Complete but conservative surgical excision is the treatment of choice.
- Benign behavior: excellent prognosis after excision; rarely metastasizes.
- Infrequent association with paraneoplastic syndrome.

ATYPICAL CARCINOID (MDNEC)
- Complete surgical excision is the treatment of choice.
- Radiotherapy and chemotherapy are of questionable benefit, except in metastatic disease.
- Malignant behavior, often with metastasis to cervical lymph nodes, lung, bone, liver, and skin.
- Prognosis is dependant on extent of disease at presentation:
  When the tumor is confined to the larynx—62% tumor free over a median of 3 years, 9 months.
  The presence of metastatic disease (either at presentation or developing subsequently) is an ominous sign, with death at intervals ranging from 1 to 6 years.
- Rarely associated with paraneoplastic syndrome.

SMALL CELL CARCINOMA (PDNEC)
- Systemic chemotherapy and therapeutic irradiation.
- Malignant behavior; metastases are commonly seen to the liver, lung, bone, lymph nodes, brain, pancreas.
- Prognosis is poor, with 2-year survival rates of 16%.
- Occasionally associated with paraneoplastic syndrome.

Additional Facts

- The differentiation of MDNEC from a medullary carcinoma of thyroid origin when the presentation is that of a cervical lymph node metastasis of occult origin is difficult, given the overlapping histologic and immunohistochemical features; other than identification of a thyroid mass with subsequent tissue confirmation of a medullary carcinoma, the differentiation can be made by serum calcitonin levels, which are almost invariably elevated in thyroid medullary carcinoma and almost always within normal limits in MDNEC.

References

Ferlito A (ed): Neuroendocrine neoplasms of the larynx. J Otorhinolaryngol Relat Spec 53:185–264, 1991.

Gnepp DR, Ferlito A, Hyams V: Primary anaplastic small cell (oat cell) carcinoma of the larynx. Cancer 51:1731–1745, 1983.

Mills SE, Cooper PH, Garland TA, Johns ME: Small cell undifferentiated carcinoma of the larynx: report of 2 patients and review of 13 additional cases. Cancer 51:116–120, 1983.

Myerowitz RL, Barnes EL, Myers E: Small cell anaplastic (oat cell) carcinoma of the larynx: report of a case and review of the literature. Laryngoscope 10:1697–1702, 1978.

Patterson SD, Yarrington CT: Carcinoid tumor of the larynx: the role of conservative therapy. Ann Otol Rhinol Laryngol 96:12–14, 1987.

Stanley RJ, Desanto LW, Weiland LH: Oncocytic and oncocytoid tumors (well-differentiated neuroendocrine carcinoma) of the larynx. Arch Otolaryngol Head Neck Surg 112:529–535, 1986.

Wenig BM, Hyams VJ, Heffner DK: Moderately differentiated neuroendocrine carcinoma of the larynx: a clinicopathologic study of 54 cases. Cancer 62:2658–2676, 1988.

Wenig BM, Gnepp DR: The spectrum of neuroendocrine carcinomas of the larynx. Semin Diagn Pathol 6:329–350, 1989.

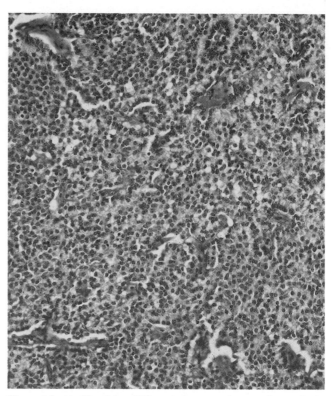

Figure 14–44. Glandular differentiation may be seen in carcinoid tumors that are composed of uniform cells with centrally located round nuclei, vesicular chromatin, and eosinophilic cytoplasm.

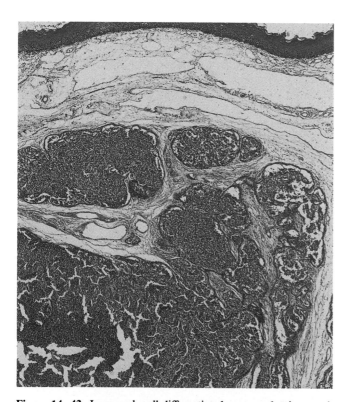

Figure 14–43. Laryngeal well-differentiated neuroendocrine carcinoma (carcinoid tumor): submucosal cellular neoplasm with lobular and solid growth patterns associated with a fibrovascular stroma.

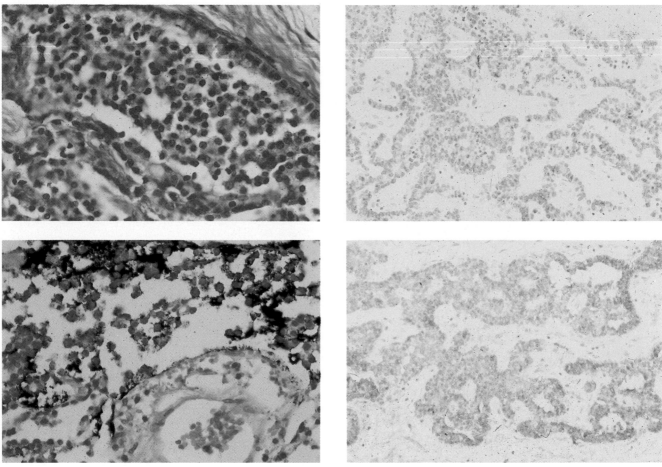

Figure 14–45. (*Top*) Carcinoid tumors are composed of uniform cells generally devoid of cellular pleomorphism, mitoses, and necrosis. (*Bottom*) Argyrophilic stain, showing the neoplastic cells to contain black cytoplasmic granules.

Figure 14–46. Immunohistochemistry of carcinoid tumors includes immunoreactivity with cytokeratin (*top*) and chromogranin (*bottom*).

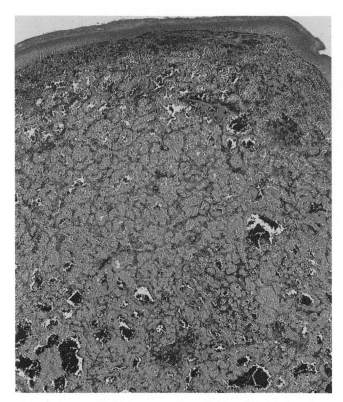

Figure 14-47. Laryngeal moderately differentiated neuroendocrine carcinoma (atypical carcinoid tumor) showing a submucosal cellular infiltrate with an organoid and glandular appearance.

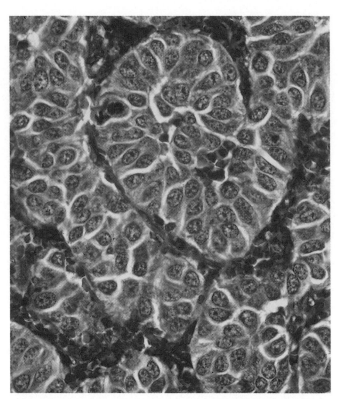

Figure 14-49. Laryngeal atypical carcinoids are characterized by mild to marked cellular pleomorphism with round to oval nuclei, vesicular to hyperchromatic chromatin and eosinophilic cytoplasm; nucleoli may be prominent and mitoses, although uncommon, can be seen.

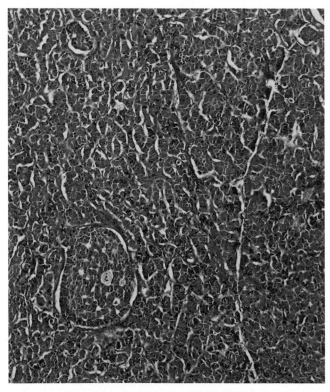

Figure 14-48. Other morphologic patterns identified in atypical carcinoids include trabecular and cribriform growth.

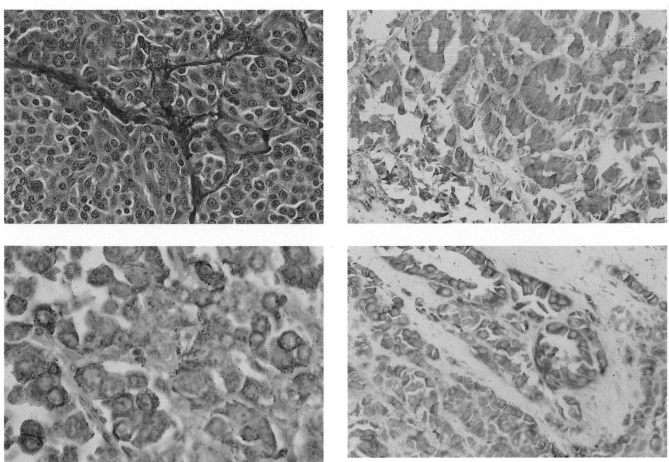

Figure 14–50. (*Top*) Organoid growth composed of pleomorphic cells characteristic of atypical carcinoids. (*Bottom*) Argyrophilic stain, showing the neoplastic cells to contain brown cytoplasmic granules.

Figure 14–51. Among the various immunohistochemical markers seen in association with atypical carcinoid tumors are cytokeratin (*top*) and chromogranin (*bottom*).

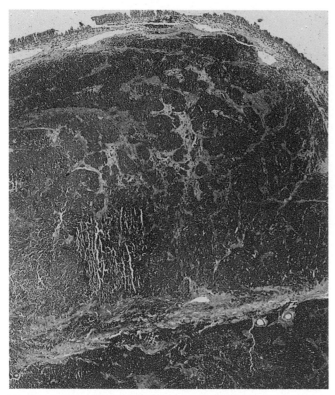

Figure 14–52. Poorly differentiated neuroendocrine carcinoma (small cell carcinoma) of the larynx showing a submucosal tumor arranged in solid nests, sheets, or ribbons.

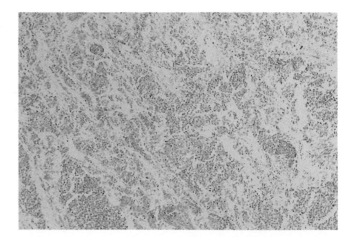

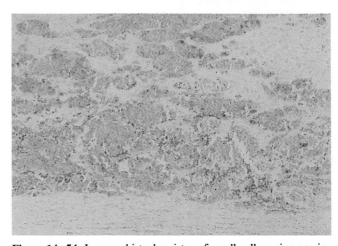

Figure 14–54. Immunohistochemistry of small cell carcinomas includes immunoreactivity with cytokeratin (*top*) and chromogranin (*bottom*); due to the poor differentiation, immunohistochemical studies may be negative, with the diagnosis based on the histologic appearance.

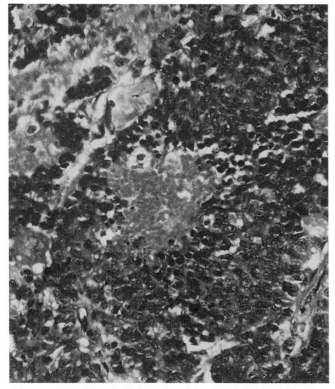

Figure 14–53. Small cell carcinoma is characterized by marked cellular pleomorphism, hyperchromatic oval to spindle nuclei, increased mitoses, and necrosis.

7. Chondrosarcoma

Definition: Malignant tumor of cartilage.

Clinical

- In general, a rare neoplasm in all head and neck sites.
- Affects males more than females; occurs in the fourth to seventh decades.
- Most common site of occurrence in the head and neck is the larynx; other sites of involvement include mandible, maxilla, maxillofacial skeleton (nose and paranasal sinuses), nasopharynx.
- The most common site in the larynx is the anterior surface of the posterior lamina of the cricoid cartilage > thyroid cartilage > arytenoid.
- Symptoms vary according to the site of origin:
  Larynx: endolaryngeal growth produces dyspnea, stridor, dysphagia, or hoarseness; extralaryngeal growth is uncommon and may produce dysphagia.
  Sinonasal: nasal obstruction, epistaxis, changes in dentition (loosening or eruption of teeth), proptosis, visual disturbances, and an expanding mass associated with pain, trismus, neural deficits.

Radiology

- Laryngeal: same as chondroma; tomograms may delineate the extent of invasiveness.
- Sinonasal: destructive lesion with single or multiple radiolucent, radiopaque, or mixed-appearing areas.

Pathology

Gross

- Smooth, lobulated, hard submucosal mass larger than 2 cm in diameter.

Histology

- Lobulated hypercellular tumor with hyperchromatic, pleomorphic nuclei and prominent nucleoli.
- Binucleate or multinucleate cells.
- Mitoses are uncommon.
- **Note:** chondrosarcomas are graded as low-grade or high-grade lesions based on the degree of cellularity, pleomorphism, multinucleated cells, and mitoses.

Differential Diagnosis

- Chondroma (Chapter 14A, #3).
- Chondromatous metaplasia/hamartomas.
- Chordoma (Chapter 9B, #7).

Treatment and Prognosis

- Laryngeal chondrosarcoma:
  Wide local (conservation) excision.
  Total laryngectomy indicated in cases with extensive cricoid involvement.
  Cured after complete excision of the tumor.
  Local recurrence occurs in approximately 25% of cases and can be managed by additional (definitive) surgery.
  Distant metastases are uncommon but can occur (lungs).
  Histologic grading (low versus high grade) has no prognostic import.
- Maxillofacial chondrosarcoma:
  Radical resection.
  Slow-growing but persistent neoplasms.
  Multiple recurrences are common.
  More lethal than laryngeal chondrosarcoma.
  Death generally related to local, uncontrolled disease with invasion and destruction of vital structures.
  Prognosis dependent on (1) site and extent of disease (chondrosarcomas of the posterior nasal cavity or nasopharynx tend to remain clinically quiescent until they reach large sizes, making resection more difficult); (2) histologic grade—high-grade chondrosarcomas have a higher incidence of metastases (lungs and bone) and are more locally aggressive; (3) adequacy of surgical resection.

Additional Facts

- Nearly all cases of laryngeal chondrosarcomas arise from hyaline rather than elastic cartilage.
- Osseous components may be identified histologically and do not impact on the diagnosis or prognosis.
- For all head and neck chondrosarcomas, radiotherapy and chemotherapy have not been demonstrated to be effective therapeutic modalities.

References

Burkey BB, Hoffman HT, Baker SR, Thornton AF, McClatchey KD: Chondrosarcoma of the head and neck. Laryngoscope 100:1301–1305, 1990.

Chaudhry AP, Robinovitch MR, Mitchell DR, Vickers RA: Chondrogenic tumors of the jaws. Am J Surg 102:403–411, 1961.

Ferlito A, Nicolai P, Montaguti A, Ceccheto A, Pennelli N: Chondrosarcoma of the larynx: review of the literature and report of three cases. Am J Otolaryngol 5:350–359, 1984.

Fu YS, Perzin KH: Non-epithelial tumors of the nasal cavity, paranasal sinuses, and nasopharynx: a clinicopathologic study. III: cartilaginous tumors (chondroma, chondrosarcoma). Cancer 34:453–463, 1974.

Hackney FL, Aragon SB, Aufdemorte TB, Holt GR, Van Sickels JE: Chondrosarcoma of the jaws: clinical findings, histopathology, and treatment. Oral Surg Oral Med Oral Pathol 71:139–143, 1991.

Hellquist H, Olofsson J, Grontoft O: Chondrosarcoma of the larynx. J Laryngol Otol 93:1037–1047, 1990.

Hyams VJ, Rabuzzi DD: Cartilaginous tumors of the larynx. Laryngoscope 80:755–767, 1970.

Nicolai P, Ferlito A, Sasaki CT, Kirchner JA: Laryngeal chondrosarcoma: incidence, pathology, biological behavior, and treatment. Ann Otol Rhinol Laryngol 99:515–523, 1990.

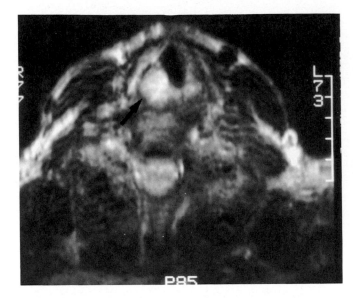

Figure 14–55. Axial T2-weighted MRI, laryngeal chondrosarcoma. The lesion is rounded, is located near the junction of the posterior right vocal cord and arytenoid cartilage, and appears bright on the T2-weighted image (*arrow*).

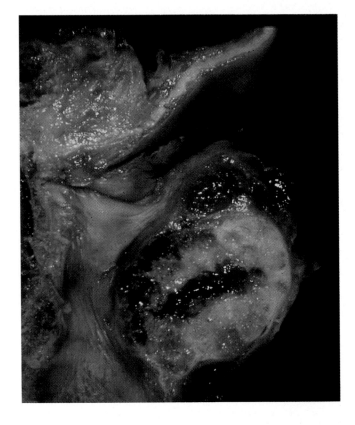

Figure 14–56. Laryngeal chondrosarcoma: a smooth, lobulated, glistening mass arising from the cricoid cartilage.

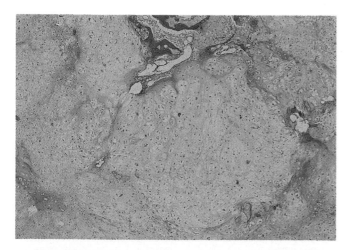

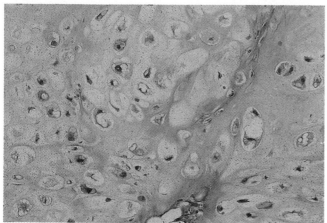

Figure 14–57. Low-grade laryngeal chondrosarcoma. (*Top*) Lobulated cellular neoplasm. (*Bottom*) The tumor is composed of enlarged chondrocytes with hyperchromatic, pleomorphic nuclei, prominent nucleoli, and binucleate cells.

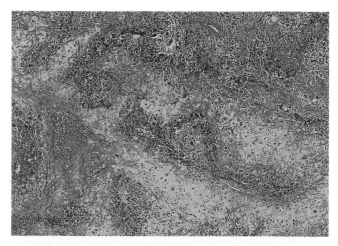

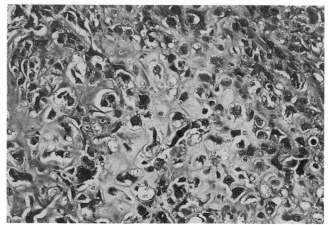

Figure 14–58. High-grade laryngeal chondrosarcoma. (*Top*) Portion of a lobulated markedly cellular neoplasm with many atypical enlarged cells with hyperchromatic nuclei and necrosis. (*Bottom*) Cellular infiltrate with hyperchromatic, pleomorphic nuclei, prominent nucleoli, multinucleated cells, and mitoses.

8. Synovial Sarcoma

Definition: Malignant neoplasm of uncertain histogenesis, primarily arising in soft tissues (paraarticular regions) in close association with a variety of joints, but uncommonly occuring within joint spaces.

Clinical

- Synovial sarcoma represents from approximately 6% to 10% of all soft tissue sarcomas; only 3% of all synovial sarcomas occur in the head and neck region.
- Affects males more than female; occurs in the adolescent and young adult population, with an average age of 25 years at the time of presentation.

- The most common sites of occurrence in the head and neck include the neck and the pharyngeal region (hypopharynx and retropharynx).
- Symptoms vary according to site of occurrence and include a neck mass with or without associated pain, dysphagia, dyspnea, hoarseness, and hemoptysis.
- There are no known predisposing risk factors.

Radiology

- Multiple, spotty opacifications that are more pronounced at the periphery than at the center of the lesion in an otherwise undistinguished soft tissue mass is a characteristic finding in about one third of cases; these opacifications represent focal calcifications and although not limited to synovial sarcoma, may assist in the radiographic differential diagnosis.

Pathology

Gross

■ Circumscribed or pseudoencapsulated spherical, lobulated, or multinodular mass, ranging in size from 1 to 10 cm.
■ Variation in color (yellow, gray, or white), consistency (soft, rubbery, firm, gritty), and appearance of the cut surface (fibrous, whorled, cystic, mucoid).

Histology

Two types:

1. biphasic—epithelioid *and* fibrous.
2. monophasic—epithelioid *or* fibrous.
   ■ Epithelioid cells—columnar, cuboidal, or polygonal cells with round to oval, vesicular nuclei, abundant pale-staining cytoplasm with distinct cell borders arranged in cords, nests, or whorls and identified lining gland-like or cystic spaces.
   ■ Spindle cells—generally represents the most prominent component; well-oriented plump cells with oval nuclei and scant cytoplasm.
   ■ Mitoses can be seen, but generally are not abundant.
   ■ Mast cells often seen and are more numerous in the spindle cell areas.
   ■ Calcification may be prominent.
   ■ Papillary areas may be seen.
   ■ Histochemistry:
     Epithelial mucin (diastase-resistant PAS-positive and mucicarmine-positive) seen within epithelial cells, pseudoglandular spaces, and intracellular areas.
     Mesenchymal mucin (colloidal iron and alcian blue, hyaluronidase-sensitive) seen in relation to the spindle cell component and myxoid areas.
   ■ Immunohistochemistry:
     Epithelioid cells: cytokeratin and epithelial membrane antigen (EMA) positive; vimentin negative.

Spindle cells: cytokeratin, EMA, and vimentin positive.

Differential Diagnosis

■ Hemangiopericytoma (Chapter 4A, #3).
■ Spindle cell carcinoma or carcinosarcoma (Chapter 14B, #2).
■ Malignant schwannoma (Chapter 9B, #6).
■ Fibrosarcoma (Chapter 4B, #7).
■ Malignant melanoma (Chapter 4B, #3).
■ Epithelioid sarcoma.
■ Papillary carcinoma of thyroid gland origin.

Treatment and Prognosis

■ Surgery, with preoperative and postoperative radiotherapy.
■ Overall prognosis is not good, with tendency to local recurrence as well as for metastatic disease (lung, lymph nodes, and bone).

Additional Facts

■ Recurrent or metastatic synovial sarcoma may demonstrate histologic variation from the primary neoplasm—a biphasic synovial sarcoma may recur or metastasize as a predominantly or exclusively monophasic (epithelioid or spindle cell) synovial sarcoma.

References

Amble FR, Olsen KD, Nascimento AG, Foote RL: Head and neck synovial sarcoma. Otolaryngol Head Neck Surg 107:631–637, 1992.

Bridge JA, Bridge RS, Borek DA, Shaffer B, Norris CW: Translocation t(x;18) in orofacial synovial sarcoma. Cancer 62:935–937, 1988.

Jernstrom P: Synovial sarcoma of the pharynx: report of a case. Am J Clin Pathol 24:957–961, 1954.

Ordonez NG, Mahfouz SM, Mackay B: Synovial sarcoma: an immunohistochemical and ultrastructural study. Hum Pathol 21:733–749, 1990.

Pruszczynski M, Manni JJ, Smedts F: Endolaryngeal synovial sarcoma: case report with immunohistochemical studies. Head Neck Surg 11:76–80, 1989.

Roth JA, Enzinger FM, Tannenbaum M: Synovial sarcoma of the neck: a follow-up study of 24 cases. Cancer 35:1243–1253, 1975.

Schmookler BM, Enzinger FM, Brannon RB: Orofacial synovial sarcoma. Cancer 1982; 50:269–276, 1982.

Varela-Duran J, Enzinger FM: Calcifying synovial sarcoma. Cancer 50:345–352, 1982.

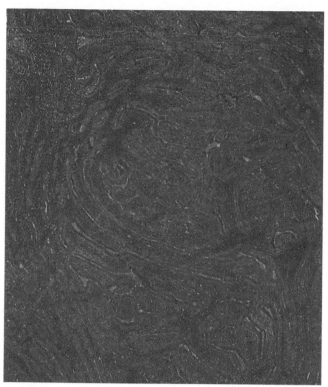

Figure 14–59. Biphasic pattern of synovial sarcoma of the hypopharynx characterized by a combination of gland- or cleft-like spaces lined by epithelioid cells admixed with a spindle-shaped cell component.

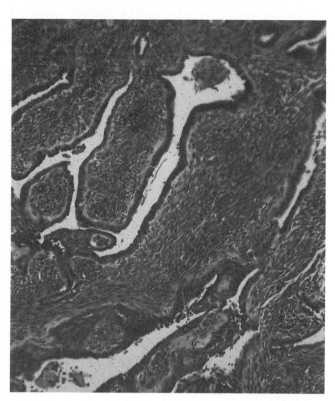

Figure 14–60. Biphasic synovial sarcoma characterized by cleft-like spaces lined by columnar- to polygonal-appearing epithelioid cells with round to oval nuclei, eosinophilic cytoplasm, and distinct cell borders demarcated from the surrounding spindle-shaped cell component.

Figure 14–61. Monophasic (fibrous) synovial sarcoma of the hypopharynx characterized by a hypercellular spindle cell population; areas of calcifications are prominently seen in the lower portion of the illustration.

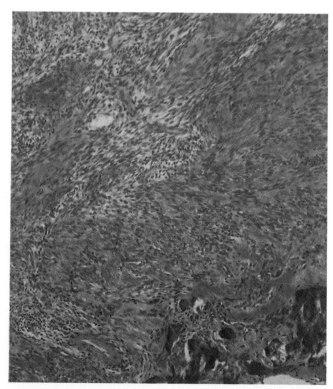

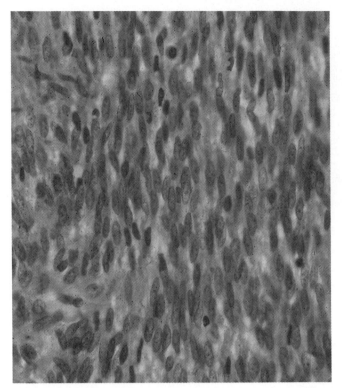

Figure 14–62. Monophasic (fibrous) synovial sarcoma composed of nondescript, fairly uniform, plump-appearing spindle-shaped cells with ovoid nuclei and indistinct cytoplasm; scattered mast cells can be seen.

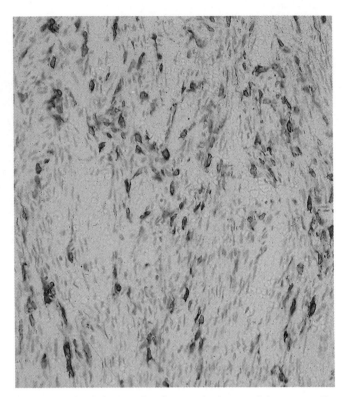

Figure 14–63. Spindle cells of monophasic synovial sarcoma display cytokeratin immunoreactivity. The typical immunohistochemical profile for synovial sarcoma includes cytokeratin reactivity in both the epithelioid and spindle cell components and vimentin reactivity in the spindle cell component but absent in the epithelial cells.

CHAPTER 15

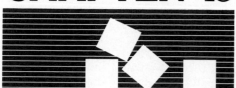

TNM Classification of Laryngeal and Hypopharyngeal Neoplasms

ANATOMIC SITES

Larynx

Supraglottis

1. Suprahyoid epiglottis.
2. Aryepiglottic fold.
3. Arytenoid.
4. Infrahyoid epiglottis.
5. Ventricular bands (false vocal cords).
6. Ventricles.

Glottis

1. True vocal cords.
2. Anterior commissure.
3. Posterior commissure.

Subglottis

Hypopharynx

1. Pharyngo-esophageal junction (posterior cricoid area).
2. Pyriform sinus.
3. Posterior pharyngeal wall.

CLASSIFICATION

1. T—extent of the primary tumor.
   - Includes both the clinical (T) and pathologic (pT) categories.
   - T designation varies according to the anatomic site involved:

TX—primary tumor cannot be assessed.
T0—no evidence of primary tumor.
Tis—carcinoma in situ.

Supraglottis

T1—tumor limited to one subsite with normal vocal cord mobility.
T2—tumor invades more than one subsite of supraglottis or glottis with normal vocal cord mobility.
T3—tumor limited to the larynx with vocal cord fixation or invades the posterior cricoid area, medial wall of the pyriform sinus, or the pre-epiglottic tissues.
T4—tumor invades through the thyroid cartilage or extends to tissues beyond the larynx (oropharynx, soft tissues of the neck).

Glottis

T1—tumor limited to the vocal cord(s), with normal vocal cord mobility; anterior and posterior commissures may be involved.
   - T1a—tumor limited to one vocal cord.
   - T1b—tumor involves both vocal cords.
T2—tumor extends to the supraglottis or subglottis, or with impaired vocal cord mobility.
T3—tumor limited to the larynx with vocal cord fixation.
T4—tumor invades through the thyroid cartilage or extends to other tissues beyond the larynx (oropharynx, soft tissues of the neck).

Subglottis

T1—tumor limited to the subglottis.

T2—tumor extends to the vocal cord(s) with normal or impaired mobility.

T3—tumor limited to the larynx with vocal cord fixation.

T4—tumor invades through the cricoid or thyroid cartilage or extends to other tissues beyond the larynx (oropharynx, soft tissues of the neck).

Hypopharynx

TX—primary tumor cannot be assessed.

T0—no evidence of primary tumor.

Tis—carcinoma in situ.

T1—tumor limited to one subsite of the hypopharynx.

T2—tumor invades more than one subsite of the hypopharynx or an adjacent site without fixation of the hemilarynx.

T3—tumor invades more than one subsite of the hypopharynx or an adjacent site with fixation of the hemilarynx.

T4—tumor invades adjacent structures (cartilage or soft tissues of the neck).

2. N—absence/presence and extent of regional lymph node metastasis; includes both the clinical (N) and pathologic (pN) categories.

NX—regional lymph nodes cannot be assessed.

N0—no regional lymph node metastasis.

N1—metastasis in a single ipsilateral lymph node, 3 cm or less in greatest dimension.

N2—metastasis in a single ipsilateral lymph node, greater than 3 cm but not greater than 6 cm in greatest dimension or metastasis in multiple ipsilateral lymph nodes, none greater than 6 cm in greatest dimension or metastasis in bilateral or contralateral lymph nodes, none greater than 6 cm in greatest dimension.

- N2a—metastasis in a single ipsilateral lymph node, greater than 3 cm but not greater than 6 cm in greatest dimension.
- N2b—metastasis in multiple ipsilateral lymph nodes, none greater than 6 cm in greatest dimension.
- N2c—metastasis in bilateral or contralateral lymph nodes, none greater than 6 cm in greatest dimension.

N3—metastasis in a lymph node greater than 6 cm in greatest dimension.

3. M—absence or presence of distant metastasis; includes both the clinical (M) and pathologic (pM) categories.

M0—no distant metastasis.

M1—distant metastasis present.

CLINICAL STAGE

Stage I—T1N0M0.

Stage II—T2N0M0.

Stage III—T3N0M0 or T1–T3N1M0.

Stage IV—T4 or N2, N3, or M1.

Reference

Spiessl B, Beahrs OH, Hermanek P, Hutter RVP, Scheibe O, Sobin LH, Wagner G (eds): TNM atlas: illustrated guide to the tnm/ptnm-classification of malignant tumours, 3rd ed. Berlin: Springer-Verlag; 1989.

SECTION ■ 4

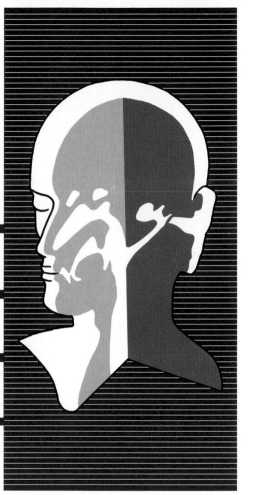

MAJOR AND MINOR SALIVARY GLANDS

CHAPTER 16

Anatomy and Histology of the Major and Minor Salivary Glands

ANATOMIC BORDERS
Parotid Glands
Submandibular (Submaxillary) Glands
Sublingual Glands
Minor Salivary Glands

HISTOLOGY
Acini
Intercalated Ducts
Striated Ducts
Excretory Ducts
Myoepithelial Cells

ANATOMIC BORDERS

Parotid Glands

Largest gland (average weight, 25 g).

Encapsulated and pyramidal-shaped, palpable between the ramus of the mandible and the mastoid process.

Artificially divided into two lobes: superficial (largest portion) and deep (situated adjacent to the lateral pharyngeal space).

■ Anterior: overlies the superficial surface of the masseter muscle.

■ Posterior: overlaps the sternocleidomastoid muscle and wraps around the lower ear.

■ Lateral or superficial: skin and dermis of the face.

■ Medial or deep: buttressed by the styloid process and its associated muscles (styloglossus, stylohyoid, stylopharyngeal) and by the carotid sheath and its contents (internal carotid artery, internal jugular vein, cranial nerves IX, X, and XII).

■ Superior: zygomatic arch.

■ Inferior: sternocleidomastoid muscle (oblique anterior border).

■ Parotid (Stensen's) duct: approximately 5 mm long; originates from the anterior portion of the parotid, coursing forward over the masseter muscle, enters the buccal fat pad piercing the buccinator muscle, and opens in the oral cavity opposite the second maxillary molar (parotid papilla).

Submandibular (Submaxillary) Glands

Each gland weighs from 10 to 15 g.

Encapsulated and walnut-shaped, located in the submandibular triangle, situated below the angle of the mandible.

Divided into superficial and deep lobes; the latter can be palpated only in the floor of the mouth.

■ Anterior: anterior belly of the digastric muscle.

■ Posterior: stylomandibular ligament, which separates it from the lower part of the parotid.

■ Lateral: in relation to the submandibular fossa on the inner surface of the body of the mandible.

■ Medial: bounded by several muscles (mylohyoid, styloglossus, hyoglossus, stylohyoid, and posterior belly of the digastric) and nerves (hypoglossal, glossopharyngeal, and lingual).

■ Superior: inferior border of the body of the mandible.

■ Inferior: skin, platysma, and deep fascia.

■ Submandibular (Wharton's) duct: runs forward along the inner surface of the mandible, in parallel with the lingual nerve passes medial to the lower border of the sublingual gland, at which point the duct may receive the major sublingual duct (Bartholin's) prior to opening in the oral cavity at the sublingual caruncle or papilla lateral to the frenulum.

Sublingual Glands

Smallest of the major salivary glands, weighing between 2 and 4 g.

Almond-shaped, located submucosally in the floor of the mouth.

- Anterior: opposite sublingual gland.
- Posterior: deep part of the submandibular gland.
- Lateral: internal aspect of the body of the mandible.
- Medial: genioglossus muscle.
- Superior: mucosa of the floor of the mouth, which it raises to form the sublingual fold.
- Inferior: mylohyoid muscle.
- Some ducts open into the oral cavity proper via tiny (Rivinus's) ducts; other ducts unite to form the common sublingual (Bartholin's) duct, which merges with the submandibular duct prior to opening in the oral cavity lateral to the frenulum.

Minor Salivary Glands

- Located throughout the submucosa of the upper aerodigestive tract.

HISTOLOGY

- Common to all salivary glands is their arborizing, epithelial ductal system, with production of saliva from the specialized secretory cells in the distal segments and delivery of these secretions via the complex branching structures to the oral cavity.
- From distal to proximal the system includes:

Acini: terminal secretory cells include serous or mucous cells, which produce the saliva.

Serous cells: pyramidal-shaped cells with a narrow apex toward the luminal aspect, round nuclei near the basal one third of the cell, and prominent eosinophilic cytoplasmic granules situated at the apical portion.

Mucous cells: pyramidal-shaped cells with basally located flattened nuclei and secretory droplets at the apical portion of the cell.

Intercalated ducts: composed of cuboidal cells with centrally located oval nuclei and scant cytoplasm.

Striated ducts: columnar cells with centrally located round nuclei that display deep basal membrane indentations, for which these ducts are named.

Excretory ducts: cellular component varies from pseudostratified columnar cells adjacent to the striated duct cells to stratified squamous cells as these cells approach the oral cavity.

Myoepithelial cells: ectodermally derived, flat, elongated cells lying at the periphery of the acinar cells and the intercalated cells in the space between the basement membrane and the basal plasma membrane; generally, myoepithelial cells are difficult to identify by light microscopy; their contractile function is similar to smooth muscle, assisting in the movement of saliva through the duct system.

- The histologic difference between the salivary glands rests with the make-up of their respective acinar cells and includes:

Parotid: entirely serous.

Submandibular: serous and mucous.

Sublingual: predominantly mucous, with serous demilunes.

Minor salivary glands: seromucous.

References

Embryology, Anatomy, Histology

Dardick I: Histogenesis and morphogenesis of salivary gland neoplasms. *In:* Ellis GL, Auclair PL, Gnepp DR, eds. Surgical pathology of the salivary glands. Philadelphia: W.B. Saunders Co., 1991; pp 108–128.

Fawcett DW: Oral cavity and associated glands. *In:* Fawcett DW, ed. Bloom and Fawcett: a textbook of histology, 11th ed. Philadelphia: W.B. Saunders Co., 1986; pp 579–601.

Hiatt JL, Sauk JJ: Embryology and anatomy of the salivary glands. *In:* Ellis GL, Auclair PL, Gnepp DR, eds. Surgical pathology of the salivary glands. Philadelphia: W.B. Saunders Co., 1991; pp 2–9.

Hollinshead WH: The face. *In:* Hollinshead WH, ed. Anatomy for surgeons, vol. 1, 3rd ed. Philadelphia: Harper & Row, 1982; Chapter 6, pp 291–323.

Hollinshead WH: The jaws, palate and tongue. *In:* Hollinshead WH, ed. Anatomy for surgeons, vol. 1, 3rd ed. Philadelphia: Harper & Row, 1982; Chapter 7, pp 325–387.

Warwick R, Williams PL: The salivary glands. *In:* Warwick R, Williams PL, eds. Gray's anatomy, 35th British ed. Philadelphia: W.B. Saunders Co., 1973; pp 1209–1214.

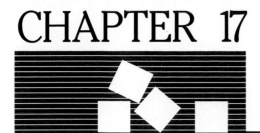

CHAPTER 17

Classification of Non-neoplastic Salivary Gland Disorders and Neoplasms of the Salivary Gland

NON-NEOPLASTIC SALIVARY GLAND DISORDERS

Table 17–1
CLASSIFICATION OF NON-NEOPLASTIC
SALIVARY GLAND DISORDERS

Developmental diseases (heterotopias, oncocytosis, hyperplasia)
Obstructive disorders (mucous retention cyst, ranula, sialolithiasis)
Necrotizing sialometaplasia
Infectious diseases (sialadenitides)
Sialadenosis and systemic diseases
Idiopathic (necrotizing sialometaplasia, cysts)
Autoimmune diseases (benign lymphoepithelial lesion, Sjögren's syndrome)
Others

Table 17–2
CLASSIFICATION OF NEOPLASMS OF
THE SALIVARY GLAND

A. Benign
 Epithelial
 Pleomorphic adenoma
 Monomorphic adenomas (papillary cystadenoma lymphomatosum or Warthin's tumor; oncocytoma; basal cell adenoma; others)
 Papillomas (sialadenoma papilliferum, inverted ductal papilloma and intraductal papilloma)
 Sebaceous neoplasms (adenoma/lymphadenoma)
 Nonepithelial
 Hemangioma
 Neurilemmoma/neurofibroma
 Lipoma
 Others
B. Malignant
 Epithelial
 Mucoepidermoid carcinoma
 Acinic cell adenocarcinoma
 Adenoid cystic carcinoma
 Malignant mixed tumor (carcinoma ex pleomorphic adenoma/carcinosarcoma

NEOPLASMS OF THE SALIVARY GLAND

B. Malignant
 Epithelial *(Continued)*
 Basal cell adenocarcinoma
 Polymorphous low-grade adenocarcinoma
 Epithelial-myoepithelial carcinoma
 Clear cell carcinoma
 Cystadenocarcinoma
 Sebaceous carcinoma/lymphadenocarcinoma
 Adenocarcinoma, not otherwise specified (NOS)
 Salivary duct carcinoma
 Squamous cell carcinoma
 Adenosquamous carcinoma
 Lymphoepithelial carcinoma (malignant lymphoepithelial lesion)
 Myoepithelial carcinoma
 Small cell carcinoma
 Oncocytic carcinoma
 Nonepithelial
 Lymphomas (non-Hodgkin's and Hodgkin's)
 Sarcomas
 Metastatic neoplasms
 Malignant melanoma
 Squamous cell carcinoma
 Renal cell carcinoma
 Thyroid carcinoma

CHAPTER 18

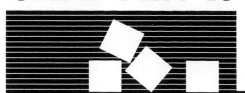

Non-neoplastic Diseases of Salivary Glands

1. SIALADENITIS
2. SIALOLITHIASIS

3. BENIGN LYMPHOEPITHELIAL LESION
   AND SJÖGREN'S SYNDROME

1. SIALADENITIS

Definition: Acute, subacute, or chronic inflammation of the salivary glands due to a variety of causes, including specific infectious agent(s), as part of a systemic disease, trauma, or secondary to stone formation.

Clinical

- Infections of the salivary glands may occur in a previously healthy gland, or may result from a decrease in the function of the gland secondary to physiologic dysfunction or to an anatomic barrier.
- Microorganisms may gain access to the gland via retrograde extension through the ductal system, lymphatic spread to intraglandular lymph nodes, or by hematogenous routes.
- Sialadenitis may be acute or chronic and result from obstructive or nonobstructive causes.
- Nonobstructive sialadenitides are generally caused by an infectious agent and are divided into acute and chronic forms.

ACUTE NONOBSTRUCTIVE SIALADENITIS

- Most commonly affects the parotid and submandibular glands.
- May be bacterial or viral.
- Bacterial—causative infectious agent is most frequently *Staphylococcus aureus;* other microorganisms implicated are *Hemophilus influenzae, Streptococcus pyogenes* and *pneumoniae, Escherichia coli,* and anaerobic organisms.
- Viral—the most common viral illness infecting the salivary glands is epidemic parotitis (mumps), the causative organism being an RNA virus in the *paramyxovirus* group; patients who are serologically negative for mumps may have infection caused by other viruses, including *coxsackie A, ECHO, Epstein-Barr virus, cytomegalovirus, parainfluenza virus type C,* and *lymphocytic choriomeningitis virus.*

CHRONIC (SPECIFIC) NONOBSTRUCTIVE SIALADENITIS

- Results from granulomatous inflammation of the salivary glands, caused by a number of diseases, including sarcoidosis, tuberculosis, actinomycosis, and cat-scratch disease.
- Granulomatous sialadenitis may occur as an isolated phenomenon, but is more commonly seen as part of a systemic process.
- Diagnosis is made by histologic appearance or identification of the causative microorganism.
- Sarcoidosis is a diagnosis of exclusion, typified by noncaseating granulomas; it may occur as an isolated process or as part of a syndrome termed *uveoparotid fever,* also known as *Heerfordt's disease,* which includes sarcoid involvement of:
  The parotid and lacrimal glands with xerostomia.
  Uveal tract inflammation with xerophthalmia.
  Cranial nerve involvement (usually the facial nerve).
- Once the diagnosis is established, treatment is directed at the causative organism; in the case of uveoparotid fever, sarcoidosis tends to resolve spontaneously and treatment is directed at the complications.

275

Chronic Obstructive Sialadenitis

■ The most common cause of obstructive or occlusive sialadenitis is stone formation (sialolithiasis).
■ Chronic sialadenitis may or may not be associated with stone formation; however, calculi are seen in nearly two thirds of patients with chronic sialadenitis.

Additional Facts

Sialadenosis

■ Non-neoplastic, noninflammatory enlargement of salivary glands (in particular, the parotid).
■ Almost always associated with a systemic disorder; occurs most commonly at the fourth decade of life or later.
■ Salivary gland enlargement is usually bilateral, is an indolent process, may be chronic and recurrent, and may be associated with pain; patients are generally afebrile.
■ Histomorphologic features include acinar enlargement with absent inflammatory cell infiltrate; histologic findings demonstrate little correlation to specific underlying disorder.

2. SIALOLITHIASIS

Definition: The occurrence of calcerous concretions within the salivary gland ducts or parenchyma as a result of mineralization of debris accumulated within duct luminae.

Clinical

■ Calculi may be seen in the ductal system of all salivary glands, but are particularly common in the submandibular (90% of cases) and parotid glands (10% of cases); sublingual or minor salivary glands are rarely affected.
■ Affects males more than females; may occur at any age, but is most frequently seen in middle-aged adults.
■ Symptoms depend on the size and location of the calculi.
  1. Submandibular gland calculi:
     Are larger than those of the parotid gland.
     Produce recurrent episodes of pain and swelling, usually in association with meals.
     May be associated with sore throat or pharyngitis refractory to antibiotic therapy.
  2. Parotid gland calculi:
     Are usually smaller than those of the submandibular gland.
     May function as a ball-valve effect, producing intermittent obstruction and symptoms; the latter include pain and swelling.
■ If the obstruction is not relieved, stasis of saliva ensues, potentially resulting in an associated bacterial infection (most often due to *Streptococcus viridans*), which is manifested by expression from the ducts of mucopurulent material (pus).

■ Calculi may be palpated or even visualized in the distal duct system; because of its deeper anatomic location, calculi within Stensen's duct are often not palpable.
■ Sialoliths may clinically simulate a neoplasm.

Radiology

■ Represents the most reliable means to detect the presence of calculi.
■ The majority of calculi are radiopaque and can be visualized by routine radiography.
■ The majority of parotid gland calculi are radiolucent and may require special oblique views of the cheek for visualization.
■ Sialography may be of assistance, but is often unnecessary, yielding limited additional information and being a potential source of inducing an infection.

Pathology

Gross

■ Enlarged, firm, nonfluctuating salivary gland.
■ Sialoliths are round to oval, white to yellow-brown, measuring from a few millimeters to several centimeters in diameter.

Histology

■ Calculi may be seen within the parenchyma or in the ducts as concentric laminations of calcification peripherally surrounded by compressed epithelium.
■ The ductal epithelium may demonstrate mucous cell, squamous, or oncocytic metaplasia.
■ Parenchymal changes may include fibrosis, chronic inflammation, and loss of acini.

Differential Diagnosis

■ Calcified cervical lymph node.
■ Phlebolith.

Treatment and Prognosis

■ Small stones can be treated conservatively by increased intake of fluids, moist heat, analgesics, and massage; such therapy may result in the passage of the stone with restoration of salivary flow.
■ Failure by conservative means or if the stone is large necessitates surgical removal of the obstruction, which varies from excisional biopsy to removal of the entire submandibular or parotid gland.
■ Antibiotics are administered in those cases that are secondarily infected.
■ Recurrent infections may occur if the cause of the obstruction is not removed.

Additional Facts

■ Calculi are formed by deposition of calcium phosphate and an organic matrix made up of various amino acids and carbohydrates around a central nidus thought to be either bacteria or inorganic material; stone development has no correlation to the serum calcium or phosphorus levels.

■ Calculi may pass spontaneously.

■ Greater involvement of the submandibular gland is thought to be due to the higher mucin content of its saliva, with more adherent properties.

■ Chronic sialadenitis more commonly affects the parotid gland, probably resulting from the anatomy of Stensen's duct, which is long and narrow, making it more susceptible to any alterations in the composition of its saliva.

■ Rarer causes of obstructive sialadenitis include stenosis, stricture, Kussmaul's disease (fibromucinous plugs in the collecting system of dehydrated patients), congenital ductal atresia, and trauma.

■ *Recurrent chronic sialadenitis* represents a group of lesions primarily affecting the parotid gland:

Characterized by recurrent attacks of swelling associated with pain involving one or both glands.

May affect children or adults.

Specific etiology remains uncertain, but predisposing factors are associated with alterations of saliva (decreased secretion, stasis, and changes in its chemical composition), creating an environment conducive to infection, with induction of ductal epithelial metaplasia resulting in obstruction and recurrent inflammation(s).

May spontaneouly resolve with puberty; however, spontaneous resolution in the adult population is not common.

References

Anneroth G, Eneroth CM, Isaacson G: Morphology of salivary calculi: the distribution of the inorganic component. J Oral Pathol 4:257–265, 1975.

Batsakis JG: Non-neoplastic diseases of salivary glands. *In:* Batsakis, JG, ed. Tumors of the head and neck: clinical and pathological considerations, 2nd ed. Baltimore: Williams & Wilkins, 1979; pp 100–120.

Blitzer A: Inflammatory and obstructive disorders of salivary glands. J Dent Res 66:675–679, 1987.

Koudelka BM: Obstructive disorders. *In:* Ellis GL, Auclair PL, Gnepp DR, eds. Surgical pathology of the salivary glands. Philadelphia: W.B. Saunders Co., 1991; pp. 26–38.

Werning JT: Infectious and systemic disorders. *In:* Ellis GL, Auclair PL, Gnepp DR, eds. Surgical pathology of the salivary glands. Philadelphia: W.B. Saunders Co., 1991; pp. 39–59.

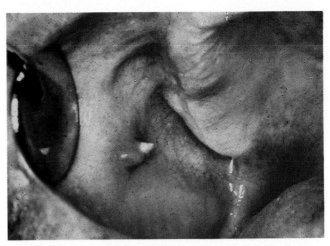

Figure 18–1. Oral cavity showing a white stone situated within the orifice of the parotid (Stensen's) duct, causing an obstructive sialadenitis.

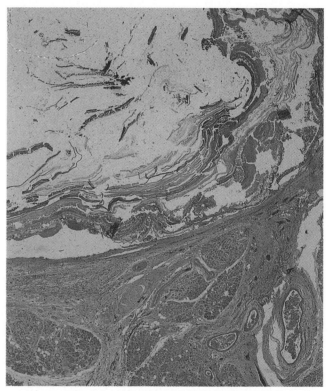

Figure 18–2. Remnant of a calculus is seen within a large duct as concentric laminations of calcification peripherally surrounded by compressed ductal epithelium and fibrotic change within adjacent salivary gland parenchyma.

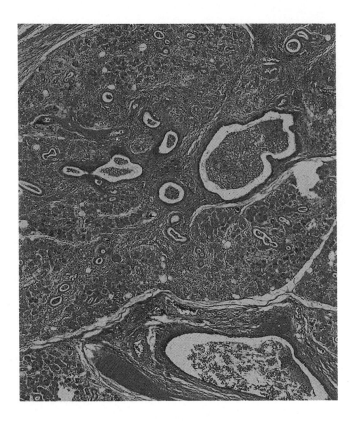

Figure 18-3. Salivary gland parenchymal changes that may result secondary to sialolithiasis include inflammation and acinar atrophy; ducts are dilated and filled with mucopurulent material.

3. BENIGN LYMPHOEPITHELIAL LESION AND SJÖGREN'S SYNDROME

Definition: Non-neoplastic unilateral or bilateral enlargement of the major or minor salivary or lacrimal glands associated with or occurring independent of an autoimmune disease and characterized by specific histopathologic findings.

Synonym: Godwin tumor.

Clinical

■ Benign lymphoepithelial lesion (BLL) encompasses a group of diseases with diverse clinical presentations but overlapping histologic features; these clinical and histologic features may be found independent of or in association with these diseases.

■ There appears to be no histopathologic differences between BLL from patients with and those without Sjögren's syndrome.

■ The diseases associated with the term benign lymphoepithelial lesion include:
Sjögren's syndrome and sicca complex.
Mickulicz's disease/syndrome.
Chronic punctate parotitis.

Benign Lymphoepithelial Lesion (BLL)

■ Affects females more than males; occurs over a wide age range, but most frequently is seen in the fifth and sixth decades of life.

■ Majority of cases involve the parotid gland; however, any salivary gland may be involved, including the submandibular glands and the minor salivary glands.

■ Presenting symptoms include firm swelling of the affected gland with or without localized pain; salivary gland involvement is usually unilateral, but bilateral involvement may be seen in up to 20% of cases.

■ May clinically simulate a neoplasm.

Sjögren's Syndrome

■ Characterized by the presence of:
Keratoconjunctivitis sicca.
Xerostomia.
Connective tissue disease, which is most often rheumatoid arthritis, but which may also include systemic lupus erythematosus, scleroderma, polyarteritis nodosa, and polymyositis.

■ Sicca complex is a variant of Sjögren's syndrome and refers to the presence of keratoconjunctivitis sicca, xerostomia, and parotid gland enlargement but the absence of a connective tissue disorder.

■ Affects females more than males; occurs most frequently in the sixth decade of life.

- Major salivary gland involvement usually is bilateral and includes diffuse, nontender enlargement .
- Minor salivary gland involvement results in the following symptoms: dry mouth; irritation of the eyes, including burning and itching; bronchitis; pneumonia; epistaxis; and otitis media.
- As a result of minor salivary gland involvement, lip biopsy is a means of establishing the diagnosis.
- Various etiologies have been suggested as the cause of Sjögren's disease, including genetic predisposition, infectious (viral) and hormonal; however, it is classified as an autoimmune disease.

Mickulicz's Disease

- Has been used synonymously with benign lymphoepithelial lesion.
- Represents asymptomatic enlargement of the (major) salivary glands or the lacrimal glands.
- Etiology is unknown.
- Terminology is appropriate for use clinically, but is not appropriate as a morphologic term.

Punctate Parotitis

- Clinical term used for cases of BLL, regardless of its association with Sjögren's syndrome.

Pathology

Gross

- Involved gland is either diffusely enlarged or demonstrates one or more well-delineated nodules, with a rubbery consistency and a smooth, tan-white to fleshy appearance.

Histology

- Progressive pathologic process, beginning as a focal mature lymphocytic reaction around salivary gland ducts with progression to a diffuse or nodular mature lymphocytic infiltration of the salivary gland parenchyma of varying severity; germinal centers may be identified but are not necessarily present.
- With increasing lymphocytic infiltration, acinar atrophy takes place, ultimately with complete replacement of acini.
- Ductal epithelial proliferation occurs with obliteration of lumina and infiltration by lymphocytes, resulting in the formation of epithelial islands (epimyoepithelial islands), which represent the hallmark of the disease.
- Deposition of extracellular eosinophilic hyalin-like or proteinaceous material can be seen in the epithelial islands in advanced disease; complete hyalinization of the epithelial islands may occur in long-standing disease.
- Although uncommon, histiocytes, plasma cells, and polymorphonuclear leukocytes may be admixed with the lymphocytic infiltrate.
- Immunohistochemistry: polyclonal lymphocytic cell population as demonstrated by reactivity with both B-cell (L26) and T-cell (UCHL) markers.

Differential Diagnosis

- Chronic, nonspecific sialadenitis (Chapter 18, #1).
- Malignant non-Hodgkin's lymphoma (Chapter 9B, #4).

Treatment and Prognosis

- Treatment is symptomatic; persistent disease or bacterial superinfection may necessitate (conservative) parotidectomy.
- Prognosis is considered good, but varies with the clinical situation; spontaneous resolution may occur, especially in children reaching puberty.
- Potential complications include:
  Development of a malignant lymphoma of B-cell lineage.
  Development of a malignant epithelial neoplasm (lymphoepithelial carcinoma).

Additional Facts

- In patients with BLL, Sjögren's syndrome may or may not be present or develop; most patients with Sjögren's syndrome have pathologic features of BLL.
- Labial salivary gland biopsy specimens are graded based on the presence of a lymphocytic infiltrate, with focus scores of greater than 1 focus/4 mm² proposed as diagnostic for the salivary gland component of Sjögren's syndrome.
- *Lymphoepithelial Carcinoma:*
  Histologic setting similar to benign lymphoepithelial lesion, except for the presence of a malignant epithelial component instead of a benign epithelial component.
  Increased incidence among Eskimos.
  Affects females more than males; most frequently seen in the fifth decade of life.
  Among Eskimos, the parotid gland is the most frequent site of occurrence; among Asians, the submandibular gland is most often involved.
  Histologic picture of the carcinomatous component ranges from low to high grade.
  Controversial whether lymphoepithelial carcinoma arises from or in association with BLL or occurs de novo; there is some evidence linking the Epstein-Barr virus (EBV) with this neoplasm, but there is equal evidence showing an absence of EBV DNA in these neoplasms.

References

Batsakis JG: Non-neoplastic diseases of salivary glands. *In:* Batsakis, JG, ed. Tumors of the head and neck: clinical and pathological considerations, 2nd ed. Baltimore: Williams & Wilkins, 1979; pp 100–120.
Batsakis JG: Lymphoepithelial lesion and Sjögren's syndrome. Ann Otol Rhinol Laryngol 96:354–355, 1987.

Batsakis JG, Bernacki EG, Rice DH, Stebler ME: Malignancy and the benign lymphoepithelial lesion. Laryngoscope 85:389–399, 1975.

Daniels TE: Benign lymphoepithelial lesion and Sjögren's syndrome. *In:* Ellis GL, Auclair PL, Gnepp DR, eds. Surgical pathology of the salivary glands. Philadelphia: W.B. Saunders Co., 1991; pp 83–106.

Daniels TE: Labial salivary gland biopsy in Sjögren's syndrome: assessment as a diagnostic criterion in 362 suspected cases. Arthritis Rheum 27:147–156, 1984.

Eversole LR, Gnepp DR, Eversole GM: Undifferentiated carcinoma. *In:* Ellis GL, Auclair PL, Gnepp DR, eds. Surgical pathology of the salivary glands. Philadelphia: W.B. Saunders Co., 1991; pp. 422–440.

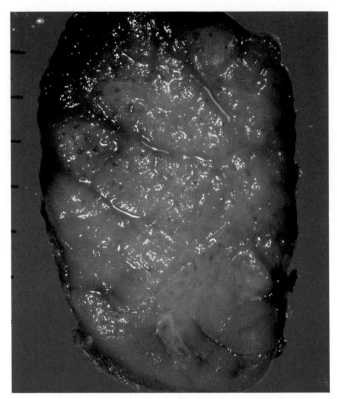

Figure 18–5. Gross appearance of BLL as seen by diffuse nodular enlargement of the parotid gland with a tan-white to fleshy appearance.

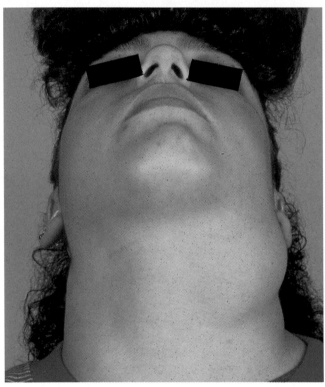

Figure 18–4. Benign lymphoepithelial lesion (BLL), presenting as a markedly enlarged left parotid gland along the mandible and lateral neck region.

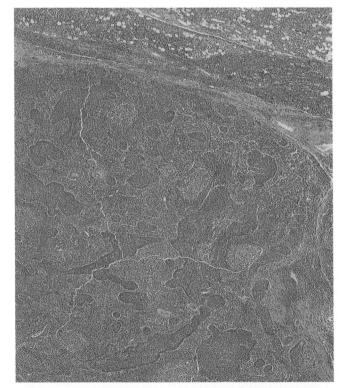

Figure 18–6. BLL. Residual salivary gland parenchyma is seen at the top, whereas most of the gland parenchyma is replaced by a mature, lymphocytic infiltrate in association with multiple germinal centers; in addition, acinar atrophy and formation of epithelial islands (epimyoepithelial islands) can be seen.

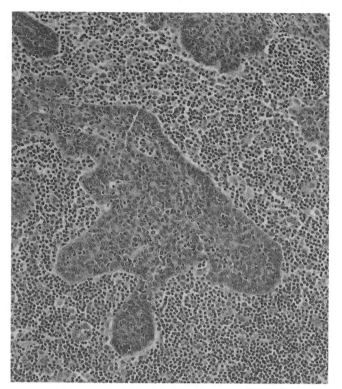

Figure 18-7. Characteristic appearance in BLL of an epimyoepithelial island, represented by lymphocytic infiltration of proliferating ductal epithelium and obliteration of ductal lumina surrounded by a severe mixed chronic inflammatory cell infiltrate.

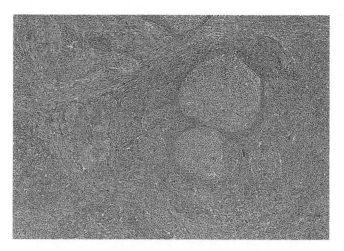

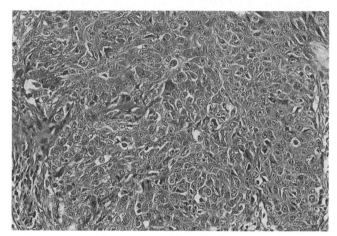

Figure 18-8. Example of lymphoepithelial carcinoma. (*Top*) Within a histologic setting similar to that of benign lymphoepithelial lesion are nests and syncytial sheets of cellular, markedly atypical-appearing epithelium. (*Bottom*) The epithelial component is composed of an undifferentiated pleomorphic cellular infiltrate with large round vesicular-appearing nuclei, prominent nucleoli, and eosinophilic cytoplasm.

CHAPTER 19

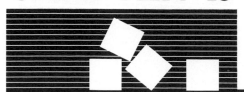

Neoplasms of the Salivary Glands

A. BENIGN NEOPLASMS
 1. Pleomorphic Adenoma
 2. Monomorphic Adenoma
   a. Warthin's Tumor
   b. Oncocytoma or Oxyphilic Adenoma
   c. Basal Cell Adenoma
   d. Canalicular Adenoma
   e. Myoepithelioma
 3. Ductal Papillomas
   a. Sialadenoma Papilliferum
   b. Intraductal Papilloma
   c. Inverted Ductal Papilloma
 4. Hemangioma, Capillary-Type
B. MALIGNANT NEOPLASMS
 1. Mucoepidermoid Carcinoma

 2. Acinic Cell Adenocarcinoma
 3. Adenoid Cystic Carcinoma
 4. Malignant Mixed Tumors of Salivary Glands
   a. Carcinoma Ex Pleomorphic Adenoma
   *b. True Malignant Mixed Tumor or
      Carcinosarcoma*
 5. Adenocarcinoma, Not Otherwise Specified
 6. Polymorphous Low-Grade Adenocarcinoma
    of Minor Salivary Glands
 7. Epithelial–Myoepithelial Cell Carcinoma of
    Intercalated Duct Origin
 8. Basal Cell Adenocarcinoma
 9. Primary Squamous Cell Carcinoma
10. Salivary Duct Carcinoma
11. Sebaceous Carcinoma

A. BENIGN NEOPLASMS

1. Pleomorphic Adenoma

Definition: Benign heterogeneous tumor of salivary gland origin composed of a variable admixture of epithelial and myoepithelial components.
Synonyms: Benign Mixed Tumor.

Clinical

- Represents the most common neoplasm of salivary glands, accounting for 40% to 70% of all neoplasms of the parotid, submandibular, and minor salivary glands; pleomorphic adenomas of the sublingual glands are rare.
- Affects females more than males; occurs over a wide age range, but is most commonly seen in the third to sixth decades of life.
- The most common site of occurrence is the tail of the parotid gland, but it may also occur in the deep lobe of the parotid, in the submandibular and sublingual glands, and in all minor salivary glands throughout the upper and lower respiratory tract.
- Involvement of minor salivary glands occurs most frequently on the palate (hard and soft), followed by the lip; the most common site of pleomorphic adenomas in the upper respiratory tract is by far the nasal cavity, followed by the nasopharynx and larynx.
- Symptoms vary according to site, but most commonly presents as a slow-growing, painless mass, present for periods up to several years; other symptoms, in particular those occurring in the minor salivary glands, may include difficulties in chewing, dysphagia, dyspnea, hoarseness, and epistaxis.
- In the parotid, the tumor typically occurs outside of the facial nerve; facial nerve involvement typified by facial nerve paralysis is rare and, if present, should cause suspicions for a malignant process.
- Arises from the distal portions of the salivary gland duct system, including intercalated ducts and acini.
- There are no known etiologic factors.

Pathology

Gross

- Firm, freely movable, unifocal mass that is encapsulated or well-demarcated, tan-white, solid in appearance, and may demonstrate cystic change; ulceration of the overlying skin does not occur.
- Tumors vary in size from a few centimeters up to large, disfiguring masses.
- Minor salivary gland tumors are polypoid or lobulated, encapsulated or well-delineated, tan-white, usually measuring 1-2 cm but capable of attaining sizes of 7 cm or more.
- Recurrent tumors tend to be multinodular.

Histology

- Admixture of epithelial, myoepithelial, and stromal components are the histologic hallmarks, with morphologic variability within a single neoplasm.
- A fibrous capsule is seen that varies in thickness; minor salivary gland pleomorphic adenomas are generally not encapsulated, but are well-demarcated.
- The epithelial component may have a variety of growth patterns, including solid, cystic, trabecular, or papillary, consisting of a proliferation of duct-lining epithelial cells and myoepithelial cells:
  The duct-lining epithelial cells that form the inner layer of acini or tubules appear flattened, cuboidal, or columnar, with round to oval nuclei and a variable amount of cytoplasm that appears eosinophilic to amphophilic.
  The myoepithelial component forms the outer layer and is spindle-shaped in appearance with hyperchromatic nuclei, and may be more than one cell layer thick.
- The stromal component, the product of myoepithelial cells, varies in appearance from myxoid to chondroid to myxochondroid, and may also appear fibrous and vascular; any one or all of these components may coexist in the same neoplasm.
- In a given tumor, any of the components may predominate so that tumors may be diagnosed as epithelial-, myoepithelial-, or stromal-predominant pleomorphic adenoma; however, all components must be identified in order to diagnose a *pleomorphic* adenoma.
- Mitoses and necrosis are uncommonly seen.
- Other potential findings include the presence of keratinization, squamous cells, mucous cells, oncocytic metaplasia, sebaceous cells, calcification, and fat.
- Extracellular, tyrosine-rich crystals may be identified, particularly in nonepithelial areas.
- Histochemistry: intraluminal epithelial mucin may be demonstrated by diastase-resistant, periodic acid–Schiff positive and mucicarmine positive material; stromal component is alcian blue positive but mucicarmine negative.
- Immunohistochemistry:

Epithelial cells: cytokeratin positive.
Myoepithelial cells: cytokeratin, S-100 protein, glial fibrillary acidic protein, actin and vimentin positive.

Differential Diagnosis

- In general, the diagnosis of pleomorphic adenoma does not present difficulties; however, in cellular tumors with a variety of growth patterns, particularly involving minor salivary glands, pleomorphic adenomas may prove difficult to differentiate from:
  Monomorphic adenomas (Chapter 19A, #2).
  Low-grade polymorphous adenocarcinoma of minor salivary gland origin (Chapter 19B, #6).
  Adenoid cystic carcinoma (Chapter 19B, #3).
- Deep-seated dermal adnexal neoplasm.
- Mesenchymal neoplasm (myxoma, myxoid lipoma, myxoid neurofibroma).

Treatment and Prognosis

- Complete surgical excision is the treatment of choice and should include an adequate margin of uninvolved tissue:
  Parotid gland tumors usually require lobectomy with preservation of the facial nerve.
  Submandibular gland tumors usually necessitate complete removal.
  Minor salivary gland involvement requires complete but conservative excision.
- Radiotherapy is not indicated because pleomorphic adenomas are radioresistant tumors.
- Incomplete excision results in recurrent tumors which:
  Are frequently multinodular.
  Tend to be hypocellular and composed predominantly of a stromal component.
- Prognosis is excellent; 5- and 10-year recurrence-free rates are 97% and 94%, respectively.
- Rare complications include malignant transformation (carcinoma ex pleomorphic adenoma) and the occurrence of so-called "benign" metastasizing mixed tumors.

Additional Facts

- Atypical histologic features include increased cellularity, cellular pleomorphism, and capsular extension; these features should not be mistaken for malignancy.
- The presence of mitoses or necrosis may be indicative of a malignant process and should prompt extensive sectioning and histologic examination of the specimen.
- Multicentric pleomorphic adenomas are rare.
- Minor salivary pleomorphic adenomas tend to be cellular and are unencapsulated; those occurring in the nasal cavity (particularly the septum) tend to have an increased plasmacytoid-appearing myoepithelial component.

References

Batsakis JG, Kraemer B, Sciubba J: The pathology of head and neck tumors: the myoepithelial cell and its participation in salivary gland neoplasia. Head Neck Surg 5:222–233, 1983.

Dardick I, van Nostrand AWP, Phillips MJ: Histogenesis of salivary gland pleomorphic adenoma (mixed tumor) with evaluation of the role of the myoepithelial cell. Hum Pathol 13:62–75, 1982.

Foote FW, Frazell EL: Tumors of the major salivary glands. Atlas of pathology, section IV, fascicle 11, 1st series. Washington, D.C.: Armed Forces Institute of Pathology, 1954.

Hickman RE, Cawson RA, Duffy SW: The prognosis of specific types of salivary gland tumors. Cancer 54:1620–1654, 1984.

Waldron CA: Mixed tumor (pleomorphic adenoma) and myoepithelioma. In: Ellis GL, Auclair PL, Gnepp DR, eds. Surgical pathology of the salivary glands. Philadelphia: W.B. Saunders Co., 1991; pp 165–186.

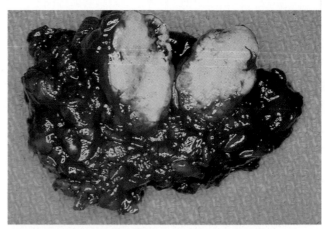

Figure 19–2. Resected gland showing an encapsulated, solid, tan-white tumor within the superficial lobe of the parotid gland.

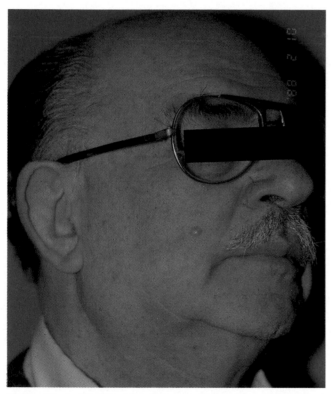

Figure 19–1. Pleomorphic adenoma of the right parotid gland, presenting as a firm, freely movable mass along the angle of the mandible.

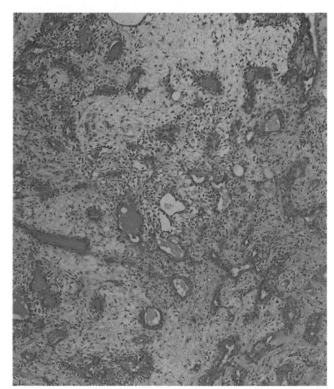

Figure 19–3. Histologic appearance of pleomorphic adenomas includes admixture of epithelial, myoepithelial, and stromal components, including the presence of acini or tubules and a myxochondroid stroma; in a given tumor, the ratio of these components varies so that any one component may dominate the histologic picture.

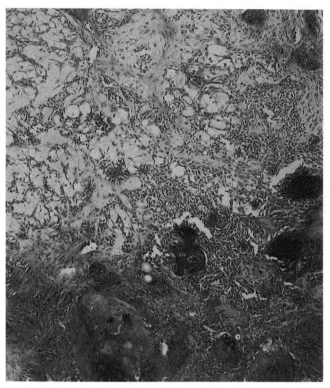

Figure 19-4. This pleomorphic adenoma has associated marked keratinization and squamous cell metaplasia, which may be mistaken for a carcinoma.

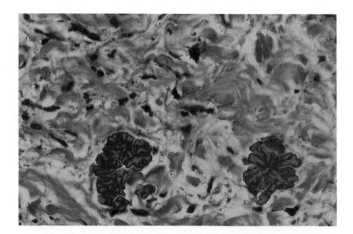

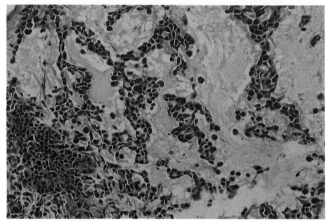

Figure 19-5. Other histologic findings that may be identified in pleomorphic adenomas include (*top*) extracellular, tyrosine-rich crystals, particularly in nonepithelial areas; and (*bottom*) prominent plasmacytoid myoepithelial component.

2. Monomorphic Adenoma

Definition: Benign tumor of salivary glands encompassing a whole group of neoplasms that are not pleomorphic adenomas; these neoplasms are characterized by a lack of the mesenchyme-like stromal component seen in pleomorphic adenomas and are composed exclusively of the epithelial component or, rarely, the myoepithelial component, arranged in a variety of morphologic patterns.

The World Health Organization classification of monomorphic adenomas includes:

Warthin's tumor or papillary cystadenoma lymphomatosum.

Oxyphilic adenoma or oncocytoma.

All others, including basal cell adenoma, canalicular adenoma, myoepithelioma, clear cell adenoma.

a. Warthin's Tumor

Definition: Benign salivary gland tumor characterized by a specific clinical profile and an easily recognizable morphologic appearance composed of papillary structures, mature lymphocytic infiltrate and cystic changes.

Synonyms: Papillary Cystadenoma Lymphomatosum; Adenolymphoma.

Clinical

- Represents from approximately 5% to 6% of all salivary gland tumors and up to 12% of benign parotid gland tumors.
- Affects males more than females; occurs over a wide age range, but is most common in the fifth to seventh decades of life.
- Almost exclusively involves the parotid gland, particularly in the superficial lobe along the inferior pole adjacent to the angle of the mandible; rare cases reported in submandibular gland, palate, lip, tonsil, larynx, and maxillary sinus.
- The most common symptom is that of a painless mass; rarely is pain an associated complaint.
- Bilateral tumors can be seen in up to 14% of cases, occurring synchronously or metachronously; unilateral, multifocal tumors may also be seen.
- The tumors take origin from the salivary gland duct epithelium.
- May be synchronously associated with pleomorphic and monomorphic adenomas, oncocytoma, basal cell adenoma, acinic cell adenocarcinoma, ductal adenocarcinoma, and adenoid cystic carcinoma.

Radiology

- CT scan: well-defined area of increased density in the posteroinferior segment of the superficial lobe of the parotid.
- Radionucleotide imaging: increased uptake of technetium-99m that does not wash out after sialogue administration; this finding plays an important role in diagnosis and is related to the presence of oncocytes and their increased mitochondrial content.

Pathology

Gross

- Encapsulated, soft and fluctuant, round to oval mass with a smooth or lobulated surface, composed of tan-brown tissue with multiple cystic spaces from which a mucoid or brown exudate may be expressed; within the cystic spaces, papillary projections are seen.
- Solid areas can be identified and are noted for a white nodular appearance, representative of lymphoid follicles.
- The tumor measures from 1 to 8 cm in diameter.

Histology

- Papillary and cystic lesion composed of epithelial and lymphoid components.
- The epithelial component that lines the papillary projections is composed of a double layer of granular eosinophilic cells called oncocytes:
  Inner or luminal cells—nonciliated, tall columnar cells with nuclei aligned toward the luminal aspect.
  Outer or basal cells—round, cuboidal, or polygonal cells with vesicular nuclei.
- The lymphoid component is mature and has lymphoid follicles with germinal centers.
- Mucus-secreting cells, goblet cells, and sebaceous glands can be seen.
- Squamous metaplasia and focal necrosis may be seen in association with secondary inflammation.
- Histochemistry: phosphotungstic acid-hematoxylin (PTAH) stains demonstrate mitochondria as seen by blue-black granules in the cytoplasm of both epithelial cell layers.
- Immunohistochemistry: cytokeratin, epithelial membrane antigen positive; S-100 protein, glial fibrillary acidic protein, and actin negative.

Differential Diagnosis

- This tumor is so characteristic that its diagnosis presents no difficulty.
- Cystadenoma (see below).
- Oncocytic papillary cystadenoma (for those cases identified in unusual sites—see below).

Treatment and Prognosis

- Complete surgical excision is the treatment of choice, and should include an adequate margin of uninvolved tissue as well as preservation of the facial nerve.
- Locally recurrent tumor may occur and is related to inadequate excision or to multicentrically occurring neoplasms.
- Transformation to malignant Warthin's tumors is exceedingly rare and may include either the epithelial (squamous cell carcinoma, mucoepidermoid carcinoma, undifferentiated carcinoma, adenocarcinoma) or lymphoid (non-Hodgkin's malignant lymphoma) component.

Additional Facts

- Presence of lymphoid component is related to embryologic development of the parotid gland:
  Ontogenically, the parotid gland is the last of the salivary glands to be encapsulated, resulting in either incorporation/entrapment of lymphoid tissue within the parotid or incorporation/entrapment of parotid ducts and acini within the periparotid lymph node epithelium.
  Supports the observation that the lymphoid component represents normal or hyperplastic lymph node structures, demonstrated by the presence of B- and T-cell markers in the lymphoid component of Warthin's tumors.

Cystadenoma

- Rare, benign salivary gland neoplasm, characterized by an adenomatous proliferation in which multiple cystic structures are seen.

■ Involves both major (parotid gland) and minor salivary glands (lips > cheek > palate).

■ Histologic appearance is characterized by the presence of multiple cysts, which vary in size and are lined by a flattened to columnar epithelium that lacks atypical features but which may be multiple cell layers thick and form papillary projections; prominent solid, extraluminal growth is unusual and should cause suspicion of a malignant neoplasm.

■ Those cystadenomas associated with oncocytic features and papillary growth are termed *oncocytic papillary cystadenomas,* which are often seen in association with minor salivary glands (larynx).

References

Auclair PL, Ellis GL, Gnepp DR: Other benign epithelial neoplasms (cystadenoma). *In:* Ellis GL, Auclair PL, Gnepp DR, eds. Surgical pathology of the salivary glands. Philadelphia: W.B. Saunders Co., 1991; pp 252–261.

Gnepp DR, Schroeder W, Heffner DK: Synchronous tumors arising in a single major salivary gland. Cancer 63:1219–1224, 1989.

Higashi T, Murahashi H, Ikuta H, Mori Y, Watanabe Y: Identification of Warthin's tumor with technetium-99m pertechnetate. Clin Nucl Med 12:796–800, 1987.

Warnock GR: Papillary cystadenoma lymphomatosum (Warthin's tumor). *In:* Ellis GL, Auclair PL, Gnepp DR, eds. Surgical pathology of the salivary glands. Philadelphia: W.B. Saunders Co., 1991; pp 187–201.

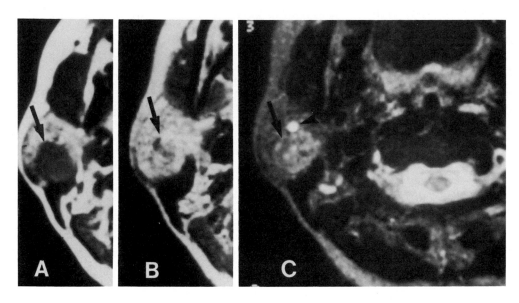

Figure 19-6. Axial MR of a Warthin's tumor: (*A*) T1-weighted, (*B*) proton-density weighted, and (*C*) T2-weighted images. Well-circumscribed mass (*arrows*) involving both the deep and superficial lobes of the right parotid gland. The mass is low intensity on T1-weighted images. Although the signal of the mass increases on proton-density and T2-weighted images, it remains nearly isointense to the parotid gland on the latter two sequences. The facial nerve divides the gland into superficial and deep lobes. The retromandibular vein (*arrowhead*) courses medial to the facial nerve. (Courtesy of Franz J. Wippold II, M.D., Mallinckrodt Institute of Radiology, St. Louis, MO.)

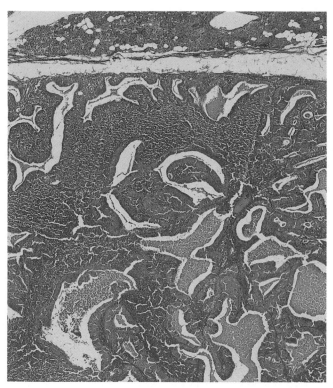

Figure 19–7. Histologic appearance of Warthin's tumor is that of a papillary and cystic lesion composed of epithelial and lymphoid components; normal parotid tissue can be seen at the top.

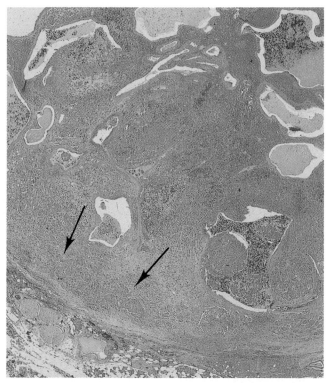

Figure 19–9. Rare example of a Warthin's tumor with malignant (carcinomatous) transformation. The typical histologic picture of Warthin's tumor is seen at the top, whereas infiltrating malignant epithelial nests can be seen throughout the lower aspect of the illustration (*arrows*).

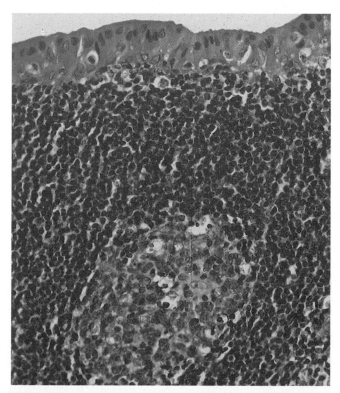

Figure 19–8. The epithelial component lining the papillary projections is composed of a double layer of granular eosinophilic cells associated with mature lymphocytic cells with an identifiable germinal center.

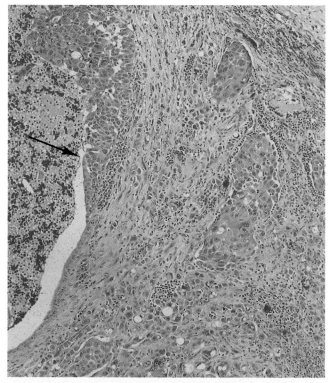

Figure 19–10. Higher power of the malignant foci in this Warthin's tumor, showing transformation of the benign oncocytic epithelium to a malignant epithelium (*arrow*), as well as nests of infiltrating, poorly differentiated carcinoma.

b. Oncocytoma or Oxyphilic Adenoma

Definition: Benign tumor of salivary gland origin composed exclusively of large epithelial cells with characteristic bright eosinophilic, granular cytoplasm (oncocytic cells).

Clinical

- Rare tumor, constituting less than 1% of all salivary gland neoplasms.
- No sex predilection; most commonly occurs in the sixth to eighth decades of life.
- Most frequently involves the parotid gland, but may also occur in the submandibular gland, as well as in minor salivary glands throughout the respiratory tract.
- Symptoms vary according to the site of occurrence, and most frequently present as a painless mass; other symptoms include nasal or airway obstruction.
- Oncocytic cells represent a cytoplasmic alteration (metaplasia) of epithelial or myoepithelial cells, with swelling of the cytoplasm by mitochondrial hyperplasia that gives the cell a characteristic granular eosinophilic appearance by light microscopy; the stimulus for the induction of oncocytic change is unknown but is generally considered age-related and is rarely seen under 50 years of age and nearly always present above 70 years old.
- Pathogenesis remains unclear; some theories support a neoplastic growth, whereas others suggest a hyperplastic/metaplastic phenomenon.

Radiology

- Similar to Warthin's tumor and as a result of the mitochondrial hyperplasia, radionucleotide imaging will demonstrate increased uptake of technetium-99m.

Pathology

Gross

- Major salivary glands: well-circumscribed, encapsulated, lobulated, solid mass with an orange to rust-colored appearance rarely measuring more than 5.0 cm in diameter.
- Minor salivary glands: unencapsulated with less well-delineated borders and with appearance and measurements similar to those of major glands; cystic change may be seen.

Histology

- Encapsulated tumor with a trabecular, cord-like, or organoid growth pattern, separated by a thin fibroconnective tissue stroma; tumors involving minor salivary glands tend to be unencapsulated with an irregular growth pattern, and may demonstrate extension into adjacent structures.
- The predominant cell is enlarged and polyhedral in shape, with a distinct cell membrane, and is char-

acterized by an abundant granular eosinophilic cytoplasm and a centrally placed, round, vesicular appearing nucleus.
- Occasionally, alveoli or acini with lumina can be seen, but duct formation is uncommon.
- Cellular pleomorphism, mitoses, and necrosis are infrequently seen.
- In place of the granular eosinophilic cytoplasm, a clear, nongranular cytoplasm may occur, giving rise to the entity *clear cell oncocytoma:*
  Other than the cytoplasmic appearance, the histology and histochemical staining are similar to those of the more conventional type of oncocytoma.
  The clear cytoplasm is due in part to fixation and tissue processing artifact, and to accumulation of glycogen within the cytoplasm.
  A metastatic renal cell carcinoma must be ruled out.
- Histochemistry: phosphotungstic acid-hematoxylin (PTAH) stains demonstrate mitochondria, as seen by blue-black granules in the cytoplasm; intracytoplasmic glycogen is demonstrated by diastase-sensitive, PAS-positive granules.
- Immunohistochemistry: cytokeratin, epithelial membrane antigen positive; S-100 protein, glial fibrillary acidic protein, and actin negative.
- Electronmicroscopy: ultrastructural characteristic that defines the oncocyte is the presence of mitochondria within the cell cytoplasm almost to the exclusion of other cell organelles; other organelles can be seen as well as basement membrane and desmosomes.

Differential Diagnosis

- Warthin's tumor (Chapter 19A, #2a).
- Pleomorphic adenoma (Chapter 19A, #1).
- Mucoepidermoid carcinoma (Chapter 19B, #1).
- Acinic cell adenocarcinoma (Chapter 19B, #2).
- Adenoid cystic carcinoma (Chapter 19B, #3).
- Clear cell carcinoma (Chapter 19B, #7).
- Metastatic renal cell carcinoma and thyroid carcinoma.

Treatment and Prognosis

- Complete surgical excision is the treatment of choice.
- Radiotherapy is not indicated because oncocytes are radioresistant.
- Prognosis is excellent after removal.
- Locally recurrent tumors are uncommon.

Additional Facts

- Controversy exists as to whether oncocytomas represent true neoplasms or a reactive (metaplastic) process; the controversy extends to the use of the term *oncocytosis* rather than *oncocytoma.*
- *Malignant oncocytomas* or *oncocytic adenocarcino-*

mas are exceedingly rare and have the following clinicopathologic features:

May arise from a long-standing, benign oncocytoma or occur de novo.

Occur predominantly but not exclusively in the parotid gland.

Affect males more than females; most frequently occur in the fifth to eighth decades of life.

Present as a mass with or without associated pain.

Histologic diagnostic criteria include increased mitotic activity with cellular pleomorphism and necrosis, absence of encapsulation, invasion into surrounding tissue, and perineural or vascular invasion and metastases (regional lymph nodes, lung, mediastinum, thyroid, and kidney).

Treatment is complete surgical excision which, if appropriate, should include a parotidectomy.

May be lethal, especially in the presence of widespread metastatic disease.

References

Blanck C, Eneroth CM, Jakobsson PA: Oncocytoma of the parotid gland: neoplasm or nodular hyperplasia? Cancer 24:919–925, 1970.

Ellis GL: "Clear cell" oncocytoma of salivary gland. Hum Pathol 19:862–867, 1988.

Ellis GL, Auclair PL, Gnepp DR, Goode RK: Other malignant epithelial neoplasms. *In:* Ellis GL, Auclair PL, Gnepp DR, eds. Surgical pathology of the salivary glands. Philadelphia: W.B. Saunders Co., 1991; pp 459–464.

Goode RK: Oncocytoma. *In:* Ellis GL, Auclair PL, Gnepp DR, eds. Surgical pathology of the salivary glands. Philadelphia: W.B. Saunders Co., 1991; pp 225–237.

Goode RK, Corio RL: Oncocytic adenocarcinoma of salivary glands. Oral Surg Oral Med Oral Pathol 65:61–66, 1988.

Sun CN, White HJ, Thompson BW: Oncocytoma (mitochondrioma) of the parotid gland: ultrastructural study of a salivary gland oncocytoma. Arch Pathol Lab Med 99:208–214, 1975.

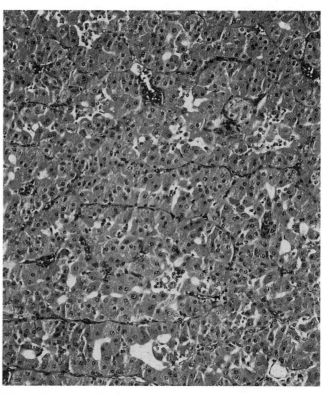

Figure 19–11. Portion of an encapsulated parotid gland oncocytoma consisting of a solid cellular tumor with an organoid and focally trabecular growth, fibrovascular stroma, and cells with a prominent eosinophilic cytoplasm.

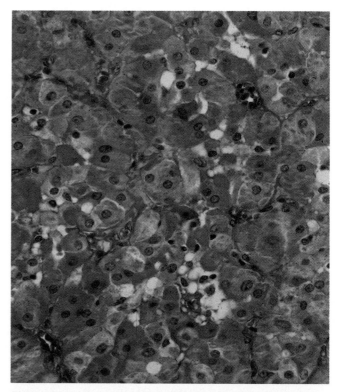

Figure 19–12. Oncocytomas are composed of enlarged, polyhedral-shaped cells characterized by an abundant granular eosinophilic cytoplasm and centrally placed, round, vesicular-appearing nuclei.

c. Basal Cell Adenoma

Definition: Histologic variant of monomorphic adenoma of salivary glands characterized by a proliferation of basaloid-appearing cells and subdivided according to morphologic pattern, including: solid, trabecular, tubular, and membranous types.

Clinical

■ Accounts for approximately 2% of all salivary gland tumors.

■ No sex predilection; occurs over a wide age range, from the fourth to ninth decades of life.

■ The most common site of occurrence is in the major salivary glands, particularly in the parotid gland (superficial lobe); involvement of minor salivary glands occurs but is uncommon.

■ Symptoms vary according to site, but most frequently presents as a freely mobile, asymptomatic mass, with a growth period ranging from months to several decades.

■ Etiology is unknown; evidence supports derivation from both ductal and myoepithelial cells.

Pathology

Gross

■ Encapsulated, tan-white to red-pink, solid mass measuring up to 4 cm in diameter.

■ Minor salivary glands: similar to those of major salivary glands except that, while well-circumscribed, they often are unencapsulated and may be associated with surface ulceration.

Histology

A. Solid Basal Cell Adenoma
   ■ Most common histologic variant.
   ■ Solid masses of basal cells composed of small, isomorphic cells with uniform, hyperchromatic, round to oval nuclei and indistinct cytoplasm.
   ■ The peripheral aspect of these nests is characterized by nuclear palisading.
   ■ A scant stroma is present, from which the epithelial islands are sharply demarcated by an intact membrane.
   ■ Squamous cells and squamous whorled eddies ("keratin pearls") can be seen as a terminal expansion of the epithelial islands.
   ■ Mitoses are generally absent.
B. Trabecular Basal Cell Adenoma
   ■ Basal cell proliferation growing in an elongated, ribbon-like (trabecular) pattern with the cell islands separated by proliferation of a prominent vascular (capillary) stroma.
C. Tubular Basal Cell Adenoma
   ■ Basal cell proliferation composed of multiple, small, duct-like structures lined by columnar-appearing cells with uniform, hyperchromatic, round to oval nuclei.

■ The tubules are well demarcated from the stroma by an intact membrane; the stroma is noteworthy for the presence of a prominent vascular pattern that consists of capillaries and venules.

■ Mitoses are generally absent.

D. Membranous Basal Cell Adenoma
   ■ In contrast to the other types, the membranous basal cell adenoma is multilobular and encapsulated in only approximately 50% of cases.
   ■ This type is characterized by the presence of thick, eosinophilic hyaline membranes surrounding and separating cell islands and creating a jigsaw-puzzle appearance; this material represents reduplicated basal lamina and its appearance is similar to that of the dermal cylindroma, prompting the synonym *dermal analogue tumor.*
   ■ The eosinophilic hyalin material can also be seen within the tumor islands and is diastase-resistant, periodic acid-Schiff positive.
   ■ Tumor nests are often separated by normal salivary gland parenchyma, giving the appearance of multifocal growth.
   ■ Epithelial nests are composed of two types of cells:
      Small cells with hyperchromatic nuclei and indistinct cytoplasm, usually seen at the periphery of the cell nests.
      Larger polygonal-shaped cells with pale-staining nuclei indistinct cytoplasm, usually more centrally located in cell nests; in addition, these cells may form squamous whorls or eddies.
   ■ Mitoses are generally absent.
   ■ Perineural invasion is not seen.

Differential Diagnosis

■ Pleomorphic adenoma (Chapter 19A, #1).

■ Ameloblastoma (Chapter 4A, #10).

■ Adenoid cystic carcinoma (solid type in particular) (Chapter 19B, #3).

■ Basal cell adenocarcinoma (Chapter 19B, #8).

Treatment and Prognosis

■ Complete surgical excision is the treatment of choice and is curative.

■ Prognosis is excellent.

■ Local recurrences are unusual, but may be seen and relate to inadequate surgical excision as a consequence of the characteristic multifocal growth pattern; membranous basal cell adenoma is the variant most commonly associated with recurrence.

Additional Facts

■ Malignant transformation of basal cell adenomas is exceedingly rare; these tumors are composed of a basal cell adenoma and adenoid cystic carcinoma and have been termed hybrid tumors.

References

Batsakis JG: Basal cell adenoma of the parotid gland. Cancer 29:226–230, 1972.

Batsakis JG, Brannon BR: Dermal analogue tumor of major salivary glands. J Laryngol Otol 95:155–164, 1981.

Batsakis JG, Brannon BR, Sciubba JJ: Monomorphic adenoma of major salivary glands: a histologic study of 96 tumours. Clin Otolaryngol 6:129–143, 1981.

Ellis GL, Gnepp DR: Membranous basal cell adenoma: dermal analogue tumor. *In:* Gnepp DR, ed. Pathology of the head and neck. New York: Churchill Livingstone, 1988; pp 586–592.

Gardner DG, Daley TD: The use of the terms monomorphic adenoma, basal cell adenoma, and canalicular adenoma as applied to salivary gland tumors. Oral Surg Oral Med Oral Pathol 56:608–615, 1983.

Kratochvil FJ: Canalicular adenoma and basal cell adenoma. *In:* Ellis GL, Auclair PL, Gnepp DR, eds. Surgical pathology of the salivary glands. Philadelphia: W.B. Saunders Co., 1991; pp 202–224.

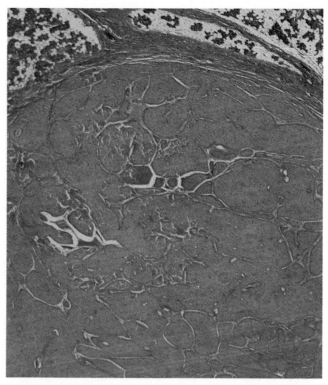

Figure 19–14. Solid basal cell adenoma: encapsulated neoplasm composed of solid cellular nests or masses, the peripheral aspect of which is characterized by nuclear palisading.

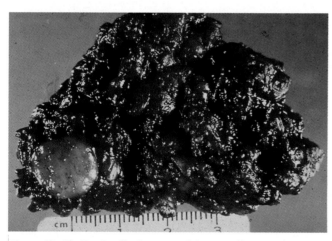

Figure 19–13. Basal cell adenoma of the parotid gland, appearing as an encapsulated, tan-white, solid mass along the lower left aspect of the resected gland.

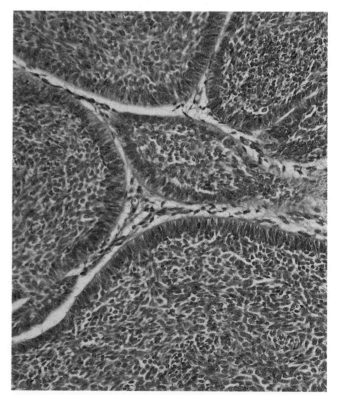

Figure 19–15. Higher power of a solid basal cell adenoma, showing the presence of small, isomorphic cells with uniform, hyperchromatic, round to oval nuclei, indistinct cytoplasm, and peripheral palisading of nuclei; scant stroma is present, from which the epithelial islands are sharply demarcated by an intact membrane.

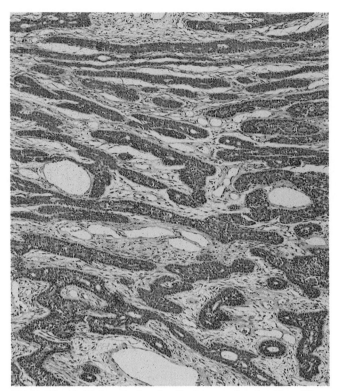

Figure 19–16. Trabecular basal cell adenoma: basal cell proliferation growing in elongated, ribbon-like (trabecular) pattern with the cell islands separated by proliferation of a prominent vascular (capillary) stroma.

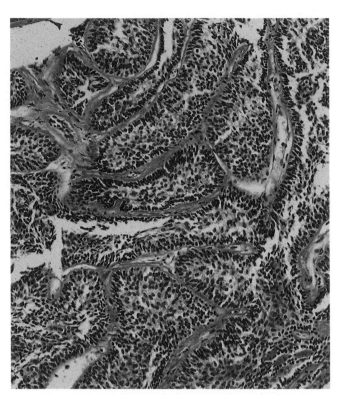

Figure 19–18. Membranous basal cell adenoma (dermal analogue tumor), characterized by the presence of thick, eosinophilic hyaline membranes surrounding and separating epithelial islands composed of small cells with hyperchromatic nuclei at the periphery of the cell nests and larger, polygonal-shaped cells with pale-staining nuclei, more centrally located in cell nests.

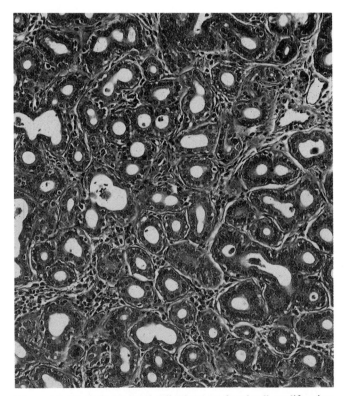

Figure 19–17. Tubular basal cell adenoma: basal cell proliferation composed of multiple, small, ductlike structures lined by cuboidal to columnar-appearing cells with uniform, hyperchromatic, round to oval nuclei, distinctly separated from a vascularized stroma by an intact membrane.

d. Canalicular Adenoma

Definition: Benign salivary gland tumor included in the monomorphic adenoma group, with predilection for the upper lip and with a distinct histomorphologic appearance.

Clinical

- Affects females more than males; occurs over a wide age range from the fourth to ninth decades of life, but most commonly occurs in the seventh decade.
- Most common site of occurrence is the upper lip; other sites of occurrence include the buccal mucosa and, infrequently, the parotid gland.
- Symptoms include gradually enlarging, nonpainful nodule; multinodular growths may be seen.
- Clinical confusion with mucocele, sebaceous cysts, and lipoma may occur.

Pathology

Gross

- Circumscribed or encapsulated, tan-pink to yellow-brown, rubbery to firm nodule measuring from 0.5 to 2 cm in diameter.
- Surface ulceration may be seen but is not common.
- Cystic spaces and a gelatinous mucoid material may be identified in transecting the tumor.

Histology

- Encapsulated or well-circumscribed neoplasm; multifocality may be seen and usually these scattered foci are small and unencapsulated.
- Basal cell proliferation with a tubular growth lined by cuboidal to columnar cells with uniform, hyperchromatic, round to oval nuclei, variable amount of eosinophilic cytoplasm and indistinct cell borders.
- The tubules are well demarcated from the stroma by an intact membrane; the stroma is noteworthy for the absence of cellularity and the presence of a prominent vascular pattern that consists of capillaries and venules.
- Mitoses are generally absent.
- Histochemistry: diastase-sensitive, PAS-positive cytoplasmic granularity is seen.

Differential Diagnosis

- Pleomorphic adenoma (Chapter 19A, #1).
- Ameloblastoma (Chapter 4A, #10).
- Cutaneous basal cell carcinoma (Chapter 25C, #1).
- Adenoid cystic carcinoma (Chapter 19B, #3).

Treatment and Prognosis

- Conservative but complete surgical excision is the treatment of choice; enucleation is not recommended.
- Recurrence after complete excision is uncommon.

Additional Facts

- The multifocal growth of this neoplasm often is devoid of a capsule, and can be mistaken for a carcinoma with invasion into the minor salivary gland parenchyma; awareness of this tendency reduces the likelihood of the erroneous diagnosis of carcinoma.
- Classification of this neoplasm within the basal cell adenoma category has been advocated; however, given the specific clinical and pathologic features, separation from this categorization is justified.

References

Bhaskar SN, Weinmann JP: Tumors of the minor salivary glands. Oral Surg Oral Med Oral Pathol 8:1278–1297, 1955.

Daley TD: Canalicular adenoma: not a basal cell adenoma. Oral Surg Oral Med Oral Pathol 57:181–188, 1984.

Daley TD: The canalicular adenoma: considerations on differential diagnosis and treatment. J Oral Maxillofac Surg 42:728–730, 1984.

Kratochvil FJ: Canalicular adenoma and basal cell adenoma. In: Ellis GL, Auclair PL, Gnepp DR, eds. Surgical pathology of the salivary glands. Philadelphia: W.B. Saunders Co., 1991; pp 202–224.

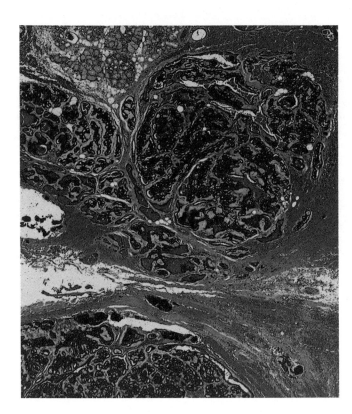

Figure 19-19. Biopsy specimen of upper lip showing multifocal, well-circumscribed nodules characteristic of canalicular adenoma; residual normal seromucous glands are seen at the top left of the illustration.

Figure 19-20. Canalicular adenomas are composed of a basal cell proliferation, forming long lumina lined by cuboidal to columnar cells with uniform, hyperchromatic, round to oval nuclei, variable amount of eosinophilic cytoplasm, and indistinct cell borders; the tubules are well demarcated from the stroma, which is noteworthy for the absence of cellularity and the presence of prominent vascularity.

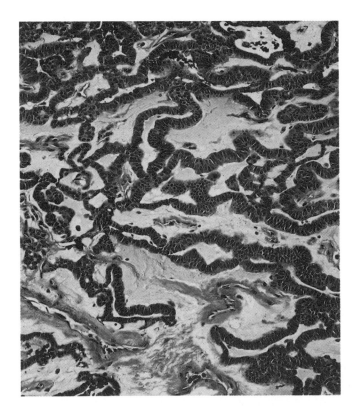

e. Myoepithelioma

Definition: Benign salivary gland tumor composed predominantly or exclusively of myoepithelial cells.

Clinical

- Accounts for less than 1% of all salivary gland neoplasms.
- No sex predilection; occurs over a wide age range, but is most commonly seen in the third to sixth decades of life.
- Primarily involves the parotid gland, but may also be seen in the submandibular gland and oral minor salivary glands (palate, retromolar region, upper lip).
- Most commonly present as a slow-growing, painless mass.

Pathology

Gross

- Well-demarcated, smooth, and bosselated lesion with a homogeneous white appearance and measuring up to 5 cm in diameter.

Histology

- Encapsulated (except for tumors originating in minor salivary glands) cellular neoplasm composed of spindle-shaped or plasmacytoid cells (hyaline cells) in a fascicular or swirling growth pattern.
- The spindle-shaped cells have uniform, centrally located nuclei with dispersed nuclear chromatin and eosinophilic granular to fibrillar appearing cytoplasm.
- The plasmacytoid cells are polygonal, with round to oval pyknotic appearing nuclei, which may be eccentrically located as a result of the accumulation of eosinophilic hyaline material in the cytoplasm; a paranuclear clear zone (hof) and methyl green pyronine staining are not seen.
- Cellular pleomorphism may be seen, but mitoses and necrosis are uncommon.
- The stroma varies from minimal in amount to loose and myxomatous in appearance; the stroma is alcian blue positive but mucicarmine negative.
- Immunohistochemistry: cytokeratin, S-100 protein, actin and glial fibrillary acidic protein (GFAP), and vimentin positive.
- Electronmicroscopy: intracytoplasmic myofibrils, desmosomes, and basal lamina.

Differential Diagnosis

- Pleomorphic adenoma (Chapter 19A, #1).
- Extracranial meningioma (Chapter 25B, #4).
- Neurilemmoma (Chapter 9A, #6) and malignant schwannoma (Chapter 9B, #6).
- Leiomyoma (Chapter 4A, #6) and leiomyosarcoma (Chapter 4B, #8).
- Extramedullary plasmacytoma (Chapter 9B, #4).
- Spindle cell carcinoma (Chapter 14B, #2).

Treatment and Prognosis

- Complete surgical excision is the treament of choice and should include a portion of surrounding uninvolved tissue; if appropriate, a superficial parotidectomy should be performed.
- Local recurrence is related to inadequate excision.

Additional Facts

- The majority of myoepitheliomas are of the spindle cell variety; prognosis is unrelated to the cell type.

Myoepithelial Carcinoma

- Malignant epithelial neoplasm with cytologic differentiation and immunohistochemical features of myoepithelial cells but without ductal or acinar differentiation.
- Extremely rare; may occur de novo or as the malignant portion of a carcinoma arising in a pleomorphic adenoma.
- Diagnosis is based on the presence of increased cellularity, cellular pleomorphism, and increased mitotic activity and invasiveness.
- Must be differentiated from spindle cell carcinoma and spindle cell sarcomas.

References

Barnes L, Appel BN, Perez H, El-Attar AM: Myoepithelioma of the head and neck: case report and review. J Surg Oncol 28:21–28, 1985.

Batsakis JG, Kraemer B, Sciubba J: The pathology of head and neck tumors: the myoepithelial cell and its participation in salivary gland neoplasia. Head Neck Surg 5:222–233, 1983.

Morinaga S, Nakajima T, Shimosato Y: Normal and neoplastic myoepithelial cells in salivary gland: an immunohistochemical study. Hum Pathol 18:1218–1226, 1989.

Sciubba JJ, Brannon R: Myoepithelioma of salivary glands: report of 23 cases. Cancer 47:562–572, 1982.

Singh R, Cawson RA: Malignant myoepithelial carcinoma (myoepithelioma) arising in a pleomorphic adenoma of the parotid gland: an immunohistochemical study and review of the literature. Oral Surg Oral Med Oral Pathol 66:65–70, 1988.

Waldron CA: Mixed tumor (pleomorphic adenoma) and myoepithelioma. In: Ellis GL, Auclair PL, Gnepp DR, eds. Surgical pathology of the salivary glands. Philadelphia: W.B. Saunders Co., 1991; pp 165–186.

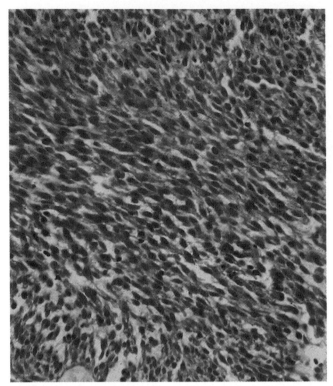

Figure 19–21. Myoepithelioma, spindle-cell pattern: cellular neoplasm composed of spindle-shaped cells in a fascicular growth pattern with uniform, centrally located nuclei, dispersed to hyperchromatic nuclear chromatin and eosinophilic granular cytoplasm; no epithelial ductal structures are seen.

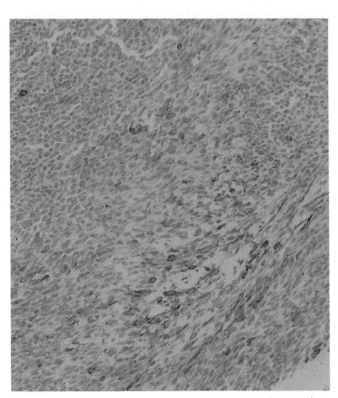

Figure 19–23. Spindle-cell myoepithelioma immunohistochemistry showing cytokeratin reactivity.

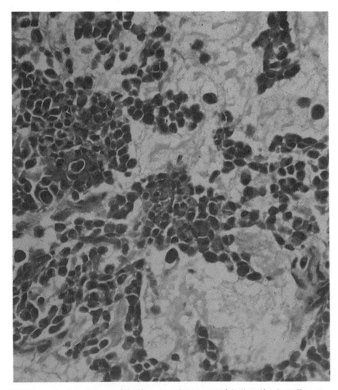

Figure 19–22. Myoepithelioma, plasmacytoid (hyaline) cells: polygonal cells with round to oval, centrally or eccentrically located nuclei and an eosinophilic cytoplasm; a paranuclear clear zone (hof) typical of true plasma cells is not seen.

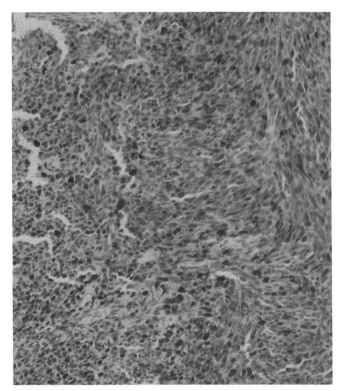

Figure 19–24. Spindle-cell myoepithelioma immunohistochemistry showing diffuse S-100 protein reactivity.

3. Ductal Papillomas

Definition: A group of benign epithelial salivary gland neoplasms with unique histologic features that allow for easy identification; classification includes three types: sialadenoma papilliferum, intraductal papilloma, and inverted ductal papilloma.

a. Sialadenoma Papilliferum

Definition: Benign salivary gland tumor so named because of its similarity to the cutaneous syringocystadenoma papilliferum.

Clinical

- Uncommon tumor.
- Affects males more than females; occurs over a wide age range but is most frequently seen in the sixth to seventh decades of life.
- The most common site of occurrence is on the palate, particularly at the junction of the hard and soft palates; other sites of involvement include the buccal mucosa, retromolar region, parotid gland, lip, and nasopharynx (adenoids).
- Asymptomatic lesions generally are discovered incidentally.
- The origin is disputed; however, evidence supports salivary gland excretory duct rather than intercalated duct origin.

Pathology

Gross

- Exophytic, papillary-appearing, tan-pink lesion measuring from a few millimeters to as large as 7.0 cm.

Histology

- Exophytic and endophytic proliferation of surface and ductal epithelium.
- The surface has a papillary growth that is composed of a stratified squamous epithelium with a fibrovascular connective tissue core.
- Merging with the surface epithelium is an endophytic proliferation of ductal epithelium forming dilated and tortuous structures; in the deeper portions, the ductal structures have papillary luminal projections and microcysts.
- The ductal epithelium is composed of two cell layers:
  Outer or luminal layer: tall columnar cells with an eosinophilic granular cytoplasm.
  Inner or basal cell: cuboidal cells with an eosinophilic granular cytoplasm.
- The stromal component consists of a predominantly plasma cell infiltrate admixed with mature lymphocytes.

Differential Diagnosis

- Papilloma of surface epithelial origin (Chapter 14A, #1).
- Inverted ductal papilloma (Chapter 19A, #3c).
- Warty dyskeratoma.
- Verrucous carcinoma (Chapter 14B, #3).
- Mucoepidermoid carcinoma (Chapter 19B, #1).

Treatment and Prognosis

- Complete conservative surgical excision is the treatment of choice and is curative.
- Malignant transformation or a malignant counterpart does not occur.

b. Intraductal Papilloma

Definition: Benign salivary gland neoplasm arising from the interlobular and excretory ducts.

Clinical

- Uncommon tumor.
- No sex predilection; primarily affects adults, occurring in the fourth to seventh decades of life.
- Intraoral minor salivary glands are most frequently involved: buccal mucosa > lips > floor of mouth > soft palate.
- Symptoms relate to a painless mass.

Pathology

Gross

- Submucosal, nonulcerated nodule measuring from 1 to 1.5 cm in diameter.

Histology

- Unicystic cavity lined by one or two layers of cuboidal or columnar epithelium that give rise to numerous papillary fronds, filling the cavity; papillations are covered by a similar epithelium.
- The papillations have a thin, fibrovascular connective tissue core.
- The epithelial component is confined to the cyst cavity, and there are no extensions into the adjacent stromal tissue.

Differential Diagnosis

- Inverted ductal papilloma (Chapter 19A, #3c).
- Papillary cystadenoma (Chapter 19A, #2a).
- Low-grade papillary adenocarcinoma of the nasopharynx (Chapter 9B, #3).

Treatment and Prognosis

- Complete conservative surgical excision is the treatment of choice and is curative.

c. *Inverted Ductal Papilloma*

Definition: Benign salivary gland neoplasm occurring in the terminal portions of excretory ducts with a characteristic inverted growth.

Clinical

- Rare neoplasm.
- No sex predilection; occurs primarily in adults over a wide age range but is most frequently seen in the sixth decade of life.
- The most common sites of occurrence are the lower lip and the buccal (vestibular) mucosa; other sites of involvement include the upper lip, floor of mouth, and soft palate.
- Generally asymptomatic; presents as a submucosal swelling.

Pathology

Gross

- Submucosal, firm nodules measuring up to 1.5 cm in diameter; a small surface pore may be seen that is contiguous to the lumen of the tumor.

Histology

- Well-demarcated, endophytic epithelial growth composed of thick, bulbous proliferations that are contiguous to but not protruding from the surface epithelium; communication with the surface by a narrow opening may be seen.
- The neoplasm consists of basaloid and squamous/epidermoid cells, between which mucous cells and microcytes may be interspersed.
- The luminal surface epithelium is composed of cuboidal or columnar cells with a papillary appearance.
- The tumor grows downward and appears to fill a luminal cavity; the endophytic growth is "pushing" into the submucosa, rather than demonstrating invasion or infiltration.
- Histochemistry: mucous cells stain positively with mucicarmine and are diastase-resistant, PAS-positive.

Differential Diagnosis

- Inverted papilloma (Chapter 4A, #1).
- Sialadenoma papilliferum (Chapter 19A, #3a).
- Mucoepidermoid carcinoma (Chapter 19B, #1).

Treatment and Prognosis

- Simple but complete local excision is the treatment of choice and is curative.

Additional Facts

- The tumor arises in the terminal portion of minor salivary gland excretory ducts and is extraglandular.

References

Abrams AM, Finck FM: Sialadenoma papilliferum: a previously unreported salivary gland tumor. Cancer 24:1057–1063, 1969.

Ellis GL, Auclair PL: Ductal papillomas. *In:* Ellis GL, Auclair PL, Gnepp DR, eds. Surgical pathology of the salivary glands. Philadelphia: W.B. Saunders Co., 1991; pp 238–251.

Regezi JA, Lloyd RV, Zarbo RJ, McClatchey KD: Minor salivary gland tumors: a histologic and immunohistochemical study. Cancer 55:108–115, 1985.

Waldron CA, El-Mofty SK, Gnepp DR: Tumors of the intraoral minor salivary glands: a demographic and histologic study of 426 cases. Oral Surg Oral Med Oral Pathol 66:323–333, 1988.

White DK, Miller MS, McDaniel RK, Rothman BN: Inverted ductal papilloma: a distinctive lesion of minor salivary gland. Cancer 49:519–524, 1982.

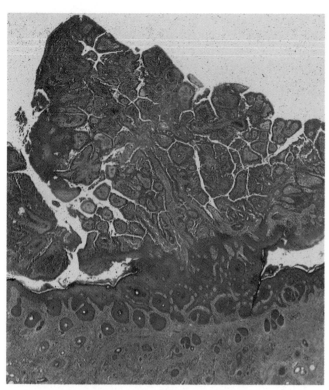

Figure 19–25. Sialadenoma papilliferum with an exophytic proliferation of surface and ductal epithelium; the surface has a papillary growth composed of a stratified squamous epithelium with a fibrovascular connective tissue core.

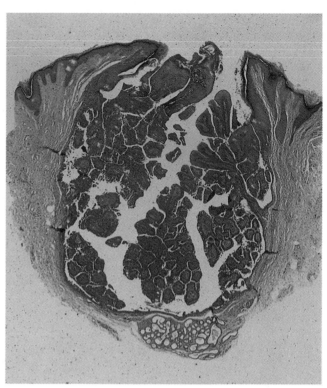

Figure 19–26. Sialadenoma papilliferum with an endophytic proliferation of ductal epithelium.

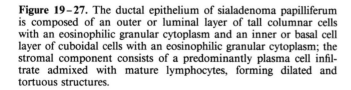

Figure 19–27. The ductal epithelium of sialadenoma papilliferum is composed of an outer or luminal layer of tall columnar cells with an eosinophilic granular cytoplasm and an inner or basal cell layer of cuboidal cells with an eosinophilic granular cytoplasm; the stromal component consists of a predominantly plasma cell infiltrate admixed with mature lymphocytes, forming dilated and tortuous structures.

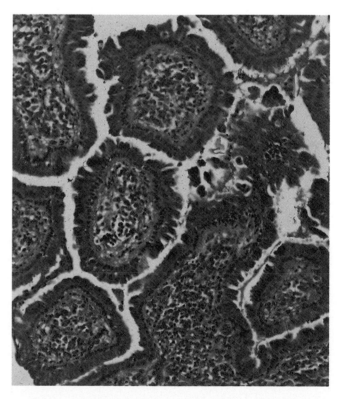

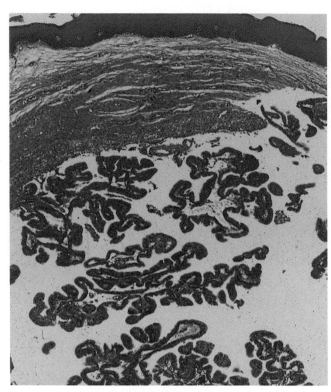

Figure 19–28. Intraductal papilloma consisting of a unicystic cavity lined by one or two layers of cuboidal or columnar epithelium, which give rise to numerous papillary fronds that have a thin fibrovascular connective tissue core.

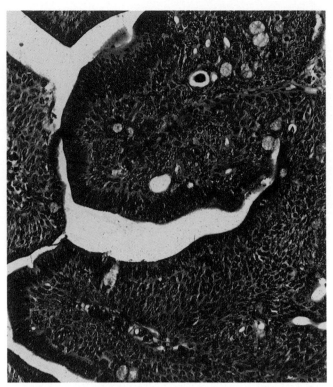

Figure 19–30. The neoplasm consists of basaloid-appearing epithelial cells composed of cuboidal or columnar cells with a papillary appearance along the luminal surface and squamous/epidermoid cells, between which mucous cells and microcytes are interspersed in the more central portions.

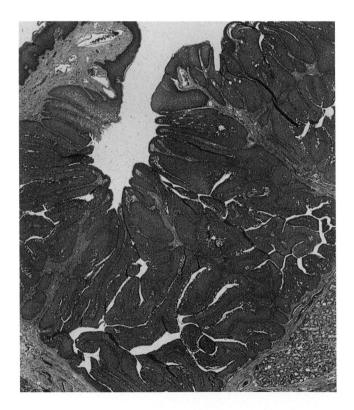

Figure 19–29. Inverted ductal papilloma: well-demarcated, endophytic epithelial growth composed of thick, bulbous proliferations contiguous with but not protruding from the surface epithelium; communication with the surface by a narrow opening is seen.

4. Hemangioma, Capillary-Type

Definition: Benign tumor of endothelial cell origin.
Synonyms: Benign hemangioendothelioma; congenital or juvenile hemangioma.

Clinical

- Accounts for less than 5% of all salivary gland tumors.
- The most common salivary gland tumor in the pediatric population, representing more than 90% of parotid gland tumors in children under 1 year old.
- Affects females more than males; may occur over a wide age range, but most frequently seen in the first decade of life.
- Almost exclusively involves the parotid gland, but occasionally the submandibular gland may be affected.
- Usually discovered at birth as a unilateral, compressible mass; rapid enlargement and facial asymmetry may be seen.
- No association with familial disorders like von Hippel-Lindau syndrome or hereditary telangiectasia.
- Intraparotid hemangiomas in adults are uncommon.

Pathology

Gross

- Lobulated, dark red tumor, measuring from 2 to 8 cm in diameter.
- Overlying skin may have a bluish discoloration, accentuated by crying episodes.

Histology

- Unencapsulated cellular neoplasm with intralobular growth and replacement of salivary gland acini.
- The tumor is composed of capillary-sized vessels, varying little in size; vascular lumina may be compressed and indistinct due to increased cellularity.
- The capillaries are lined by two or more layers of endothelial cells that have oval to spindle-shaped nuclei and eosinophilic granular cytoplasm.
- Mitoses are frequently seen and may be numerous.
- Peri- and intraneural invasion may be identified.
- Histochemistry: reticulin stain delineates the outlines of the vascular sheath, within which is the endothelial cell proliferation.
- Immunohistochemistry: factor VIII-related antigen, *Ulex europaeus* and CD34 positive.

Differential Diagnosis

- Lymphangioma/cystic hygroma (Chapter 9A, #3).
- Malignant hemangioendothelioma.

Treatment and Prognosis

- Complete surgical excision with preservation of the facial nerve is the treatment of choice.
- In infants (capillary hemangioma), in the absence of an enlarging neoplasm with compromise of the external ear canal or facial distortion, surgical intervention may be delayed until an older age; delay in surgery may allow for spontaneous regression.
- Malignant transformation does not occur.

Additional Facts

- The presence of increased mitotic activity and neural invasion do not render a diagnosis of malignancy and have no impact on behavior.
- The facial nerve in infants is in a more superficial location than in an older age; therefore, surgical intervention in infancy may be associated with a greater incidence of damage to the facial nerve.
- Cavernous hemangiomas may be identified in salivary glands and are noted for the following:
  Seen in older children and adults.
  Primarily involve the parotid gland.
  Involve the extralobular connective tissue.
  Characterized by the presence of dilated, thin-walled vessels lined by flattened endothelial cells.
  Unlike the capillary hemangioma, the cavernous type does not regress and therefore requires complete surgical excision.

References

McDaniel RK: Benign mesenchymal neoplasms. *In:* Ellis GL, Auclair PL, Gnepp DR, eds. Surgical pathology of the salivary glands. Philadelphia: W.B. Saunders Co., 1991; pp 489–492.

Peel RL, Gnepp DR: Diseases of the salivary glands. *In:* Barnes L, ed. Surgical pathology of the head and neck. New York: Marcel Dekker, 1985; pp 574–579.

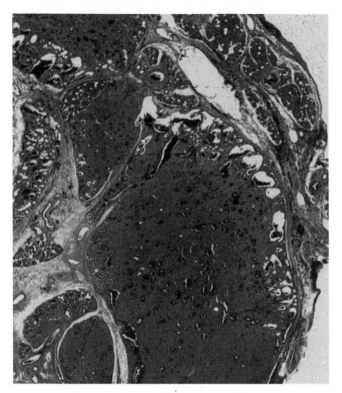

Figure 19–31. Hemangioma of the parotid gland consisting of an unencapsulated cellular neoplasm with intralobular growth replacing salivary gland acini.

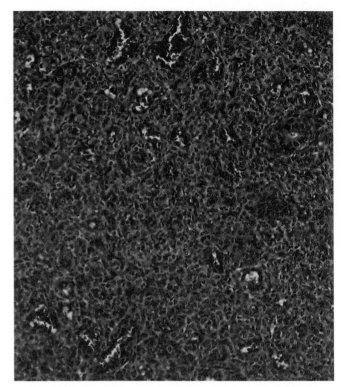

Figure 19–32. The tumor is composed of capillary-sized vessels varying little in size lined by two or more layers of endothelial cells that have oval to spindle-shaped nuclei and eosinophilic granular cytoplasm; vascular lumina are compressed and indistinct due to increased cellularity.

B. MALIGNANT NEOPLASMS

1. Mucoepidermoid Carcinoma

Definition: Malignant epithelial salivary gland neoplasm, composed of a variable admixture of both epidermoid and mucus-secreting cells.

Clinical

■ The most common malignant salivary gland tumor and, second to pleomorphic adenoma, the most frequently occurring neoplasm among all salivary gland tumors.

■ Represents approximately 30% of all malignant salivary gland tumors but less than 10% of all salivary gland neoplasms.

■ In the pediatric age group, mucoepidermoid carcinoma represents the most common malignant salivary gland neoplasm.

■ No sex predilection; occurs over a wide age range, but is most frequently seen in the third to sixth decades of life.

■ Occurs in both the major and minor salivary glands, with the majority identified in the parotid gland; the most common minor salivary gland involvement occurs in the palate.

■ Mucoepidermoid carcinomas are divided into low, intermediate, and high grades, and clinical presentation varies accordingly:

Low and intermediate-grades: slow-growing, painless mass.

High-grade: rapidly enlarging, painful mass.

■ Arise from the ductular epithelium proximal to and including the striated ducts and the extralobular excretory ducts.

■ Etiology may be related to prior therapeutic radiotherapy, with latent periods from the time of radiation to the head and neck to the development of a mucoepidermoid carcinoma of 7 to 32 years.

■ On rare occasions, intraosseous primary or "central" mucoepidermoid carcinomas may occur, which:

Occur in women more frequently than men.

Affect the mandible and maxilla.

Histologically resemble the salivary gland mucoepidermoid carcinoma.

Occur in the presence of intact cortical plates.

Pathology

Gross

- Unencapsulated or incompletely encapsulated, round to oval, predominantly solid, tan-white to pink mass, measuring up to 4.0 cm in greatest dimension.
- Low-grade tumors characteristically have identifiable cystic spaces filled with clear to blood-tinged fluid/mucus.
- High-grade tumors characteristically are infiltrative, predominantly solid, and more often have associated necrosis and hemorrhage.

Histology

- Characteristic of all grades of mucoepidermoid carcinoma is the presence of mucous cells, epidermoid cells, and intermediate cells; these cellular components vary according to the histologic grade.

Low-Grade

- Characteristically are cystic and have large numbers of mucous cells admixed with less numerous but easily identifiable epidermoid and intermediate cells.
- Mucous cells are identified lining cystic spaces or admixed within nests or solid areas with epidermoid cells, are large or balloon-shaped with distinct cell borders, and are composed of pale-staining or foamy-appearing cytoplasm with peripherally placed, small, dark-staining nuclei.
- Epidermoid cells form nests or solid areas in conjunction with the mucous cells, have a pavement-like arrangement, and are polygonal-shaped with vesicular nuclei and abundant eosinophilic cytoplasm; individual cell keratinization may be seen; however, keratin (squamous) pearls, extensive keratinization, and intercellular bridges do not predominate.
- Extracellular mucous pools or "cysts" may be seen which may infiltrate adjacent salivary gland or connective tissue.
- Intermediate cells are round to oval, contain small, dark-staining nuclei, and have scanty, eosinophilic cytoplasm.
- Cellular pleomorphism, mitoses, necrosis, and hemorrhage are generally absent.
- A variable degree of local invasion may be seen; however, neural invasion is not normally a component of the low-grade mucoepidermoid carcinoma.
- Clear cells, composed of round to oval cells with distinct cell borders, peripherally placed, small, dark nuclei, and their hallmark clear cytoplasm may be seen and, on infrequent occasions, may predominate.

Intermediate-Grade

- Cysts can be seen, but in comparison to the low-grade tumor, are less numerous and smaller in size.
- Have a greater tendency to be more cellular and form solid nests than the low-grade cancers.
- Shift in ratio of mucous cells to epidermoid and intermediate cells, with a larger percentage of the latter cells identified.
- As compared to the low-grade cancers, there is increased cellular pleomorphism and mitotic activity, with an increased tendency toward local invasive growth; nuclear atypia may be seen focally, but is not necessary for the diagnosis.

High-Grade

- Characterized by a solid, neoplastic cellular proliferation composed almost exclusively of epidermoid and intermediate cells, with only limited numbers of identifiable mucous cells, which may require liberal tissue sampling in order to be detected.
- The presence of cellular atypia/pleomorphism, nucleoli, increased mitotic activity, necrosis, hemorrhage, and invasive growth are readily identifiable.

Features Common to All Grades

- Histochemistry:
  Mucous cells: intracytoplasmic diastase-resistant, PAS-positive, and mucicarmine positive.
  Epidermoid cells: faintly PAS positive and no mucicarmine staining.
  Intermediate cells: may contain cytoplasmic mucin or diastase-sensitive, PAS-positive granules.
  Clear cells: usually only focal mucin staining is seen.
- Immunohistochemistry: cytokeratin positive; S-100 protein, glial fibrillary acidic protein, and actin negative.

Differential Diagnosis

Dependent on grade involved but includes:
- Cystadenoma (Chapter 19A, #2a).
- Acinic cell adenocarcinoma (Chapter 19B, #2).
- Primary or metastatic squamous cell carcinoma (Chapter 19B, #9).
- Adenosquamous carcinoma (Chapter 14B, #5).
- Clear cell carcinoma (Chapter 19B, #7).
- Metastatic renal cell carcinoma.

Treatment and Prognosis

Low-Grade and Intermediate-Grade

- Wide local surgical excision is the treatment of choice; in parotid-based neoplasms, preservation of the facial nerve, if feasible, is recommended.
- Palatal-based lesions that are small (2 cm) and do not involve bone can be managed by wide local excision.
- Unless clinically suspicious, neck dissections are not indicated.
- May recur locally if incompletely excised, but metastatic disease infrequently occurs.
- Some advocate postoperative irradiation (6000 to 6500 rads) for intermediate-grade tumors because

of their tendency to infiltrate, resulting in positive resection margins.

■ Excellent prognosis, with approximately 90% 5-year survival rates.

High-Grade

■ Treatment depends on the clinical stage, but in general, wide-block surgical excision is the treatment of choice, which may necessitate sacrifice of the facial nerve (parotid gland tumors) or the hypoglossal and lingual nerves (submandibular tumors); radical palatectomy is required for palatal-based large lesions with involvement of bone.

■ Associated with high rates of recurrence and metastasis and, because of the frequency of metastasis to regional lymph nodes, neck dissections are usually included in the surgical management.

■ Postoperative irradiation (6000 to 6500 rads).

■ Other than regional lymph nodes, favored metastatic sites include skin/subcutaneous tissue, lungs, and bone.

■ Overall 5 year survival rates are approximately 40%.

Additional Facts

■ The majority of mucoepidermoid carcinomas in the pediatric population are low grade.

■ Depending on the histologic appearance (grade), metastatic foci may include both mucous and epidermoid cellular components.

■ The absence of keratin (squamous) pearls, extensive keratinization, and intercellular bridges assist in separating mucoepidermoid carcinoma from squamous cell or adenosquamous carcinoma.

■ Extravasation of mucus into the surrounding tissue may elicit an inflammatory reaction, including giant cells.

References

Auclair PL, Ellis GL: Mucoepidermoid carcinoma. *In:* Ellis GL, Auclair PL, Gnepp DR, eds. Surgical pathology of the salivary glands. Philadelphia: W.B. Saunders Co., 1991; pp 269–298.

Foote FW, Frazell EL: Tumors of major salivary glands. Cancer 6:1065–1133, 1953.

Nascimento AG, Amaral AL, Prado LA, Kligerman J, Silveira RP: Mucoepidermoid carcinoma of salivary glands: a clinicopathologic study of 46 cases. Head Neck Surg 8:409–417, 1986.

Schneider AB, Favus MJ, Stachura ME, Arnold MJ, Frohman LA: Salivary gland neoplasms as a late consequence of head and neck irradiation. Ann Intern Med 87:160–164, 1977.

Spitz MR, Batsakis JG: Major salivary gland carcinoma: descriptive epidemiology and survival of 498 patients. Arch Otolaryngol Head Neck Surg 110:45–48, 1984.

Stewart FW, Foote FW, Becker WF: Mucoepidermoid tumors of salivary glands. Ann Surg 122:820–844, 1945.

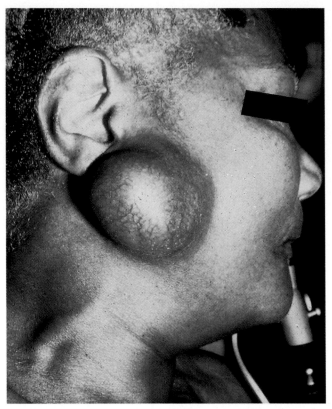

Figure 19–33. Low-grade mucoepidermoid carcinoma, presenting in this woman as a slowly enlarging, painless mass of her right parotid gland.

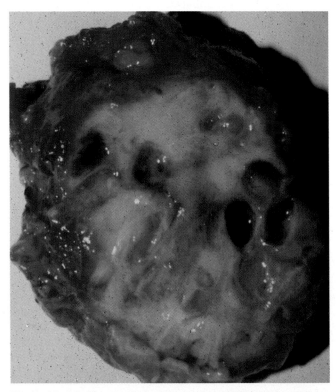

Figure 19–34. The resected and transected specimen reveals an incompletely encapsulated, round to oval, predominantly solid and partially cystic neoplasm; cystic spaces were filled with clear to blood-tinged fluid.

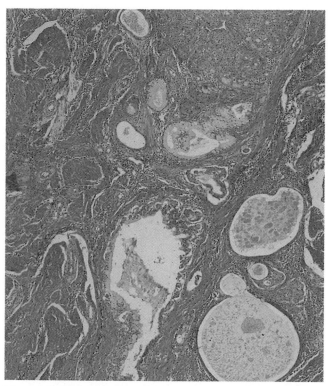

Figure 19–35. Histologic appearance of low-grade mucoepidermoid carcinoma characteristically consists of multiple cysts with large numbers of mucous cells admixed with less numerous but easily identifiable epidermoid cells.

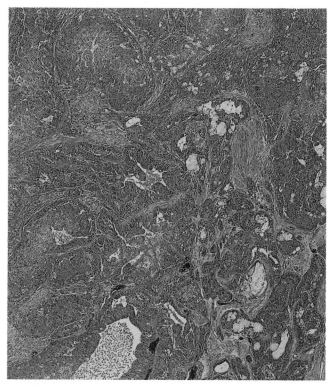

Figure 19–37. Intermediate-grade mucoepidermoid carcinoma: cysts can be seen, but in comparison to the low-grade tumor are less numerous and smaller in size; this grade is more cellular and forms solid nests, as compared to the low-grade cancers.

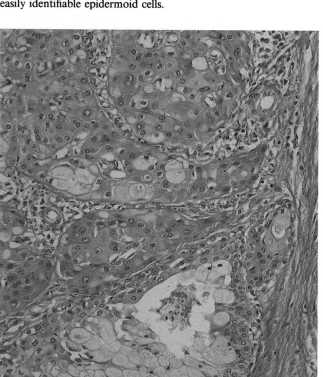

Figure 19–36. Mucous cells are identified lining cystic spaces or admixed within nests or solid areas with epidermoid cells; the epidermoid cells form nests or solid areas in conjunction with the mucous cells. Intermediate cells composed of small, dark-staining nuclei and scanty, eosinophilic cytoplasm can be seen lying peripheral to mucous cells in the lower portion of the illustration.

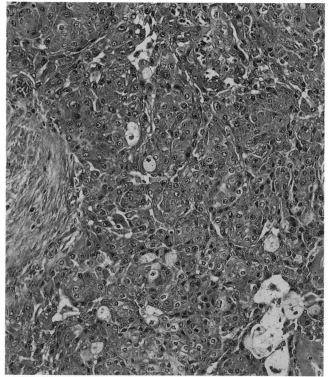

Figure 19–38. Intermediate-grade mucoepidermoid carcinoma: shift in ratio of mucous cells to epidermoid and intermediate cells, with a larger percentage of the latter cells identified; in comparison to the low-grade cancers, there is increased cellular pleomorphism and mitotic activity.

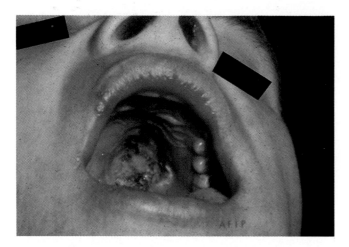

Figure 19–39. High-grade mucoepidermoid carcinoma, presenting as a large, ulcerating, and partially necrotic mass along the hard palate.

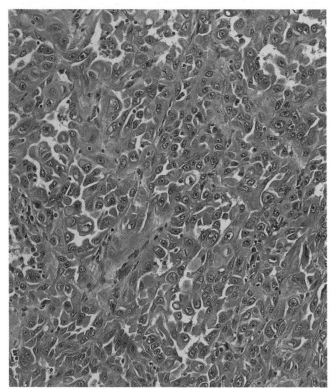

Figure 19–40. High-grade mucoepidermoid carcinoma: characterized by a solid neoplastic cellular proliferation composed almost exclusively of epidermoid and intermediate cells, with only limited numbers of identifiable mucous cells.

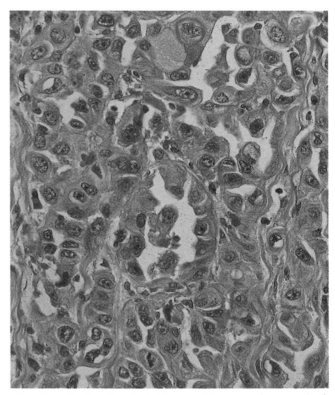

Figure 19–41. Cellular atypia/pleomorphism, prominent nucleoli, increased mitotic activity, and scattered mucous cells are characteristic findings in high-grade mucoepidermoid carcinoma.

2. Acinic Cell Adenocarcinoma

Definition: Low-grade malignant epithelial salivary gland neoplasm, characterized by a variety of histologic growth patterns and the tendency to recapitulate the appearance of normal serous acinous cells.

Clinical

- Represents approximately 18% of all malignant salivary gland neoplasms and 6.5% of all salivary gland neoplasms.
- Affects females more than males; most frequently occurs in the fourth and fifth decades of life.
- More than 90% arise in the parotid gland; may also be identified in the submandibular and sublingual glands, as well as in minor salivary glands throughout the upper respiratory tract.
- In the pediatric age group, acinic cell adenocarcinoma represents the second most common malignant salivary gland neoplasm next to mucoepidermoid carcinoma.
- Bilateral parotid gland involvement may occur in up to 3% of cases.
- The most common symptom is a solitary mass with or without associated pain; slow-growing neoplasm as seen by the clinical presentation of a mass is often present for several years.
- Thought to arise from distal portions of the salivary duct system; specifically, the intercalated duct reserve/stem cells or from the terminal salivary gland tubules.

Pathology

Gross

- Well-demarcated or encapsulated, round or multilobulated, soft to rubbery, tan-gray to yellow or pink mass, usually measuring less than 3.0 cm in greatest diameter, but occasionally may reach sizes up to 13 cm.
- Most neoplasms have a homogeneous appearance, but may be cystic and hemorrhagic.
- Recurrent neoplasms are less well-demarcated and tend to be multinodular in appearance.

Histology

- Circumscribed tumor, characterized by a variety of growth patterns including solid, microcystic, papillary-cystic, and follicular:
  Solid and microcystic: most common patterns; consist of· either sheets of tumor cells in an organoid arrangement or numerous small cystic spaces.
  Papillary-cystic and follicular: least common patterns; consist of variably sized cystic spaces that are associated with papillary projections supported by a fibrovascular core or follicular spaces which resemble thyroid parenchyma

and contain eosinophilic proteinaceous material lined by cuboidal to columnar cells.
- These neoplasms are also noteworthy for their cytologic variations, including:
  Acinic cells: polyhedral in shape, with small, dark, eccentrically placed nuclei and characteristic abundant basophilic granular cytoplasm; these cells predominate in well-differentiated tumors.
  Intercalated duct cells: cuboidal or columnar, with centrally placed, small, dark nuclei and eosinophilic to amphophilic cytoplasm.
  Vacuolated cells: contain cytoplasmic vacuoles, which may be numerous and small, or few and large, distending the cell membranes; in salivary gland neoplasms, these cells are fairly distinctive for acinic cell adenocarcinoma.
  Clear cells: round to oval cells with distinct cell borders, peripherally placed, small, dark nuclei and the hallmark clear cytoplasm; result from fixation or tissue processing.
  Nonspecific glandular cells: lack specific features seen in the other cell types, but tend to be more cellular and pleomorphic, with a syncytial growth as a result of having indistinct cell borders.
- Cellular pleomorphism and mitotic activity are absent.
- Typically, the stroma is scant, but occasionally may may be dense and hyalinized.
- A prominent lymphoid component with germinal centers may be seen.
- Histochemistry: diastase-resistant, PAS-positive material is seen in all cell types; mucicarmine and alcian blue are usually negative.
- Immunohistochemistry: cytokeratin positive; variable immunoreactivity is seen with S-100 protein and vimentin.

Differential Diagnosis

- Neoplasms containing clear cells, including:
  Oncocytoma (Chapter 19A, #2b).
  Mucoepidermoid carcinoma (Chapter 19B, #1).
  Epithelial-myoepithelial cell carcinoma (Chapter 19B, #7).
  Metastatic renal cell carcinoma or papillary carcinoma of thyroid gland origin.

Treatment and Prognosis

- Complete surgical excision is the treatment of choice and may consist of either conservative parotidectomy when the tumor is limited to the superficial lobe, or total parotidectomy when the deep lobe of the parotid is involved.
- These are indolent neoplasms, generally cured by complete surgical removal; however:
  12% of tumors may recur locally.
  8% may metastasize.
  6% of patients die as a result of the neoplasm.

■ Most recurrences and metastases occur within 5 years of the initial therapy.
■ Prognosis is best determined by the clinical stage.

Additional Facts

■ Despite attempts to separate acinic cell adenocarcinomas into low- and high-grade, the histologic pattern and cytologic appearance do not correlate with either a favorable or poor clinical outcome.
■ Factors that may correlate to either recurrence or metastases include:
Large size and infiltrative growth.
Multinodularity.
Cellular atypia/anaplasia and increased mitotic activity.
Stromal hyalinization.
■ Involvement of minor salivary glands infrequently occurs, but is associated with a better prognosis as compared to those arising in the parotid gland.

References

Abrams AM, Cornyn J, Scofield HH, Hansen LS: Acinic cell adenocarcinoma of the major salivary glands: a clinicopathologic study of 77 cases. Cancer 18:1145–1162, 1965.

Dardick I, Byard RW, Carnegie JA: A review of the proliferative capacity of major salivary glands and the relationship to current concepts of neoplasia in salivary glands. Oral Surg Oral Med Oral Pathol 69:53–67, 1990.

Ellis GL, Corio RL: Acinic cell adenocarcinoma: a clinicopathologic study of 294 cases. Cancer 52:542–549, 1983.

Ellis GL, Auclair PL: Acinic cell adenocarcinoma. *In:* Ellis GL, Auclair PL, Gnepp DR, eds. Surgical pathology of the salivary glands. Philadelphia: W.B. Saunders Co., 1991; pp 299–317.

Godwin JT, Foote FW, Frazell EL: Acinic cell adenocarcinoma of the parotid gland: report of twenty-seven cases. Am J Pathol 30:465–477, 1954.

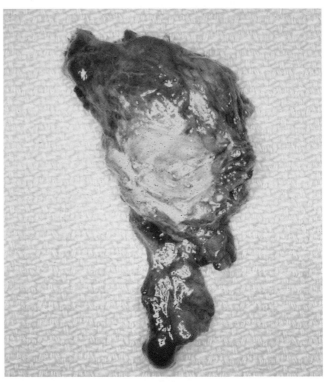

Figure 19–42. Acinic cell adenocarcinoma of the parotid, appearing as a well-demarcated but infiltrating tan-gray to yellow mass in the central portion of the resected specimen.

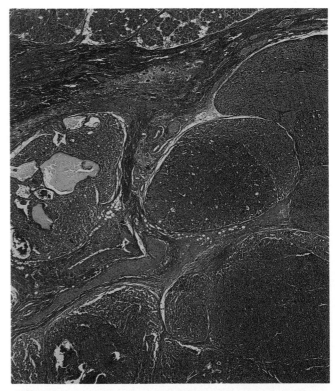

Figure 19–43. Acinic cell adenocarcinoma: circumscribed but unencapsulated tumor nodules characterized by solid, microcystic, papillary-cystic and follicular growth patterns; residual parotid gland parenchyma can be seen at the top.

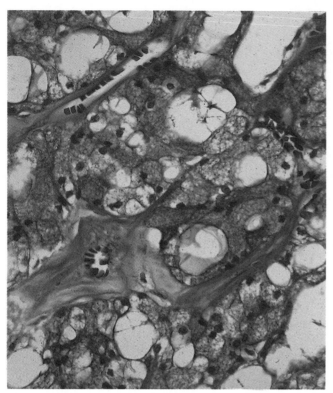

Figure 19–44. Acinic cell adenocarcinomas are composed of cells that appear polyhedral in shape, with small, dark, eccentrically placed nuclei and characteristic abundant basophilic granular cytoplasm.

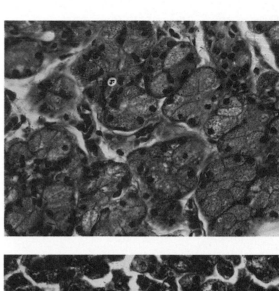

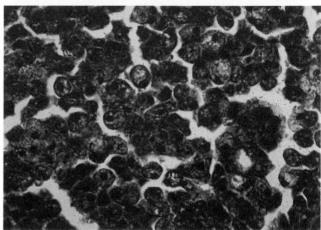

Figure 19–45. (*Top*) characteristic cellular composition of acinic cell adenocarcinomas that recapitulate the normal salivary gland acinous cells (*bottom*).

3. Adenoid Cystic Carcinoma

Definition: Malignant epithelial salivary gland neoplasm, characterized by its histologic appearance, tendency to invade nerves, and protracted but nonetheless relentless clinical course.

Clinical

- Represents approximately 12% of all malignant salivary gland neoplasms.
- No sex predilection; occurs over a wide age range and is most commonly seen in the fifth to seventh decades of life, but is uncommonly encountered prior to the third decade of life.
- In major salivary glands, primarily involves the parotid and submandibular glands, representing up to 5% of all parotid gland neoplasms and approximately 15% of submandibular gland neoplasms.
- Adenoid cystic carcinoma is the most frequently encountered malignant neoplasm of the submandibular gland.
- May involve the minor salivary glands throughout the upper respiratory tract, where it most frequently involves the palate; other sites of involvement include the tongue, ceruminal glands of the external auditory canal, as well as representing 50% of all lacrimal gland neoplasms.
- Symptoms vary according to the site involved, but the most common complaint is that of a mass with or without associated pain or cranial nerve paralysis; other symptoms include airway obstruction, epistaxis, otalgia, and hoarseness.
- Although still the subject of controversy, adenoid cystic carcinomas are believed to arise from the peripheral segments of the salivary duct system, which include the intercalated ducts and acini.

Pathology

Gross

■ Circumscribed, unencapsulated or partly encapsulated, solid, rubbery to firm, tan-white to gray-pink mass measuring from 2 to 4 cm in greatest dimension.

Histology

■ Unencapsulated, infiltrating neoplasm with varied growth patterns, consisting of cribriform, tubular/ductular, trabecular or solid; individual neoplasms may have a single growth, but characteristically are composed of multiple patterns, any one of which may predominate.

Cribriform type

■ Considered the classic pattern.
■ Arrangement of cells in a "Swiss cheese" configuration, with many oval or circular spaces.
■ Spaces contain basophilic mucinous substance or hyalinized eosinophilic material.

Tubular type

■ Cells are arranged in ducts or tubules.
■ Ducts or tubules contain faintly eosinophilic mucinous material.

Solid type

■ Neoplastic cells arranged in sheets or nests of varying size and shape.
■ Little tendency to form cystic spaces, tubules, or ducts.

Common to All Types

■ Neoplastic cells common to all growth patterns, consisting of fairly uniform-sized cells with small, hyperchromatic nuclei, scant cytoplasm, and indistinct cell borders.
■ The interstitial stroma, from which the epithelial component is sharply demarcated, varies in appearance from myxoid to hyalinized.
■ The cystic spaces seen in the cribriform or classic type are pseudocysts, which are extracellular and lined by replicated basement membrane; true glands infrequently may be seen.
■ Common to all histologic variants is the proclivity to peri- and intraneural invasion.
■ Histochemistry: pseudocysts contain diastase-resistant, PAS-positive, and mucicarmine-positive material.
■ Immunohistochemistry demonstrates two cell populations: ductal cells—cytokeratin, S-100 protein, epithelial membrane antigen (EMA), and carcinoembryonic antigen (CEA) positive; myoepithelial cells—cytokeratin, S-100 protein, actin (muscle specific), and glial fibrillary acidic protein positive.

Differential Diagnosis

■ Pleomorphic adenoma (Chapter 19A, #1).
■ Monomorphic adenoma (basal cell and membranous adenoma) (Chapter 19A, #2).
■ Polymorphous low-grade adenocarcinoma (Chapter 19B, #6).
■ Basal cell adenocarcinoma (Chapter 19B, #8).
■ Salivary duct carcinoma (Chapter 19B, #10).

Treatment and Prognosis

■ Wide local surgical excision is the treatment of choice; problems confronting their surgical removal relate to the infiltrative nature of these neoplasms, with the tendency to extend along nerve segments and further compounded by their deceptively circumscribed, macroscopic appearance.
■ Recurrence rates are high and directly relate to inadequate surgical excision.
■ Regional lymph node metastases are uncommon; therefore, neck dissection at the time of surgical removal of the primary tumor is not warranted.
■ Distant metastases generally occur late in the disease course, following multiple local recurrences; metastatic disease primarily occurs to lungs, lymph nodes, and bone, and although prolonged survivals may occur after metastases, death usually follows within 1 year of identification of metastatic foci.
■ Adenoid cystic carcinomas are radiosensitive, and radiotherapy is particularly useful in controlling microscopic disease after initial surgery, in treating locally recurrent disease, or as palliation management in unresectable tumors; radiotherapy is not curative.
■ Although the short-term prognosis is generally good, corresponding to the slow growth that leads to prolonged survivals, the long-term prognosis is poor; these facts are reflected in the 5- and 20-year survival rates of adenoid cystic carcinomas of all head and neck sites of 75% and 13%, respectively.
■ Factors affecting prognosis include:
  Location of primary tumor: major salivary gland adenoid cystic carcinomas have a better prognosis than their minor salivary gland counterparts.
  Size of the primary tumor: the smaller the primary neoplasm, the more complete the resection and the better the prognosis.
  Symptoms of facial nerve paralysis may be associated with a worse prognosis and a quicker demise of the patient.
  Histologic pattern: this parameter remains controversial as to its efficacy, with the best prognosis thought to occur in those neoplasms with a predominant tubular pattern; the worst prognosis is thought to be associated with predominantly solid neoplasms (predominance defined as representing more than 50% of the overall pattern); cribriform predominance has an intermediate prognosis.

Failure of local disease control following initial surgery, recurrent and metastatic disease.

Additional Facts

■ EMA and CEA staining is seen in equal proportion and intensity in the true luminal cells of adenoid cystic carcinoma.
■ Myoepithelial cellular components are found in:
Pseudocyst lining cells of the cribriform type.
Nonluminal cells of the tubular type.
As cellular components of the solid and cribriform types.

References

Batsakis JG: Neoplasms of the minor and "lesser" major salivary glands. *In:* Batsakis, JG, ed. Tumors of the head and neck: Clinical and pathological considerations, 2nd ed. Baltimore: Williams & Wilkins, 1979; pp 76–84.

Chen JC, Gnepp DR, Bedrossian CWM: Adenoid cystic carcinoma arising in salivary glands: an immunohistochemical study. Oral Surg Oral Med Oral Pathol 65:316–326, 1988.

Foote FW, Frazell EL: Tumors of major salivary glands. Cancer 6:1065–1133, 1953.

Perzin KH, Gullane P, Clairmont AC: Adenoid cystic carcinoma arising in salivary glands: a correlation of histologic features and clinical course. Cancer 42:265–282, 1978.

Tomich CE: Adenoid cystic carcinoma. *In:* Ellis GL, Auclair PL, Gnepp DR, eds. Surgical pathology of the salivary glands. Philadelphia: W.B. Saunders Co., 1991; pp 333–349.

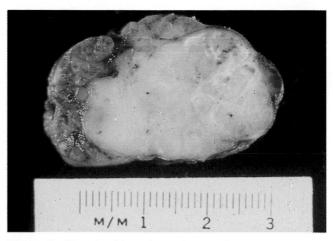

Figure 19-47. Adenoid cystic carcinoma of the submandibular gland, appearing as a circumscribed, unencapsulated, and infiltrating solid tan-white mass.

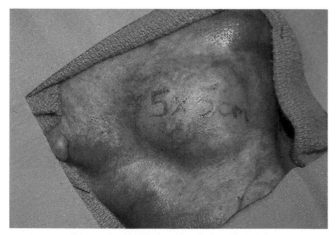

Figure 19-46. Large, bulging, and painful adenoid cystic carcinoma of the right submandibular gland; the patient's lower ear lobe can be seen to the left and the chin to the upper right.

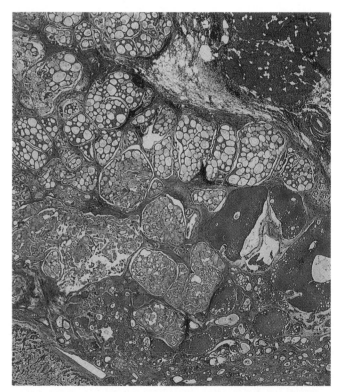

Figure 19-48. Adenoid cystic carcinoma: infiltrating neoplasm with varied growth patterns consisting of cribriform, solid, tubular/ductular, and trabecular; hyalinized eosinophilic material can be seen associated with the tumor nests.

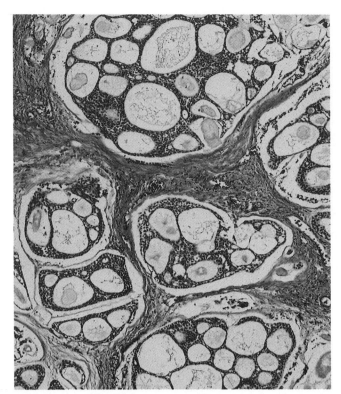

Figure 19–49. Adenoid cystic carcinoma: cribriform growth pattern with a "Swiss cheese" configuration of oval or circular spaces; neoplastic cells are small with hyperchromatic nuclei, scant cytoplasm, and indistinct cell borders.

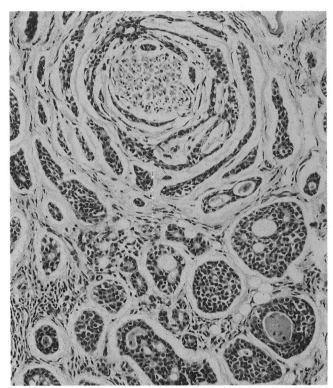

Figure 19–51. Adenoid cystic carcinoma composed of solid nests and tubules with characteristic neurotropism (*top*).

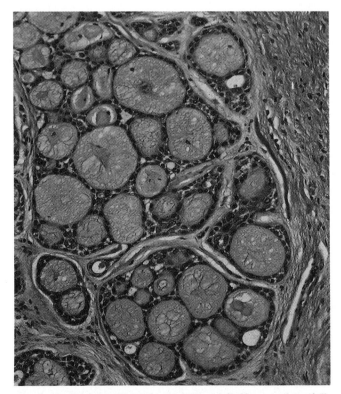

Figure 19–50. Adenoid cystic carcinoma: cribriform and partially tubular growth with spaces containing basophilic mucinous substance ("blue-goo").

4. Malignant Mixed Tumors of Salivary Glands

This term includes two separate malignant neoplasms:
1. Carcinoma ex pleomorphic adenoma.
2. True malignant mixed tumor or carcinosarcoma.

a. Carcinoma Ex Pleomorphic Adenoma

Definition: Malignant *epithelial* salivary gland neoplasm, containing a carcinoma arising from or within a preexisting (primary or recurrent) pleomorphic adenoma.

Synonym: Carcinoma arising in a mixed tumor.

Clinical

- Accounts for approximately 7% of all malignant salivary gland neoplasms, 4% to 6% of all mixed tumors (benign and malignant combined), and 2% to 4% of all salivary gland neoplasms.
- Of the two neoplasms included under the designation of malignant mixed tumor, more than 90% fall within the category of carcinoma ex pleomorphic adenoma.
- No sex predilection; may be seen over a wide age range, but most frequently occurs in the sixth and seventh decades of life (approximately one decade older than patients with pleomorphic adenomas).
- Occurs most commonly in the parotid gland > submandibular gland > minor salivary glands (the palate being the most commonly involved minor salivary gland site).
- Typical clinical presentation is that of a long-standing, painless, nonenlarging or slowly enlarging mass suddenly undergoing rapid enlargement over a 3- to 6-month period; associated symptoms may include pain, facial nerve paralysis, and soft tissue fixation.
- Although less frequent, malignant transformation, as clinically evident by a rapidly enlarging mass, may occur in the absence of a previous history of a pleomorphic adenoma and with histologic confirmation proving the existence of the pleomorphic adenoma component.
- The time period for malignant transformation of a pleomorphic adenoma (initial or recurrent) may be from 2 to 50 years, but on average is approximately 20 years; the risk of malignant transformation increases with the duration of the tumor.

Pathology

Gross

- Many similarities to pleomorphic adenoma.
- Features that should alert the physician to the possible presence of a malignant neoplasm include poor circumscription or infiltration, hemorrhage, necrosis, and cystic change.
- The presence of any of these features should prompt liberal sectioning of the neoplasm for histologic evaluation.

Histology

- In order to render the diagnosis of a carcinoma ex pleomorphic adenoma, residual histologic evidence of a pleomorphic adenoma must be present.
- Destructive infiltrative growth is the most reliable histologic criterion for the diagnosis.
- The carcinoma is most often an adenocarcinoma of varying differentiation, followed in frequency by undifferentiated carcinoma; other, less frequently identified carcinomatous components include squamous cell carcinoma, mucoepidermoid carcinoma, adenoid cystic carcinoma, myoepithelial carcinoma, polymorphous low-grade adenocarcinoma, and acinic cell adenocarcinoma.
- In the absence of an unequivocal carcinoma or in cases with equivocal cytologic features for carcinoma, the following features lend support to the presence of malignant transformation:
  Micronecrosis and hemorrhage.
  Infiltrative margins.
  Excessive hyalinization.
  Dystrophic calcification and ossification.
  Vascular or neural invasion.
- Pleomorphic/monomorphic adenomas may be very cellular and demonstrate cellular pleomorphism, but generally lack the features detailed above.
- The malignant component may be confined within the capsule and devoid of an invasive growth; such neoplasms are designated noninvasive carcinoma ex pleomorphic adenoma (carcinoma in situ).

Differential Diagnosis

- Cellular pleomorphic adenoma or monomorphic adenoma (Chapter 19A, #1,2).
- True malignant mixed tumor (see below).

Treatment and Prognosis

- Wide surgical excision is the treatment of choice and may necessitate radical parotidectomy with sacrifice of the facial nerve.
- These neoplasms are associated with both high recurrence and metastatic rates; metastases most frequently occur to regional lymph nodes, lungs, brain, and bone (vertebral column).
- If clinical evidence supports nodal metastases, then neck dissection can be performed.
- Radiotherapy and chemotherapy are of questionable benefit.
- Noninvasive carcinoma ex pleomorphic adenomas have survival rates similar to those of benign mixed tumors.
- Invasive carcinoma ex pleomorphic adenomas have 5-year survival rates between 25% and 65% and 15-year survival rates between 10% and 35%.
- Recurrence of tumor generally carries a poor prognosis; after the discovery of metastatic disease, death usually follows within 1 year.

■ Factors adversely affecting prognosis include:
Origin in a major salivary gland.
Recurrent or metastatic disease.
Penetration of the capsule.
Neural invasion.

Additional Facts

■ There is no correlation between the number of recurrences of the pleomorphic adenoma and the development of malignant transformation.

■ In carcinoma ex pleomorphic adenomas occurring in cases without a prior history of a salivary gland tumor, it is possible that the pleomorphic adenoma was present for long periods but was too small to be symptomatic or detected clinically.

■ Another category of salivary gland neoplasms that is included within the spectrum of malignant mixed tumors is the *metastasizing mixed tumor:*

Extremely rare neoplasm, characterized histologically by the presence of a tumor that conforms with all the morphologic criteria of a pleomorphic adenoma but which metastasizes; metastatic foci are histologically similar to the primary and recurrent neoplasms.

Primary neoplasm most frequently originates in the parotid; other sites include the submandibular gland and sinonasal seromucous glands.

Typically, multiple recurrent benign mixed tumors are seen within the area of the primary tumor prior to the development of metastases, which occur either at the time of a recurrent tumor or from years to decades later.

Metastatic spread is by both hematogenous and lymphatic routes, with metastatic foci seen in bone (femur, humerus, pelvis, ribs, calvarium), lung, kidney, retroperitoneum, skin, and lymph nodes.

Treatment is complete surgical excision of all tumor foci.

Prognosis is generally good, even with metastatic disease; however, death may occur from metastatic disease, thereby, justifying inclusion of these neoplasms within the spectrum of malignant mixed tumors.

Reasons for metastases remain unproven, but repeated surgical manipulation(s) may represent a primary factor in introducing neoplastic foci into vascular channels, resulting in metastatic disease.

b. True Malignant Mixed Tumor or Carcinosarcoma

Definition: Malignant salivary gland neoplasm, consisting of an admixture of malignant epithelial **and** malignant mesenchymal elements.

Clinical

■ Rare salivary gland neoplasm.

■ No sex predilection; most commonly seen in the sixth decade of life.

■ May occur in both major and minor salivary glands, including the parotid, submandibular, and sublingual glands and the oral cavity (palate).

■ Most common symptoms relate to an enlarging mass with recent increase in size, with or without associated pain or facial nerve paralysis.

■ Generally arise de novo; however, have been associated with previously excised benign mixed tumors, recurrent mixed tumor, and recurring benign mixed tumors treated by radiotherapy.

Pathology

Gross

■ Poorly circumscribed, infiltrative lesion, with a tan-gray to yellow appearance, measuring from 2 to 9 cm in diameter.

■ Cut section may show cystic areas, hemorrhage, and calcification.

Histology

■ Biphasic appearance composed of carcinomatous and sarcomatous elements.

■ Carcinomatous component: epithelial component is usually a moderately to poorly differentiated ductal carcinoma, but may be an undifferentiated carcinoma or an epidermoid carcinoma.

■ Sarcomatous component: typically represents the predominant tissue type and is usually a chondrosarcoma; other malignant mesenchymal elements may include osteosarcoma, fibrosarcoma, malignant fibrous histiocytoma and, rarely, liposarcoma.

■ Rarely, nonmalignant osteoid may be seen.

Differential Diagnosis

■ Spindle cell carcinoma (Chapter 14B, #2).
■ Synovial sarcoma (Chapter 14B, #8).

Treatment and Prognosis

■ Complete surgical excision is the treatment of choice; because these neoplasms are locally infiltrative and destructive, radical surgery is usually necessary.

■ Radiotherapy and lymph node dissection for palpable disease are also advocated.

■ The role of chemotherapy is still unproven, but is used in cases with distant metastases.

■ Metastases that include both histologic components occur frequently and most often metastasize to the lungs, followed by cervical and hilar lymph nodes; metastases to liver, bone, and brain also occur.

■ These are highly lethal neoplasms, with mean survival of patients dying from their disease of less than 30 months.

Additional Facts

■ These neoplasms are considered to take origin from epithelial cells; support of the epithelial histogenesis includes:

Pleomorphic adenomas, consisting of an admixture of both epithelial- and mesenchymal-appearing tissue originate from epithelial and myoepithelial cells.

The sarcomatous element in the carcinosarcoma is nearly always a chondrosarcoma and less often an osteosarcoma, both of which represent the mesenchymal-like elements seen in pleomorphic adenomas.

References

Gerughty RM, Scofield HH, Brown FM, Hennigar GR: Malignant mixed tumors of salivary gland origin. Cancer 24:471–486, 1969.

Gnepp DR, Wenig BM: Malignant mixed tumors. *In:* Ellis GL, Auclair PL, Gnepp DR, eds. Surgical pathology of the salivary glands. Philadelphia: W.B. Saunders Co., 1991; pp 350–368.

LiVolsi VA, Perzin KH: Malignant mixed tumors arising in salivary glands: I. Carcinomas arising in benign mixed tumors: a clinicopathologic study. Cancer 39:2209–2239, 1977.

Stephen J, Batsakis JG, Luna MA, von der Heyden U, Byers RM: True malignant mixed tumors (carcinosarcoma) of salivary glands. Oral Surg Oral Med Oral Pathol 61:597–602, 1986.

Wenig BM, Hitchcock CC, Ellis GL, Gnepp DR: Metastasizing mixed tumor of salivary glands: a clinicopathologic and flow cytometric analysis. Am J Surg Pathol 16:845–858, 1992.

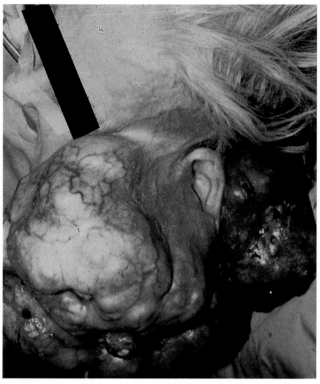

Figure 19–52. Carcinoma ex pleomorphic adenoma presenting as a huge, fungating, and necrotic mass completely obliterating and distorting normal facial structures.

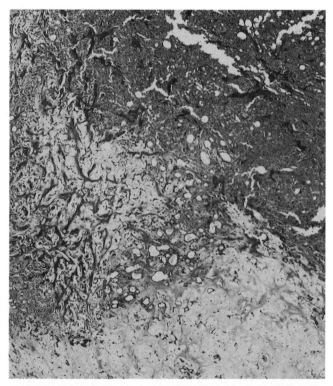

Figure 19–53. Carcinoma ex pleomorphic adenoma: residual histologic evidence of a pleomorphic adenoma, in the lower portion of the illustration, is seen by the presence of benign epithelial structures within a myxochondroid matrix; the upper portion of the illustration demonstrates a solid and cellular malignant infiltrate.

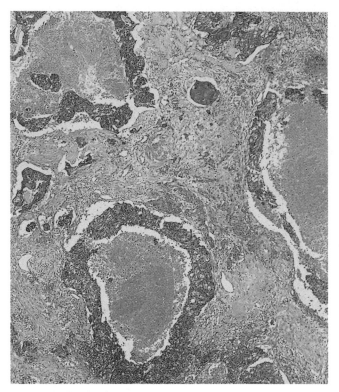

Figure 19–54. Carcinoma ex pleomorphic adenoma with infiltrating malignant epithelial nests having morphologic features of an undifferentiated carcinoma and demonstrating comedonecrosis within the center of the lobules.

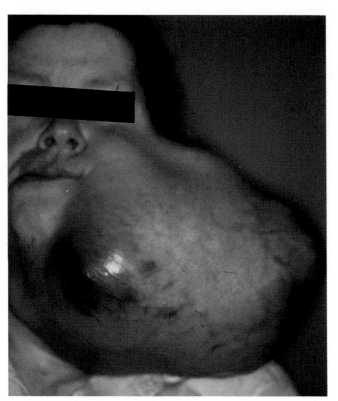

Figure 19–56. Woman presenting with a huge, true malignant mixed tumor causing facial distortion; the neoplasm originated in the parotid gland.

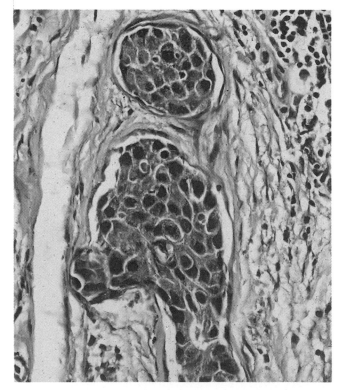

Figure 19–55. Carcinoma ex pleomorphic adenoma in which the carcinomatous component invades into vascular structures.

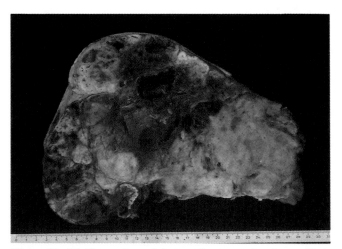

Figure 19–57. Cut section of the neoplasm reveals a hemorrhagic and partially necrotic mass with a solid, cystic, and lobular appearance.

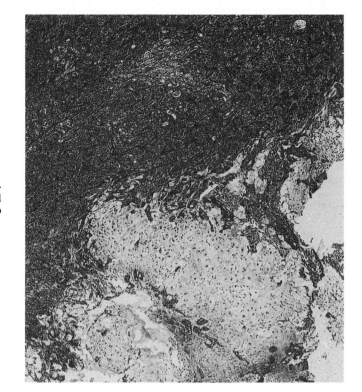

Figure 19–58. True malignant mixed tumor demonstrating a biphasic appearance, composed of carcinomatous (undifferentiated carcinoma) and sarcomatous (chondrosarcoma) elements at the top and lower portions of the illustration, respectively.

5. Adenocarcinoma, Not Otherwise Specified

Definition: Malignant epithelial salivary gland neoplasm with adenocarcinomatous features but without other specific histologic features, allowing for a more definitive classification.

Clinical

■ Considered one of the more common malignant salivary gland neoplasms, and the third most common behind mucoepidermoid carcinoma and acinic cell adenocarcinoma.

■ Affects females more than males; occurs over a wide age range, but is most frequently seen in the fifth to eighth decades of life.

■ The most common site of occurrence is in the parotid gland; other sites of involvement include submandibular and sublingual glands and the intraoral minor salivary glands, particularly along the palate.

■ Symptoms relate to a solitary mass with or without associated pain, cranial nerve paralysis, or cutaneous involvement.

Pathology

Gross

■ Poorly demarcated and infiltrating, firm to hard, tan-white mass measuring from 2 to 10 cm in diameter.

■ Hemorrhage, necrosis, and cystic change may be seen.

Histology

■ These neoplasms display histologic heterogeneity, but common to all growth patterns and cytologic appearances is the presence of glands and an absence of epidermoid differentiation; in higher grade neoplasms, the glandular features may require diligent searching or may be represented by primitive attempts at gland or duct formation.

■ These neoplasms are infiltrative with varied growth patterns, including solid or sheetlike, tubular, nests, and cordlike.

■ Cytologic diversification is also seen and ranges from cells having a uniform appearance and distinct cell borders to markedly pleomorphic cells with indistinct cell borders; a clear-cell population may be prominent.

■ Histologic grading into low (grade I), intermediate (grade II), and high (grade III) is based on degree of gland formation (differentiation), cellular pleomorphism, and mitotic activity:

Low-grade: well circumscribed but at least focally invasive, numerous gland or ductlike structures, relatively uniform cytomorphologic features with little cellular pleomorphism, few mitoses.

Intermediate-grade: glands or ductlike structures are readily seen, but in comparison to low-grade tumors, there is greater cellular pleomorphism and more mitoses.

High-grade: generally grow in solid sheets of cells, marked by anaplastic cytologic features, numerous mitoses, necrosis, and hemorrhage; the presence of glandular differentiation may require extensive searching or the use of special stains.

■ Papillary structures or large cystic spaces are generally not seen.

■ May contain areas with features of adenoid cystic carcinoma or acinic cell adenocarcinoma; however, these foci are very limited and do not justify exclusion from classification as adenocarcinoma, not otherwise specified.

■ Histochemistry: the presence of intracytoplasmic mucin is seen with mucicarmine staining.

■ Immunohistochemistry: cytokeratin positive.

Differential Diagnosis

■ Benign mixed tumor or other adenomas (Chapter 19A, #1).

■ Epithelial-myoepithelial cell carcinoma (Chapter 19B, #7).

■ Clear cell adenocarcinoma (Chapter 19B, #7).

■ Polymorphous low-grade adenocarcinoma (Chapter 19B, #6).

■ High-grade mucoepidermoid carcinoma (Chapter 19B, #1).

■ Metastatic adenocarcinoma.

Treatment and Prognosis

■ Complete surgical excision is the treatment of choice, and the extent of the surgery is dependent on the location and clinical stage of disease (subtotal versus total glandectomy).

■ Neck dissection is dependent on the presence of overt neck disease or the clinical suspicion of nodal involvement.

■ Postoperative radiotherapy may be of benefit in higher stage neoplasms.

■ Local recurrence of tumor is not uncommon; metastatic disease occurs in approximately 25% of patients, with cervical lymph nodes and the lungs the most commonly affected sites, but bone, skin, and abdominal sites may also be involved.

■ The most accurate factor in predicting survival is the clinical stage, with 15-year cure rates of 67%, 35%, and 8% seen for stages I, II, and III, respectively; other factors correlating with prognosis include:

Histologic grade: the lower the grade, the lower the rate of local recurrence(s) or metastatic disease.

Site of involvement: survival rates decrease in order with involvement of intraoral salivary glands, the parotid gland, and the submandibular gland.

Additional Facts

■ A higher percentage of submandibular gland adenocarcinomas are high-grade neoplasms as compared to parotid-based neoplasms, accounting for the greater likelihood of submandibular adenocarcinomas metastasizing to regional lymph nodes than lesions of the parotid gland or intraoral minor salivary glands.

■ Poorly differentiated carcinomas that lack glandular differentiation are classified as *undifferentiated carcinoma*, which include:

Lymphoepithelial carcinoma.

Large cell type of undifferentiated carcinoma.

Small cell type of undifferentiated carcinoma.

References

Auclair PL, Ellis GL: Adenocarcinoma, not otherwise specified. *In:* Ellis GL, Auclair PL, Gnepp DR, eds. Surgical pathology of the salivary glands. Philadelphia: W.B. Saunders Co., 1991; pp 318–332.

Eversole LR, Gnepp DR, Eversole GM: Undifferentiated carcinoma. *In:* Ellis GL, Auclair PL, Gnepp DR, eds. Surgical pathology of the salivary glands. Philadelphia: W.B. Saunders Co., 1991; pp. 422–440.

Hamilton-Dutoit SJ, Therkildsen MH, Nielsen NH, Jensen H, Hart Hansen JP, Pallesen G: Undifferentiated carcinoma of the salivary gland in Greenland Eskimos: demonstration of Epstein-Barr virus DNA by in situ nucleic acid hybridization. Hum Pathol 22:811–815, 1991.

Spiro RH, Huvos AG, Strong EW: Adenocarcinoma of salivary gland origin: clinicopathologic study of 204 patients. Am J Surg 144:423–431, 1982.

Weiss LM, Gaffey MJ, Shibata D: Lymphoepithelioma-like carcinoma and its relationship to Epstein-Barr virus. Am J Clin Pathol 96:156–158, 1991.

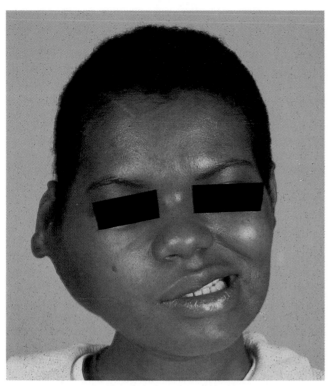

Figure 19–59. Adenocarcinoma, not otherwise specified (NOS), presenting in this young woman as a right parotid gland mass with facial distortion and evidence of facial nerve paralysis.

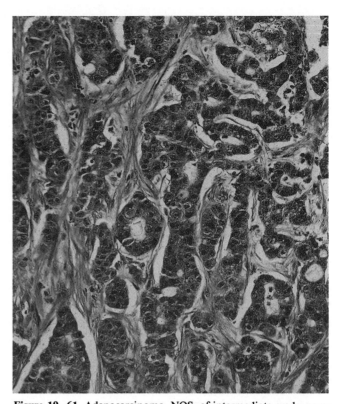

Figure 19–61. Adenocarcinoma, NOS, of intermediate grade, composed of glands and ductlike structures with cellular pleomorphism, prominent eosinophilic nucleoli and scattered mitoses; pleomorphism and mitoses are greater than those of low-grade tumors, but not as prominent as seen in higher grade tumors, which generally grow in solid sheets of cells without prominent glandular differentiation and marked by anaplasia, necrosis, and hemorrhage.

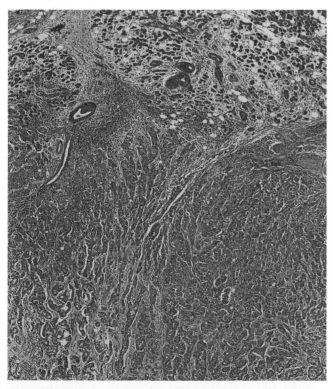

Figure 19–60. Adenocarcinoma, NOS, showing an infiltrating neoplasm with glandular and trabecular growth.

6. Polymorphous Low-Grade Adenocarcinoma of Minor Salivary Glands

Definition: A malignant neoplasm arising from minor salivary glands, characterized by a varied or polymorphous histomorphology and an indolent behavior.

Synonyms: Terminal duct carcinoma; lobular carcinoma.

Clinical

- Affects females more than males; occurs over a wide age range, but is most frequently seen in the seventh decade of life.
- The tumor is almost exclusively identified in the oral cavity, where the palate represents the most frequent site of occurrence; in descending order of frequency, the other intraoral sites include the buccal mucosa > lip > retromolar pad > cheek > tongue > maxillary area > mandibular mucosal area > posterior trigone region.
- Involvement of non-oral sites is rare and includes the nasal cavity and nasopharynx.
- The most common symptom is a painless mass or swelling, occasionally associated with bleeding, increase in size, or discomfort; other less frequently identified symptoms include otalgia, odynophagia, tinnitus, and airway obstruction.
- The duration of symptoms is quite variable, ranging from as short as 2 weeks to a 20- to 30-year history of a mass lesion.
- No predisposing factors associated with this neoplasm are known to exist.

Pathology

Gross

- The tumors are polypoid or raised, round to oval, mucosal-covered masses ranging in size from 1.0 to 6.0 cm in greatest dimension.
- In general, the mucosa remains intact; however, scattered surface ulceration may occur.

Histology

- Well-circumscribed but unencapsulated tumor characterized by morphologic diversity, cytologic uniformity, and infiltrative growth.
- The polymorphic nature of these lesions refers to the variety of growth patterns, which include solid, glandular, cribriform, ductular, tubular, trabecular, or cystic; these patterns may be identified within the same lesion and from lesion to lesion.
- A pattern of cell growth in which the cells are arranged in a single row, termed "Indian-file," can be seen and is often located at the periphery of the tumor; occasionally, a focal papillary pattern can be identified.
- The tumor is composed of cuboidal to columnar isomorphic cells with indistinct cell borders that have uniform ovoid to spindle-shaped nuclei and

small and inconspicuous nucleoli; the nuclear chromatin pattern varies from vesicular to stippled, but basophilic nuclei can also be identified.

- Scant to moderate amounts of eosinophilic to amphophilic cytoplasm can be seen, and occasionally clear cytoplasmic changes predominate.
- The tumor stroma varies from mucoid to hyaline to mucohyaline, and in some cases tumor nests are separated by a fibrovascular stroma.
- Neurotropism (peri- and intraneural) is found in the majority of tumors; perivascular invasion can also be seen, with tumor nests often arranged in concentric fashion around these structures.
- In addition, the tumor may infiltrate the surface epithelium, residual minor salivary glands, or connective tissue components (bone, cartilage, muscle, and adipose tissue).
- Mitotic figures are rare, and necrosis is not seen.
- Other changes that may be identified include intratubular calcifications (psammoma-like bodies), pseudoepitheliomatous hyperplasia of the surface epithelium, and squamous metaplasia within the tumor; the latter can be identified after fine-needle aspiration biopsy of their tumors.
- Histochemistry: intraluminal mucin can be identified by diastase-resistant, PAS-positive material; however, only focal intracytoplasmic mucin is seen.
- Immunohistochemistry: cytokeratin, epithelial membrane antigen (EMA), and S-100 protein are consistently positive, with immunoreactivity in both the luminal and nonluminal cells; carcinoembryonic antigen (CEA) and muscle-specific actin are variably immunoreactive; glial fibrillary acidic protein (GFAP) immunoreactivity may be seen.
- Electronmicroscopy: glandular differentiation, junctional complexes (desmosomes, tight junctions), lumina, microvilli.

Differential Diagnosis

- Pleomorphic adenoma (benign mixed tumor) (Chapter 19A, #1).
- Monomorphic adenomas (Chapter 19A, #2).
- Adenoid cystic carcinoma (Chapter 19B, #3).

Treatment and Prognosis

- Conservative but complete surgical excision is the treatment of choice; radical neck dissections are unwarranted, unless there is clinical evidence of cervical lymph node metastases.
- Postoperative radiotherapy and chemotherapy have been used, but there is no evidence to substantiate any benefit of these modalities in conjunction with surgery.
- This is a slow-growing, indolent, malignant neoplasm that has a good prognosis after complete surgical excision; it can recur over long periods of time and may even metastasize to regional cervical lymph nodes, but distant metastases do not occur

and death attributable to polymorphous low-grade adenocarcinoma is extemely rare.

Additional Facts

■ The terminology of "terminal duct" carcinoma was used to emphasize the proposed histogenesis of the tumor, thought to be the progenitor cell of the distal or terminal duct portions of the salivary gland unit, that is, the intercalated duct reserve cell; "lobular" carcinoma was used because these salivary gland adenocarcinomas demonstrated areas of an infiltrative, Indian-file growth pattern identical to that of the lobular carcinoma of the breast.

■ Polymorphous low-grade adenocarcinoma is a tumor of minor salivary glands and has not been identified in major salivary glands, except as the malignant epithelial component in carcinoma ex pleomorphic adenoma.

■ The antigenic profile of polymorphous low-grade adenocarcinoma is consistent with its proposed derivation from the intercalated duct region of the salivary duct system, supporting the presence of at least two populations of tumor cells, including those that form ductal structures and those with myoepithelial features.

■ Low-grade papillary adenocarcinoma of minor salivary gland origin has been considered a variant of the polymorphous low-grade adenocarcinoma; however, based on differences in morphology and, more importantly, the biologic behavior (local recurrence, cervical lymph node and distant metastases, and mortalities directly related to the neoplasm), these neoplasms represent distinct entities and the low-grade papillary adenocarcinoma is grouped under *papillary cystadenocarcinomas:*
Group of malignant epithelial neoplasms charac-
terized by large cystic spaces with epithelial lining with or without a papillary growth.

Majority are considered low grade, but intermediate grade cystadenocarcinomas may be identified.

■ Some consider polymorphous low-grade adenocarcinoma the low-grade variant of adenoid cystic carcinoma, based on the morphologic similarities as well as common derivation from the intercalated duct region; however, cytologic, immunohistochemical, and biologic differences do not support this contention.

References

Batsakis JG, Pinkston GR, Luna MA, Byers RM, Sciubba JJ, Tillery GW: Adenocarcinoma of the oral cavity: a clinicopathologic study of terminal duct carcinomas. J Laryngol Otol 97:825–835, 1983.

Ellis GL, Auclair PL, Gnepp DR, Goode RK: Other malignant epithelial neoplasms. *In:* Ellis GL, Auclair PL, Gnepp DR, eds. Surgical pathology of the salivary glands. Philadelphia: W.B. Saunders Co., 1991; pp 464–470.

Evans HL, Batsakis JG: Polymorphous low-grade adenocarcinoma of minor salivary glands: a study of 14 cases of a distinctive neoplasm. Cancer 53:935–942, 1984.

Freedman PD, Lumerman H: Lobular carcinoma of intraoral minor salivary glands. Oral Surg Oral Med Oral Pathol 56:157–165, 1983.

Mills SE, Garland TA, Allen MS: Low-grade papillary adenocarcinoma of palatal minor salivary glands. Am J Surg Pathol 8:367–374, 1985.

Regezi JA, Zarbo RJ, Stewart JCB, Courtney RM: Polymorphous low-grade adenocarcinoma of minor salivary glands: a comparative histologic and immunohistochemical study. Oral Surg Oral Med Oral Pathol 71:469–475, 1991.

Slootweg PJ, Muller H: Low-grade adenocarcinoma of the oral cavity: a comparison between the terminal duct and the papillary type. J Craniomaxillofac Surg 15:359–364, 1987.

Wenig BM, Gnepp DR: Polymorphous low-grade adenocarcinoma of minor salivary glands. *In:* Ellis GL, Auclair PL, Gnepp DR, eds. Surgical pathology of the salivary glands. Philadelphia: W.B. Saunders Co., 1991; pp 390–411.

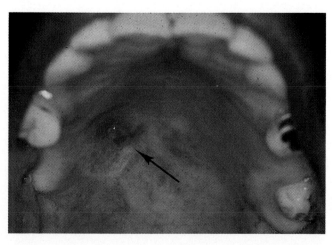

Figure 19–62. Polymorphous, low-grade adenocarcinoma (PLGA) of minor salivary glands, presenting as a mucosal-covered, irregular area on the hard palate (*arrow*).

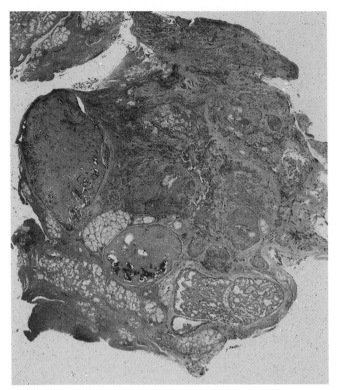

Figure 19–63. As the name implies, PLGA have a polymorphous growth, composed of solid, glandular, cribriform, tubular, trabecular, and cystic patterns of growth.

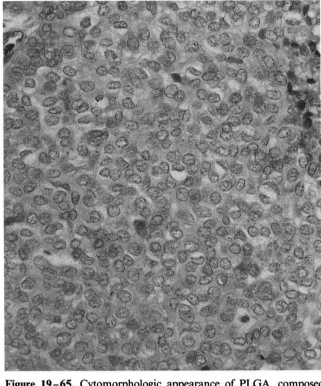

Figure 19–65. Cytomorphologic appearance of PLGA, composed of isomorphic cells with indistinct cell borders, uniform ovoid to spindle-shaped nuclei, and small, inconspicuous nucleoli; the nuclear chromatin pattern varies from vesicular to stippled, but basophilic nuclei can also be identified.

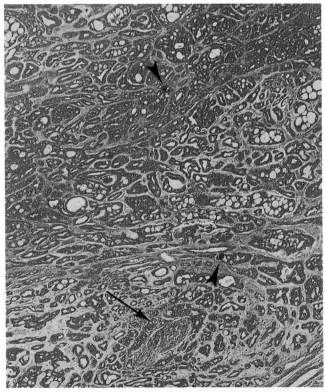

Figure 19–64. PLGA demonstrating cribriform, tubular, ductular, and trabecular patterns, as well as the neurotropism (*arrow*) and intratubular calcifications (psammoma-like bodies; *arrowheads*).

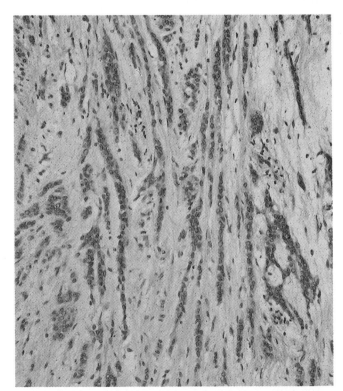

Figure 19–66. An Indian-file pattern can be seen, which is often located at the periphery of the tumor and initially resulted in the terminology for these neoplasms as lobular carcinoma because of the histologic resemblance to lobular carcinoma of the breast.

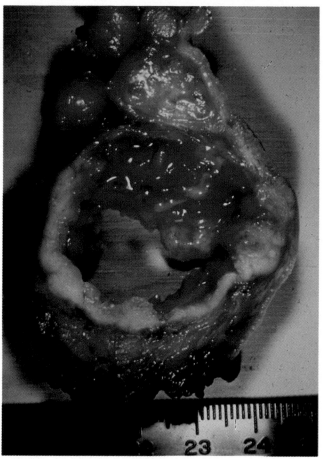

Figure 19–67. Papillary cystadenocarcinoma of the parotid gland, showing large, cystic spaces lined by solid white tissue focally with a papillary-like appearance.

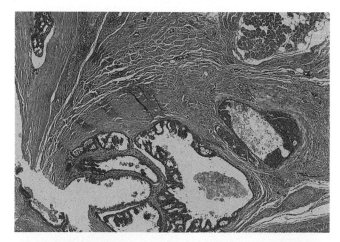

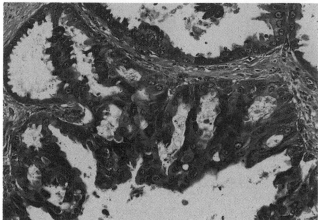

Figure 19–68. Papillary cystadenocarcinoma. (*Top*) Infiltrating cystic spaces lined by epithelium with a papillary and cribriform glandular appearance as well as one cystic space with a solid-appearing epithelial component; residual parotid parenchyma is seen at the top. (*Bottom*) Cystic spaces lined by a single- or multilayered epithelium with a complex glandular growth composed of pleomorphic cells with oval, vesicular to basophilic nuclei, prominent nucleoli, and eosinophilic cytoplasm.

7. Epithelial–Myoepithelial Cell Carcinoma of Intercalated Duct Origin

Definition: Low-grade malignant salivary gland neoplasm, characterized by the presence of two cell types, including clear cells.

Synonyms: Clear cell adenoma/carcinoma; glycogen-rich clear cell adenoma/carcinoma; tubular carcinoma.

Clinical

■ Represents less than 1% of all salivary gland neoplasms.

■ Affects females more than males; may occur over a wide age range, but is most frequently encountered in the seventh and eighth decades of life.

■ More than 80% of these neoplasms occur in the parotid gland; other sites of involvement include the submandibular gland and the minor salivary glands throughout the upper respiratory tract.

■ Symptoms vary from an asymptomatic mass to a mass associated with pain or facial nerve paralysis.

■ As its name indicates, these neoplasms take origin from the intercalated duct segment of the salivary duct system, with histologic and immunohistochemical evidence supporting epithelial and myoepithelial differentiation.

Pathology

Gross

- Encapsulated or circumscribed, solid, tan-white to yellow mass measuring from 1 to 8 cm in diameter.
- Minor salivary gland involvement may be associated with mucosal ulceration.

Histology

- Multinodular tumor that may or may not be encapsulated; infiltration is seen by extension of tumor through the capsule, if present, or into surrounding salivary gland parenchyma in unencapsulated tumors.
- Tumor nests frequently have an organoid arrangement, but may also have a cystic, papillary, or solid appearance.
- Histologic hallmark is the presence of two cell types, identified in varying proportions in any given tumor:
  Inner cell layer (epithelial): dark-staining, cuboidal to columnar cells with central or basally placed nuclei and scant eosinophilic cytoplasm.
  Outer cell layer (myoepithelial): polyhedral-shaped cells with eccentrically placed nuclei and abundant clear cytoplasm.
- Cell nests are separated by basement membrane, which may be thickened, creating a hyalinized appearance.
- Mitoses are rarely seen and necrosis or neural or vascular invasion may occasionally be identified.
- Histochemistry:
  Inner cells have diastase-resistant, PAS-positive intracytoplasmic material.
  Outer (clear) cells have diastase-sensitive, PAS-positive intracytoplasmic material; mucicarmine stains are negative.
- Immunohistochemistry:
  Inner cells: cytokeratin and EMA positive; S-100 protein is variably immunoreactive.
  Outer (clear) cells: S-100 protein, GFAP, and actin (muscle-specific) positive; cytokeratin is variably reactive.

Differential Diagnosis

- Clear cell oncocytoma (Chapter 19A, #2b).
- Mucoepidermoid carcinoma (Chapter 19B, #1).
- Acinic cell adenocarcinoma (Chapter 19B, #2).
- Clear cell carcinoma (see below).
- Metastatic tumors composed of clear cells: renal cell carcinoma and thyroid carcinoma.

Treatment and Prognosis

- Complete surgical excision is the treatment of choice and often is curative.
- Local recurrence is not an infrequent occurrence; however, metastatic tumor may occur but is unusual.

- Metastases occur to regional lymph nodes, lungs, and kidney.
- In general, the prognosis is excellent; however, deaths may occur, restricted to, but not always seen in, cases with metastatic tumor.

Additional Facts

- A spectrum of morphologic appearance may be seen, such that the typical bicellular features with epithelial-lined lumens may be seen at one end of the spectrum, whereas at the other extreme, the neoplasm may be totally composed of solid masses of clear cells, without evidence of lumina or luminal-lining cells.
- Given the spectrum of morphologic appearances, it appears reasonable to classify many of the neoplasms designated as clear cell tumors under epithelial-myoepithelial cell carcinoma; this is true assuming that the clear cell components are not part of other salivary gland neoplasms (acinic cell or mucoepidermoid carcinomas) or metastatic tumors that are composed partly or exclusively of clear cells.
- Despite incorporation within the classification of epithelial-myoepithelial cell carcinoma, a group of epithelial salivary gland neoplasms composed exclusively of clear cells are identified, termed *clear cell carcinomas,* and have the following features:
  Distinct from epithelial-myoepithelial cell carcinoma.
  No sex predilection; primarily identified in the sixth to eighth decades of life.
  Occur most frequently in intraoral sites (palate is the most common location); other sites of involvement include the parotid and submandibular glands.
  Histologic picture is dominated by cells with clear cytoplasm that contain glycogen (diastase-sensitive, PAS-positive) in solid, nested, cord-like, and organoid growth patterns; infiltration into adjacent tissue is characteristically seen.
  Considered malignant, albeit low grade; associated with a good prognosis after complete surgical excision.

References

Batsakis JG, Regezi JA: Selected controversial lesions of salivary tissue. Otolaryngol Clin North Am 10:309–328, 1977.
Corio RL, Sciubba JJ, Brannon RB, Batsakis JG: Epithelial-myoepithelial carcinoma of intercalated duct origin. Oral Surg Oral Med Oral Pathol 53:280–287, 1982.
Corio RL: Epithelial-myoepithelial carcinoma. In: Ellis GL, Auclair PL, Gnepp DR, eds. Surgical pathology of the salivary glands. Philadelphia: W.B. Saunders Co., 1991; pp 412–421.
Donath K, Seifert G, Schmitz R: Zur diagnose und ultrastruktur des tubulären speichelgangcarcinoms: epithelial-myoepitheliales schaltstuckcarcinom. Virchows Arch [A] 356:16–31, 1972.
Ellis GL, Auclair PL: Clear cell carcinoma. In: Ellis GL, Auclair PL, Gnepp DR, eds. Surgical pathology of the salivary glands. Philadelphia: W.B. Saunders Co., 1991; pp 379–389.
Luna MA, Ordonez NG, MacKay B, Batsakis JG, Guillamondegui O: Salivary epithelial-myoepithelial carcinoma of intercalated ducts: a clinical, electron microscopy, and immunocytochemical study. Oral Surg Oral Med Oral Pathol 59:482–490, 1985.

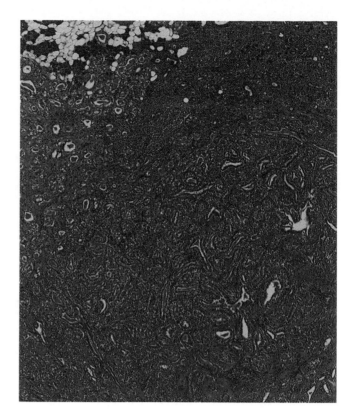

Figure 19–69. Epithelial-myoepithelial cell carcinoma (EMC) of intercalated duct origin: infiltration neoplasm with extension of tumor into the surrounding salivary gland parenchyma and with a predominantly solid appearance and a vague, organoid configuration.

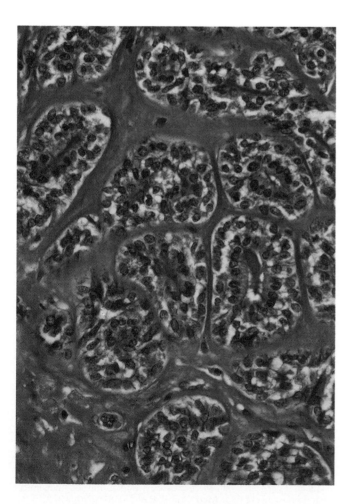

Figure 19–70. Histologic hallmark of EMC is the presence of tumor nests composed of two cell types: an inner cell layer (epithelial) with dark-staining, cuboidal to columnar cells, central or basally placed nuclei and scant eosinophilic cytoplasm, and the outer cell layer (myoepithelial), composed of polyhedral-shaped cells with eccentrically placed nuclei and abundant clear cytoplasm. Cell nests are separated by a thickened, hyalinized basement membrane.

8. Basal Cell Adenocarcinoma

Definition: Epithelial neoplasm of salivary glands that has features of basal cell adenoma but growth characteristics of a malignant neoplasm.

Clinical

■ Uncommon salivary gland neoplasm.
■ No sex predilection; occurs over a wide age range, but is most frequently seen in the sixth decade of life.
■ The parotid gland is most frequently affected; the other site of occurrence is the submandibular gland.
■ Symptoms relate to a mass with or without associated pain or tenderness.

Pathology

Gross

■ Circumscribed, solid, tan-white mass, varying in size from 0.7 to 4 cm in diameter.

Histology

■ Morphologic similarity to basal cell adenoma, especially of the membranous type.
■ Variably sized nodules or islands of tumor cells growing in solid, trabecular, membranous, or tubular patterns; a variety of morphologic patterns can be seen in any given neoplasm, with subtyping based on the predominant pattern.
■ The cytologic appearance is composed of uniform, basaloid epithelial cells consisting of two cell types:
  Small, round cell with dark (basophilic) nuclei, scant cytoplasm, and indistinct cell borders.
  Large, round to polygonal to elongated cell with pale-staining basophilic nuclei, eosinophilic to amphophilic cytoplasm, and indistinct cell borders.
■ The cellular components may be seen in equal proportion or one cell type may predominate; in the former, the small dark cells are generally located peripheral to the larger cells.
■ Eosinophilic, hyalinized, PAS-positive basal lamina can be seen either as intercellular droplets or as perinodule membranes.
■ Cytologic blandness may predominate, and although cellular pleomorphism, increased mitotic activity, and necrosis may be seen, they are not consistently identified nor diagnostic for a carcinoma.

■ The histologic hallmark for the diagnosis of adenocarcinoma rests on the identification of infiltration as manifested by:
  Invasion of adjacent structures (salivary gland parenchyma, soft tissue structures).
  Vascular invasion.
  Peri- or intraneural invasion.
■ Peripheral palisading of nuclei may be seen, but is less prominent as compared to basal cell adenoma.
■ Tubules, lumens, squamous differentiation, and cystic or cribriform patterns may be present.
■ Histochemistry: in general, PAS- and mucicarmine-positive material is absent or minimally present within the basal cell adenocarcinoma; PAS-positive material may be seen within tubular lumens.

Differential Diagnosis

■ Basal cell adenoma (Chapter 19A, #2c).
■ Adenoid cystic carcinoma (Chapter 19B, #3).
■ Polymorphous low-grade adenocarcinoma (Chapter 19B, #6).

Treatment and Prognosis

■ Complete surgical excision is the treatment of choice and may include parotidectomy.
■ Unless lymph node involvement is clinically evident, neck dissection appears unwarranted.
■ Local recurrences and metastases may occur, but are infrequent; metastatic disease involves regional lymph nodes and, rarely, the lungs.
■ Prognosis is generally excellent; rarely will death be directly caused by the neoplasm.

Additional Facts

■ Comparisons of the age distribution and frequency between basal cell adenoma and basal cell adenocarcinoma are essentially the same; therefore, it is unlikely that the basal cell adenocarcinoma has arisen from a preexisting basal cell adenoma.
■ Concomitant dermal eccrine cylindroma may be identified, suggesting a salivary gland–skin adnexal diathesis.

References

Ellis GL, Wiscovitch JG: Basal cell adenocarcinoma of the major salivary glands. Oral Surg Oral Med Oral Pathol 69:461–469, 1990.
Ellis GL, Auclair PL. Basal cell adenocarcinoma. *In:* Ellis GL, Auclair PL, Gnepp DR, eds. Surgical pathology of the salivary glands. Philadelphia: W.B. Saunders Co., 1991; pp 441–454.

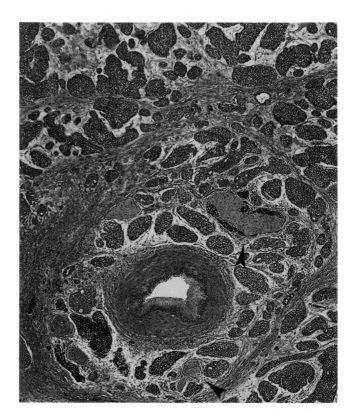

Figure 19–71. Portion of an infiltrating basal cell adenocarcinoma of the parotid gland composed of solid nodules of tumor demonstrating peri- and intraneural invasion (*arrowheads*) as well as perivascular infiltration.

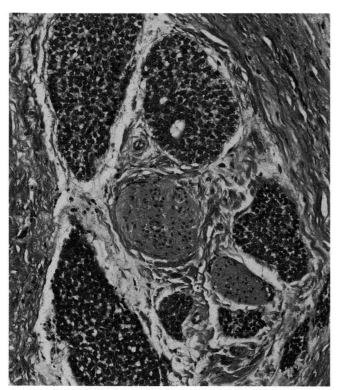

Figure 19–72. The cellular component seen in basal cell adenocarcinomas consists of a variable admixture of small, round cells with basophilic nuclei, scant cytoplasm, and indistinct cell borders and large round to polygonal to elongated cells with pale-staining basophilic nuclei, eosinophilic to amphophilic cytoplasm, and indistinct cell borders; tumor nests are grouped around nerves.

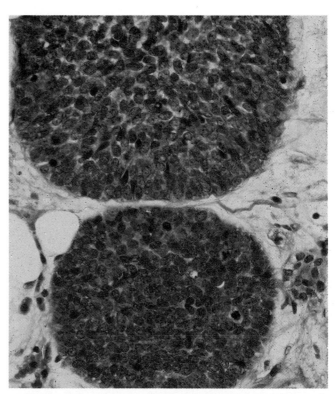

Figure 19–73. In contrast to basal cell adenomas, the adenocarcinomas either lack peripheral palisading of nuclei, or it is less prominently seen, and increased mitotic activity is present.

9. Primary Squamous Cell Carcinoma

Definition: Malignant epithelial neoplasm of major salivary glands, composed of squamous cells with the diagnosis contingent on the absence of clinical or historical evidence of a squamous cell carcinoma in another (head and neck) site.

Clinical

- Represents less than 2% of all primary epithelial (benign and malignant) major and minor salivary gland neoplasms.
- Affects males more than females; occurs over a wide age range, but most frequently is identified in the seventh and eighth decades of life.
- Primarily identified in the parotid gland, but may also be seen in the submandibular gland and, rarely, in the sublingual gland.
- The most common symptom is a mass lesion with or without pain or cranial nerve paralysis.
- Etiology may be related to prior radiotherapy to the head and neck.

Pathology

Gross

- Ulcerated and fixed, unencapsulated, firm to hard, gray to white mass, usually measuring more than 3 cm in diameter.

Histology

- Infiltrating, well to moderately differentiated squamous cell carcinoma similar to those occurring in other sites.
- Tissue invasion produces a desmoplastic response, giving the neoplasm a trabecular or nested appearance.
- Intracellular keratin, keratin pearl formation, and intercellular bridges are seen.
- A marked chronic inflammatory cell infiltrate occasionally may be associated with the invasive tumor nests.
- Special stains for epithelial mucin are negative, but should be performed in order to rule out the presence of a high-grade mucoepidermoid carcinoma.

Differential Diagnosis

- Ductal squamous metaplasia.
- High-grade mucoepidermoid carcinoma (Chapter 19B, #1).
- Metastatic squamous cell carcinoma.

Treatment and Prognosis

- Complete surgical excision (parotidectomy) is the treatment of choice and, if possible, with preservation of the facial nerve; however, direct involvement of the nerve is not uncommon, necessitating its resection.
- Neck dissection is indicated only in the presence of clinically evident or suspected nodal involvement.
- Radiotherapy may be beneficial in controlling local disease or may also improve survival.
- Treatment failure, as manifested by local recurrence or metastatic disease, is a common occurrence.
- Five- and 10-year survival rates are 24% and 18%, respectively.
- Prognosis does not correlate to the histology; poor prognosis correlates with the presence of ulceration or fixation, older patients, and a higher stage tumor.

Additional Facts

- Given the number of lymph nodes normally identified in the area of the submandibular gland, prior to rendering a diagnosis of primary submandibular squamous cell carcinoma, exclusion of secondary involvement of the submandibular gland from extension of a squamous carcinoma to the lymph nodes must be accomplished.

References

Auclair PL, Ellis GL: Primary squamous cell carcinoma. *In:* Ellis GL, Auclair PL, Gnepp DR, eds. Surgical pathology of the salivary glands. Philadelphia: W.B. Saunders Co., 1991; pp 369–378.

Batsakis JG, McClatchey KD, Johns M, Regezi J: Primary squamous cell carcinoma of parotid gland. Arch Otolaryngol Head Neck Surg 102:355–357, 1976.

Foote FW, Frazell EL: Tumors of the major salivary glands. Cancer 6:1065–1133, 1953.

Shemen LJ, Huvos AG, Spiro RH: Squamous cell carcinoma of salivary gland origin. Head Neck Surg 9:235–240, 1987.

Spitz MR, Batsakis JG: Major salivary gland carcinoma: descriptive epidemiology and survival of 498 patients. Arch Otolaryngol Head Neck Surg 110:45–48, 1984.

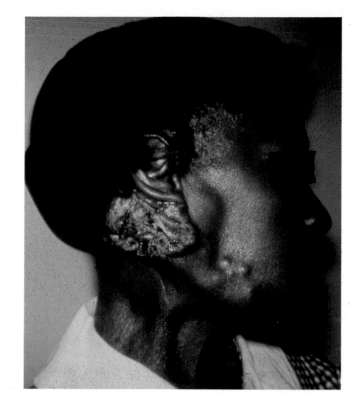

Figure 19-74. Primary squamous cell carcinoma of the parotid, presenting as an ulcerated and necrotic, firm mass extending behind the ear, with separate tumor nodules just anterior to the gland, and associated with facial nerve invasion and paralysis. From this appearance and obvious cutaneous involvement, a primary cutaneous carcinoma cannot be ruled out and is clinically the most likely origin.

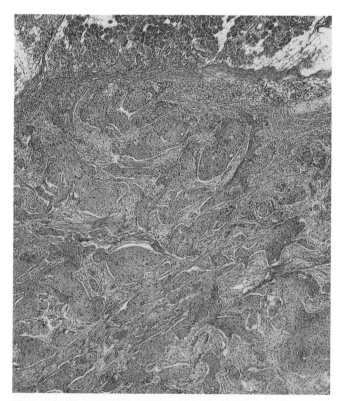

Figure 19-75. Infiltrating, moderately differentiated squamous cell carcinoma associated with a desmoplastic response, giving the neoplasm a trabecular or nested appearance.

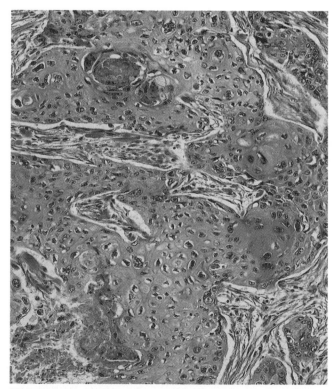

Figure 19-76. Parotid gland squamous cell carcinoma, morphologically similar to those occurring in other sites.

10. Salivary Duct Carcinoma

Definition: High-grade malignant epithelial salivary gland neoplasm arising from the excretory ducts and histologically resembling ductal carcinoma of the breast.

Clinical

- Uncommon type of salivary gland neoplasm.
- Affects males more than females; most frequently identified in the sixth to eighth decades of life.
- The parotid gland (related to Stensen's duct) is the most common site of occurrence; the submandibular and minor salivary glands also may be involved.
- Symptoms relate to a rapidly enlarging mass with or without associated pain or facial nerve paralysis.

Pathology

Gross

- Circumscribed to infiltrating, tan-white to gray-yellow, solid mass measuring from 1 to more than 6 cm in diameter.
- Cystic spaces filled with necrotic material may be identified.

Histology

- Intraductal or infiltrating neoplasm with a variety of growth patterns, including cell nests with central necrosis (comedonecrosis), cribriform, solid, cystic, and papillary; multiple growth patterns can be seen in any given tumor.
- The cells are large, with hyperchromatic, pleomorphic nuclei and eosinophilic cytoplasm; eosinophilic nucleoli may be prominent.
- Increased mitotic activity and necrosis are commonly seen.
- Vascular and neural invasion frequently is present, as is invasion of salivary gland parenchyma and surrounding soft tissue structures.
- Histochemistry: intracytoplasmic diastase-sensitive, PAS-positive material can be seen; mucicarmine is negative.
- Immunohistochemistry: cytokeratin positive and variable reactivity with epithelial membrane antigen; S-100 protein negative.

Differential Diagnosis

- Mucoepidermoid carcinoma (Chapter 19B, #1).
- Acinic cell adenocarcinoma (Chapter 19B, #2).
- Papillary cystadenocarcinoma (Chapter 19B, #6).
- Metastatic carcinoma including breast and prostatic origin.

Treatment and Prognosis

- Complete (aggressive) surgical excision is the treatment of choice, usually in association with radical neck dissection and postoperative radiotherapy.
- These neoplasms are frequently associated with metastatic disease, particularly to the regional lymph nodes, lungs, bone, and brain.
- Mortality rates attributed to this neoplasm are high, and tumors more than 3 cm in diameter are associated with greater morbidity and mortality.

References

Ellis GL, Auclair PL, Gnepp DR, Goode RK: Other malignant epithelial neoplasms. *In:* Ellis GL, Auclair PL, Gnepp DR, eds. Surgical pathology of the salivary glands. Philadelphia: W.B. Saunders Co., 1991; pp 476–480.

Garland TA, Innes DJ, Fechner RE: Salivary duct carcinoma: an analysis of four cases with review of the literature. Am J Clin Pathol 81:436–441, 1984.

Hui KK, Batsakis JG, Luna MA, MacKay B, Byers RM: Salivary duct adenocarcinoma: a high grade malignancy. J Laryngol Otol 100:105–114, 1986.

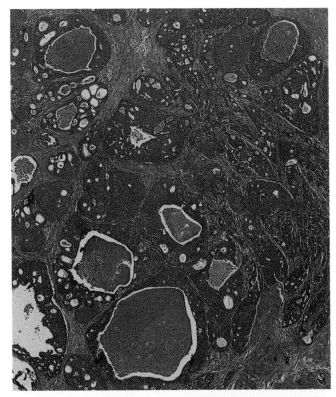

Figure 19–77. Salivary duct carcinoma: intraductal and infiltrating neoplasm, demonstrating a variety of growth patterns, including cell nests with central necrosis (comedonecrosis), cribriform, solid, and cystic.

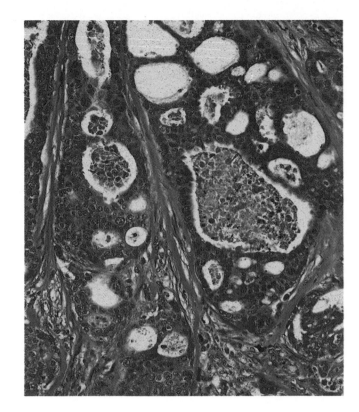

Figure 19–78. The cytologic appearance of salivary duct carcinoma consists of large cells with hyperchromatic, pleomorphic nuclei, prominent eosinophilic nucleoli, and eosinophilic cytoplasm; mitotic activity and necrosis are commonly seen.

11. Sebaceous Carcinoma

Definition: Malignant epithelial salivary gland neoplasm composed of sebaceous cells of varying maturity.

Clinical

■ Uncommon neoplasm, representing less than 0.5% of all salivary gland neoplasms.
■ No sex predilection; bimodal age distribution with peak incidences in the third and the seventh and eighth decades.
■ Overwhelming majority occur in the parotid gland; rare cases identified in the oral cavity and vallecula.
■ Most common symptom is a painful mass with or without facial nerve paralysis; cutaneous fixation may be present.

Pathology

Gross

■ Well-circumscribed or partially encapsulated, yellow to tan-white mass, measuring from 0.5 to 8.5 cm in diameter.

Histology

■ Encapsulation may be present, but these lesions demonstrate a pushing or infiltrative margin with a sheet-like or nested growth pattern.
■ Cytologic features are characterized by large cells with hyperchromatic nuclei and abundant clear to eosinophilic cytoplasm.
■ Cellular pleomorphism with cytologic atypia and cellular necrosis is seen; perineural invasion can be identified, but vascular invasion is uncommon.
■ Oncocytes and foreign body giant cells may rarely be seen.

Differential Diagnosis

■ Sebaceous adenoma.
■ Metastatic sebaceous carcinoma from orbital or cutaneous sites.

Treatment and Prognosis

■ Surgical excision (subtotal or total parotidectomy) is the treatment of choice.
■ These appear to represent low-grade neoplasms; however, local recurrence may occur, and 5-year survival rate is reported to be approximately 62%.

■ Metastatic disease (regional lymph node or to distant sites) may develop late in the disease course.

Additional Facts

■ Included in the classification of malignant sebaceous neoplasms of salivary glands is the *sebaceous lymphadenocarcinoma:*

Malignant counterpart of and arises from sebaceous lymphadenoma.

Rarest sebaceous tumor of salivary glands.

Histologically composed of sebaceous lymphadenoma (sebaceous cell nests admixed with salivary ducts in a lymphoid background with or without germinal centers) admixed with cytologic features of malignant sebaceous cells or poorly differentiated carcinoma.

■ Sebaceous carcinoma of salivary glands appears to be a more aggressive neoplasm than its counterpart in the orbit.

■ Sebaceous cell differentiation may be associated with other salivary gland neoplasms, including pleomorphic adenomas, oncocytomas, Warthin's tumors, basal cell adenoma, mucoepidermoid carcinoma, acinic cell adenocarcinoma, and adenoid cystic carcinoma.

References

Ellis GL, Auclair PL, Gnepp DR, Goode RK: Other malignant epithelial neoplasms. *In:* Ellis GL, Auclair PL, Gnepp DR, eds. Surgical pathology of the salivary glands. Philadelphia: W.B. Saunders Co., 1991; pp 470–476.

Gnepp DR: Sebaceous neoplasms of salivary gland origin: a review. Pathol Ann 18(pt 1):71–102, 1983.

Gnepp DR, Brannon R: Sebaceous neoplasms of salivary gland origin: report of 21 cases. Cancer 53:2155–2170, 1984.

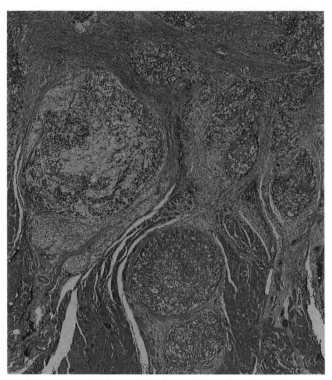

Figure 19–80. Sebaceous carcinoma of the parotid gland, composed of cell nests and sheet-like growth with invasion of skeletal muscle.

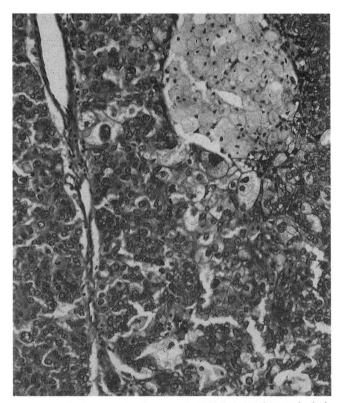

Figure 19–81. Cytologic features of sebaceous carcinoma include basaloid-appearing cells with pleomorphic, hyperchromatic nuclei, clear to eosinophilic cytoplasm, and mitoses; admixed with the pleomorphic cell infiltrate is a nest of more mature appearing cells with abundant cytoplasm and small, hyperchromatic, eccentrically located nuclei.

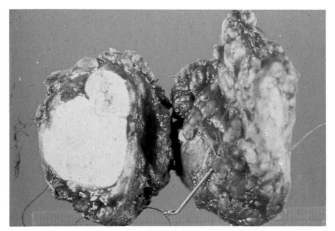

Figure 19–79. Sebaceous carcinoma of the parotid gland, presenting as a well-circumscribed but infiltrating, yellow to tan-white mass.

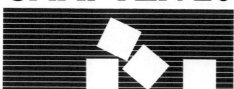

CHAPTER 20

Immunohistochemistry of Salivary Gland Tumors

IMMUNOHISTOCHEMISTRY OF NORMAL SALIVARY GLAND STRUCTURES AND NEOPLASMS

■ In general, the light microscopic features of salivary gland neoplasms are distinctive, such that use of immunohistochemistry is not necessarily required in order to arrive at a diagnosis.

■ The immunohistochemical antigenic profile expressed by the normal salivary gland component may be different from those of neoplasms arising

from these components; this phenomenon is explained by neoplastic modification of the cell.

■ The cellular make-up of salivary gland neoplasms demonstrates interrelating histogenesis, such that all cellular constituents in the salivary duct system potentially may contribute to the development of a given neoplasm; therefore, the immunohistochemi-

Table 20-1
Immunohistochemistry of Normal Salivary Gland Structures and Neoplasms

	CK	EMA	CEA	S-100 Protein	Actin	GFAP	Vim	Amyl
Normal Gland Components								
Excretory ducts	+	+	+	0	±	0	0	0
Striated ducts	+	+	+	0	±	0	0	0
Intercalated ducts	+	+	+	+	±	0	0	0
Acinous cells	+	+	+	0	0	0	0	+
Myoepithelial cells	+	0	0	+	+	0	0	0
Tumors								
Pleomorphic adenoma	+	+	+	+	+	+	+	+
	(D+M)	(D)	(D)	(M)	(M)	(M)	(M)	
Oncocytoma	+			0	0			
Myoepithelioma	+			+	+	+	+	0
Mucoepidermoid carcinoma	+	+	+	0	0	0	0	+
Acinic cell adenocarcinoma	+	+	+	+	+	+	+	+
Adenoid cystic carcinoma	+	+	+	+	+	+	+	+
	(D+M)	(D)	(D)	(D+M)	(M)	(M)	(M)	
Polymorphous low-grade adenocarcinoma	+	+	+v	+	+v	±	+	
	(D+M)	(D)	(D)	(D+M)	(M)			
Salivary duct carcinoma	+	+	+	0	0	0	0	
Epithelial-myoepithelial cell carcinoma	+	+	+	+	+			+
	(D+M)	(D)	(D)	(D+M)	(M)			(D)
Adenocarcinoma not otherwise specified	+	+	+	±	0	0		±

CK—cytokeratin; EMA—epithelial membrane antigen; CEA—carcinoembryonic antigen; Actin—muscle specific actin; GFAP—glial fibrillary acidic protein; Vim—vimentin; Amyl—salivary amylase; D—ductal cell; M—myoepithelial cell; V—variably reactive.

cal antigenic profile of salivary gland neoplasms may vary for histologically identical tumors or may demonstrate similar findings for tumors of different classification.

■ Tumors derived from the proximal segments of the salivary duct system devoid of myoepithelial cells have been excluded from those salivary gland tumors associated with myoepithelial differentiation; this neat separation may not hold true based on the complexity and heterogeneity of the salivary gland duct system; Table 20–1 reflects some of the immunohistochemical findings seen in association with salivary gland components and neoplasms but, given recent advances in the study of the salivary duct epithelia, should not be considered as definitive features.

References

Immunohistochemistry of Normal Salivary Gland Structures and Its Neoplasms

Batsakis JG, Ordonez NG, Ro J, Meis JM, Bruner JM: S-100 protein and myoepithelial neoplasms. J Laryngol Otol 100:687–698, 1986.

Chen JC, Gnepp DR, Bedrossian CWM: Adenoid cystic carcinoma of the salivary glands: an immunohistochemical analysis. Oral Surg Oral Med Oral Pathol 65:316–326, 1988.

Dardick I: Histogenesis and morphogenesis of salivary gland neoplasms. In: Ellis GL, Auclair PL, Gnepp DR, eds. Surgical pathology of the salivary glands. Philadelphia: W.B. Saunders Company, 1991; pp 108–128.

Ellis GL, Auclair PL: Acinic cell adenocarcinoma. In: Ellis GL, Auclair PL, Gnepp DR, eds. Surgical pathology of the salivary glands. Philadelphia: W.B. Saunders Company, 1991; pp 299–317.

Goode RK: Oncocytoma. In: Ellis GL, Auclair PL, Gnepp DR, eds. Surgical pathology of the salivary glands. Philadelphia: W.B. Saunders Company, 1991; pp 225–237.

Kahn HJ, Baumal R, Marks A, Dardick I, van Nostrand AWP: Myoepithelial cells in salivary gland tumors: an immunohistochemical study. Arch Pathol Lab Med 109:190–195, 1985.

Luna MA, Ordonez NG, MacKay B, Batsakis JG, Guillamondegui O: Salivary epithelial-myoepithelial carcinoma of intercalated ducts: a clinical, electron microscopy, and immunocytochemical study. Oral Surg Oral Med Oral Pathol 59:482–490, 1985.

Nakazato Y, Ishida Y, Takahashi K, Suzuki K: Immunohistochemical distribution of S-100 protein and glial fibrillary acidic protein in normal and neoplastic salivary glands. Virchows Arch [A] 405:299–310, 1985.

Nakazato Y, Ishizeki J, Takahashi K, Yamaguchi H, Kamei T, Mori T: Localization of S-100 protein and glial fibrillary acidic protein-related antigen in pleomorphic adenoma of salivary glands. Lab Invest 46:621–626, 1982.

Regezi JA, Lloyd RV, Zarbo RJ, McClatchey KD: Minor salivary gland tumors: a histologic and immunohistochemical study. Cancer 55:108–115, 1985.

Stead RH, Qizilbash AH, Kontozoglou T, Daya AD, Riddel RH: An immunohistochemical study of pleomorphic adenomas of salivary gland: glial fibrillary acidic protein-like immunoreactivity identifies a major myoepithelial component. Hum Pathol 19:32–40, 1988.

Waldron CA: Mixed tumor (pleomorphic adenoma) and myoepithelioma. In: Ellis GL, Auclair PL, Gnepp DR, eds. Surgical pathology of the salivary glands. Philadelphia: W.B. Saunders Company, 1991; pp 165–186.

Wenig BM, Gnepp DR: Polymorphous low-grade adenocarcinoma of minor salivary glands. In: Ellis GL, Auclair PL, Gnepp DR, eds. Surgical pathology of the salivary glands. Philadelphia: W.B. Saunders Company, 1991; pp 290–411.

Wick MR, Abenoza P, Manivel JC: Diagnostic immunohistopathology. In: Gnepp DR, ed. Pathology of the head and neck. New York: Churchill Livingstone, 1988; pp 191–261.

Zarbo RJ, Regezi JA, Batsakis JG: S-100 protein in salivary gland tumors: an immunohistochemical study of 129 cases. Head Neck Surg 8:268–275, 1986.

Zarbo RJ, Regezi JA, Hatfield JS, Maisel H, et al: Immunoreactive glial fibrillary acidic protein in normal and neoplastic salivary glands: a combined immunohistochemical and immunoblot study. Surg Pathol 1:55–63, 1988.

CHAPTER 21

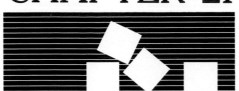

TNM Classification of Salivary Gland Neoplasms

ANATOMIC SITES
Classification

CLINICAL STAGE

ANATOMIC SITES

■ Classification applies only to carcinoma of the major salivary glands (parotid, submandibular, and sublingual), and does not apply to carcinomas arising in the minor salivary glands of the upper respiratory tract.

Classification

1. T—extent of the primary tumor; includes both the clinical (T) and pathologic (pT) categories.
   TX—primary tumor cannot be assessed.
   T0—no evidence of primary tumor.
   T1—tumor 2 cm or less in greatest dimension.
   T2—tumor more than 2 cm but not more than 4 cm in greatest dimension.
   T3—tumor more than 4 cm but not more than 6 cm in greatest dimension.
   T4—tumor more than 6 cm in greatest dimension.
      ■ T4a—Tumor more than 6 cm in greatest dimension, without significant local extension.
      ■ T4b—Tumor more than 6 cm in greatest dimension with significant local extension.
2. N—absence/presence and extent of regional lymph node metastasis; includes both the clinical (N) and pathologic (pN) categories.
   NX—regional lymph nodes cannot be assessed.
   N0—No regional lymph node metastasis.
   N1—metastasis in a single ipsilateral lymph node, 3 cm or less in greatest dimension.
   N2—metastasis in a single ipsilateral lymph node, more than 3 cm but not more than 6 cm in greatest dimension **or** metastasis in multiple ipsilateral lymph nodes, none more than 6 cm in greatest dimension **or** metastasis in bilateral or contralateral lymph nodes, none more than 6 cm in greatest dimension.
      ■ N2a—metastasis in a single ipsilateral lymph node, more than 3 cm but not more than 6 cm in greatest dimension.
      ■ N2b—metastasis in multiple ipsilateral lymph nodes, none more than 6 cm in greatest dimension.
      ■ N2c—metastasis in bilateral or contralateral lymph nodes, none more than 6 cm in greatest dimension.
   N3—metastasis in a lymph node more than 6 cm in greatest dimension.
3. M—absence or presence of distant metastasis; includes both the clinical (M) and pathologic (pM) categories.
   Mx—not assessed.
   M0—no distant metastasis.
   M1—distant metastasis present.
4. R—residual tumor.
   R0—no residual tumor.
   R1—microscopic residual tumor.
   R2—macroscopic residual tumor.

CLINICAL STAGE

Stage I—T1N0M0 or T2N0M0.
Stage II—T3N0M0.
Stage III—T1N1M0 or T2N1M0 or any T4, N0M0.
Stage IV—T3N1M0 or any T4,N1M0.
         —Any T, any N, M1.

Reference

TNM Classification

Spiessl B, Beahrs OH, Hermanek P, Hutter RVP, Scheibe O, Sobin LH, Wagner G (eds): TNM atlas: illustrated guide to the TNM/PTNM-classification of malignant tumours, 3rd ed. Berlin: Springer-Verlag, 1989.

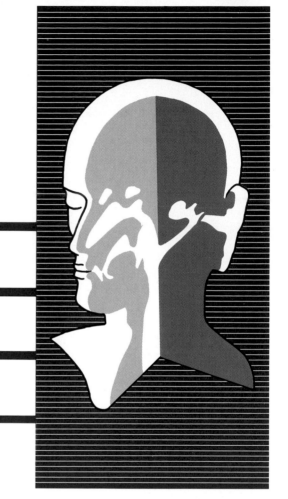

CHAPTER 22

Anatomy and Histology

ANATOMIC BORDERS

External Ear

- Consists of the auricle (pinna) and entire external auditory canal, and is limited medially by the external aspect of the tympanic membrane.

Middle Ear (Tympanic Cavity)

- Contents include the ossicles, eustacian tube, tympanic cavity proper, epitympanic recess, mastoid cavity, and the chorda tympani of the facial nerve (VII n.); the middle ear as well as the external ear function as conduits for sound conduction for the auditory part of the internal ear.
- Lateral: internal aspect of the tympanic membrane and squamous portion of the temporal bone.
- Medial: petrous portion of the temporal bone.
- Superior (roof): tegmen tympani, a thin plate of bone that separates the middle ear space from the cranial cavity.
- Inferior (floor): thin plate of bone separating the tympanic cavity from the superior bulb of the internal jugular vein.
- Anterior: thin plate of bone separating the tympanic cavity from the carotid canal that houses the internal carotid artery.
- Posterior: petrous portion of the temporal bone containing the mastoid antrum and mastoid air cells.

Internal Ear

- Embedded within the petrous portion of the temporal bone and consists of the structures of the membranous and osseous labyrinth, and the internal auditory canal, in which the vestibulocochlear nerve (VIII n.) runs.
- The internal ear is the sense organ for hearing and balance.

HISTOLOGY

External Ear

- The auricle is essentially a cutaneous structure, composed of keratinizing, stratified squamous epithelium with associated adnexal structures, including hair follicles, sebaceous glands, and eccrine sweat glands; its subcutaneous tissue is composed of fibroconnective tissue, fat, and elastic-type fibrocartilage, which gives the auricle its structural support.
- Like the auricle, the external auditory canal is lined by keratinizing squamous epithelium that runs throughout the canal and covers the external aspect of the tympanic membrane.
- The outer third of the external canal is noteworthy, in addition to the other adnexal structures, for the presence of modified apocrine glands, called ceruminal glands, that replace the eccrine glands seen in the auricle.
- Ceruminal glands:
  Produce cerumen.
  Are arranged in clusters composed of cuboidal cells with eosinophilic cytoplasm, often containing a granular, golden-yellow pigment.
  Have secretory droplets along the luminal border.
  Are absent in the inner portion of the external auditory canal, as are the other adnexal structures.
- The inner two thirds of the external auditory canal contain bone rather than cartilage.

Middle Ear

- Lining is composed of respiratory epithelium, varying from ciliated epithelium (eustacian tube) to a flat, single, cuboidal epithelium (tympanic cavity and mastoid); the epithelium lining the eustacian tube becomes pseudostratified as it approaches the pharyngeal end.

■ The eustacian tubes contain a lymphoid component, particularly in children, that is referred to as Gerlach's tubal tonsil.

■ The ossicular articulations are typical synovial joints.

Internal Ear

■ The complexity of the histology of the inner ear precludes description; the reader is referred to specific texts that detail the inner ear histoanatomy.

References

Embryology, Anatomy, and Histology

Fawcett DW: The ear. *In:* Fawcett DW, ed. Bloom and Fawcett: a textbook of histology, 11th ed. Philadelphia: W.B. Saunders Co., 1986; pp 961–986.

Hollinshead WH: The ear. *In:* Hollinshead WH, ed. Anatomy for surgeons, vol. 1, 3rd ed. Philadelphia: Harper & Row, 1982; pp 159–221.

Moore KL: The ear. *In:* Moore ML, ed. The developing human: clinically oriented embryology, 4th ed. Philadelphia: W.B. Saunders Co., 1988; pp 412–420.

Schuknecht HF: Anatomy. *In:* Schuknecht HF, ed. Pathology of the ear. Cambridge, MA.: Harvard University Press, 1974; pp 21–96.

Warwick R, Williams PL: The auditory and vestibular apparatus. *In:* Warwick R, Williams PL, eds. Gray's anatomy, 35th British ed. Philadelphia: W.B. Saunders Co., 1973; pp 1134–1158.

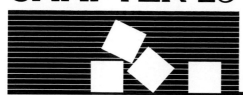

CHAPTER 23

Classification of Non-neoplastic Lesions and Neoplasms of the Ear

NON-NEOPLASTIC LESIONS
NEOPLASMS

Table 23–1
CLASSIFICATION OF NON-NEOPLASTIC
LESIONS OF THE EAR

External ear
 Developmental (first branchial cleft anomalies; accessory tragi)
 Hamartomas
 Idiopathic cystic chondromalacia
 Chondrodermatitis nodularis helicis chronica
 Angiolymphoid hyperplasia with eosinophilia/Kimura's disease
 Infectious (malignant external otitis)
 Systemic diseases (relapsing polychondritis; gout)
 Keloid
 Epidermal and sebaceous cysts
 Exostosis
Middle and inner ear, including temporal bone
 Developmental and congenital anomalies
 Infectious (otitis media)
 Otic or aural polyp
 Cholesteatoma
 Otosclerosis
 Eosinophilic granuloma
 Heterotopias (central nervous system tissue; salivary gland), teratoma, and choristoma

Table 23–2
CLASSIFICATION OF NEOPLASMS OF THE EAR

I. External ear
 A. Benign
  1. Epithelial/neuroectodermal/mesenchymal
   Ceruminal gland neoplasms
   Keratoacanthoma
   Squamous papilloma
   Melanocytic nevi
   Dermal adnexal neoplasms
   Pilomatrixoma (calcifying epithelioma of Malherbe)
   Neurilemmoma/neurofibroma
   Chondroma; osteoma
   Hemangioma

Table 23–2
CLASSIFICATION OF NEOPLASMS OF THE EAR
Continued

 B. Malignant
  1. Epithelial/neuroectodermal/mesenchymal
   Basal cell carcinoma
   Squamous cell carcinoma ("conventional" and spindle-cell types)
   Verrucous carcinoma
   Ceruminal gland adenocarcinomas
   Malignant melanoma
   Merkel cell carcinoma
   Atypical fibroxanthoma (superficial malignant fibrous histiocytoma)
   Vascular (angiosarcoma; Kaposi's sarcoma)
II. Middle and inner ear
 A. Benign
  1. Epithelial
   Middle ear adenoma
   Middle ear papilloma
  2. Neuroectodermal/mesenchymal
   Jugulotympanic paraganglioma
   Meningioma
   Acoustic neuroma
   Others
 B. Malignant
  1. Epithelial
   Middle ear adenocarcinoma
   Primary squamous cell carcinoma
   Temporal bone adenocarcinoma of endolymphatic sac origin
  2. Mesenchymal
   Rhabdomyosarcoma
   Lymphoproliferative (malignant lymphoma; plasmacytoma)
  3. Metastatic neoplasms:
   Squamous cell carcinoma from other head and neck sites
   Breast carcinoma; pulmonary adenocarcinoma; malignant melanoma; renal cell carcinoma; others

CHAPTER 24

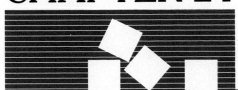

Non-neoplastic Diseases of the Ear

A. EXTERNAL EAR

1. Idiopathic Cystic Chondromalacia of the Auricular Cartilage

Definition: Cystic degeneration of the auricular cartilage of unknown etiology.
Synonyms: Pseudocyst of the auricle.

Clinical

- Affects males more than females (rarely seen in women); generally affects young and middle-aged adults.
- Can occur along any portion of the auricle, with the most common site adjacent to the helix.
- Symptoms are those of a unilateral, painless swelling along the anterior pinna.
- Although trauma has been implicated in causing these lesions, there is no definitive connection to a prior traumatic event and the cause for this condition remains unknown.

Pathology

Gross

- Fluid-filled, distended mass.

Histology

- Changes are restricted to the cartilage, within which irregularly shaped cystic areas are seen; the cysts lack a cell lining and generally are devoid of content.
- A granulation tissue reaction composed of fibrovascular tissue and scattered chronic inflammatory cells can be seen in association with the cysts.
- Surrounding cartilage is unremarkable.

Differential Diagnosis

- Relapsing polychondritis (Chapter 24A, #3).

Treatment and Prognosis

- Complete surgical excsion is the treatment of choice and is curative.

Reference

Heffner DK, Hyams VJ: Cystic chondromalacia (endochondral pseudocyst) of the auricle. Arch Pathol Lab Med 110:740–743, 1986.

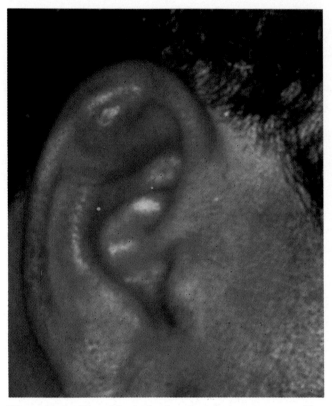

Figure 24–1. Idiopathic cystic chondromalacia, seen as swelling along the anterior pinna.

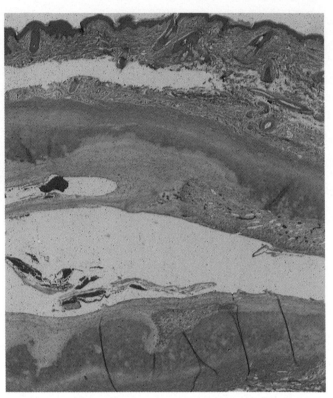

Figure 24–2. Idiopathic cystic chondromalacia with pathologic changes restricted to the cartilage, within which irregular-shaped cystic areas are seen devoid of an epithelial cell lining and associated with a granulation tissue reaction composed of fibrovascular tissue and scattered chronic inflammatory cells.

2. Chondrodermatitis Nodularis Helicis Chronica

Definition: Non-neoplastic ulcerative lesion of the auricle.
Synonyms: Winkler's disease or nodule.

Clinical

- Affects males more than females (considered uncommon in women); most commonly occurs in late middle-aged and older age groups.
- Most frequently occurs along the superior portion of the helix; lateral helical, antihelical, and antitragal involvement also is seen.
- Spontaneously occurring unilateral painful nodule is the most common clinical presentation; manipulation of the lesion results in intense pain.
- Etiology remains unknown; however, a combination of solar damage and minor trauma with vascular compromise may play a causative role.

Pathology

Gross

- Raised, discrete oval nodule with central ulceration, reaching but not exceeding 1 to 1.5 cm in diameter.

Histology

- Central portion of the involved epidermis is ulcerated, with adjacent epithelium showing acanthosis, hyper- and parakeratosis, and pseudoepitheliomatous hyperplasia.
- The base of the ulcer shows granulation tissue, edema, fibrinoid necrosis, and an acute or chronic inflammatory cell infiltrate.
- The granulation tissue and inflammatory process usually extends to and involves the perichondrium and cartilage.

Differential Diagnosis

■ Basal cell carcinoma (Chapter 25C, #1).
■ Squamous cell carcinoma (Chapter 25C, #2).

Treatment and Prognosis

■ Complete surgical excision is the treatment of choice and is curative.
■ Trials with injection of glucocorticoids directly into the lesion have been shown to be effective in eradicating the lesion.

Additional Facts

■ Pain is thought to result from the perichondrial involvement.

References

Bard JW: Chondrodermatitis nodularis chronica helicis. Dermatologica 163:376–384, 1981.

Goette DK: Chondrodermatitis nodularis chronica helicis: a perforating necrobiotic granuloma. J Am Acad Dermatol 2:148–154, 1980.

Metzger SA, Goodman ML: Chondrodermatitis helicis: a clinical re-evaluation and pathological review. Laryngoscope 86:1402–1412, 1976.

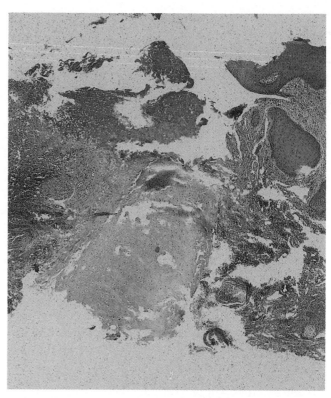

Figure 24–4. Histologic picture of CNHC with ulcerated epithelium, fibrinoid necrosis, associated granulation tissue, and an inflammatory cell infiltrate; this process extends to the subjacent perichondrium.

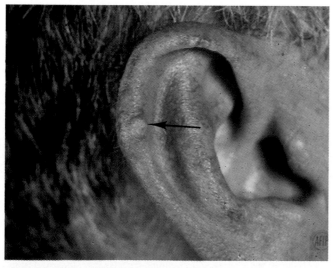

Figure 24–3. Chondrodermatitis nodularis helicis chronica (CNHC), presenting as a raised, oval nodule with central ulceration along the anterior pinna *(arrow)*.

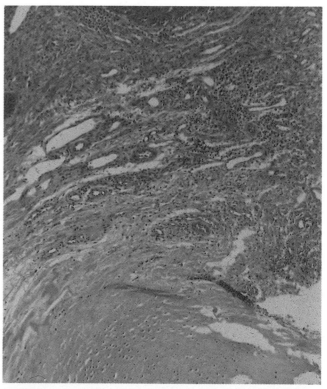

Figure 24–5. CNHC demonstrating the granulation tissue and inflammatory cell process extending to and involving perichondrium.

3. Relapsing Polychondritis

Definition: Rare, systemic, relapsing disease, characterized by progressive degeneration of cartilaginous structures throughout the body.

Clinical

■ No sex predilection; occurs in all age groups.
■ May affect any cartilage tissue in the body.
■ As the name implies, the disease manifestations relapse with both severity and frequency of occurrence, and are markedly variable.
■ In descending order of frequency, involvement and clinical presentation include:
1. Auricular chondritis: uni- or bilateral diffuse, painful swelling of the ear, which is warm to touch and red in color.
2. Arthritis: large and small joints may be affected, which may take the form of mono- or polyarticular involvement.
3. Respiratory tract chondritis: hoarseness, airway obstruction, pneumonia.
4. Nasal chondritis: crusting and nasal obstruction.
5. Audiovestibular disturbances: conductive or sensorineural hearing loss.
■ Noncartilaginous sites of involvement include:
Ocular: inflammation of the sclera, iris, uvea, or conjunctiva.
Cardiovascular: aortic insufficiency and aortic aneurysms.
■ Progression of disease may result in "cauliflower" ears and "saddle" nose deformities.
■ In association with relapsing polychondritis, some patients suffer from other diseases, including systemic lupus erythematosus, rheumatoid arthritis, scleroderma, glomerulonephritis, endocrine dysfunctions, and ulcerative colitis.
■ There are no characteristic laboratory findings seen in association with relapsing polychondritis, and the most common abnormalities include elevated erythrocyte sedimentation rate, leukocytosis, and anemia; the arthritis is seronegative.
■ The etiology is thought to be autoimmune, as demonstrated by the presence of circulating antibodies to type II collagen (only present in cartilage) in patients with this disease; immune complexes of immunoglobulins and complement have been detected in the biopsy specimens taken from inflamed cartilage of involved ears.
■ There is no evidence to support either hereditary or familial predisposition.

Pathology

Histology

■ On hematoxylin and eosin stained sections, there is a loss of the normal cartilage basophilia, replaced by an acidophilic appearance.
■ The perichondrium is infiltrated by a mixture of polymorphonuclear leukocytes, lymphocytes, plasma cells, and eosinophils, resulting in a loss of the normally distinct perichondrial–cartilaginous interface.
■ In advanced cases, granulation tissue, fibrosis, and scarring with cartilage destruction can be seen.

Differential Diagnosis

■ External otitis (Chapter 24A, #5).
■ Acute (infectious) perichondritis.
■ Gout.
■ Systemic vasculitides (Wegener's granulomatosis) (Chapter 3, #8).
■ Rheumatoid arthritis.

Treatment and Prognosis

■ In the acute stages of disease, corticosteroids are used.
■ Immunosuppressive agents may be used in patients with severe disease.
■ Prognosis is variable and unpredictable, with some patients having a prolonged course and others suffering from a more aggressive and fulminant disease.
■ Death may occur and is most often the result of respiratory tract or cardiovascular system involvement.

Additional Facts

■ Arthritic involvement of the costochondral, sternoclavicular, and sternomanubrial joints is common.
■ Increased titers to rheumatoid factor and antinuclear antibodies can be seen in a small percentage of patients.
■ The diagnosis of relapsing polychondritis can be made in the presence of more than three 3 of the following:
Bilateral auricular chondritis.
Nasal chondritis.
Respiratory tract chondritis.
Audiovestibular disease (conductive or sensorineural hearing loss).
Seronegative arthritis.
Ocular inflammation.

References

Barnes L: Relapsing polychondritis. *In:* Barnes L, ed. Surgical pathology of the head and neck. New York: Marcel Dekker, 1985; pp 903–908.

Hughes RAC, Berry CL, Seifert M, Lessof MH: Relapsing polychondritis: three cases with a clinico-pathological study and literature review. Q J Med 41:363–380, 1972.

McCaffrey TV, McDonald TJ, McCaffrey LA: Head and neck manifestations of relapsing polychondritis: review of 29 cases. Otolaryngology 86:473–478, 1978.

McCune WJ, Schiller AL, Dynesius-Trentham RA, Trentham DE: Type II collagen-induced auricular chondritis. Arthritis Rheum 25:266–273, 1982.

Moloney JR: Relapsing polychondritis: its otolaryngological manifestations. J Laryngol Otol 92:9–15, 1978.

Valenzuela R, Cooperrider PA, Gogate P, Deodhar SD, Bergfeld WF: Relapsing polychondritis: immunomicroscopic findings in cartilage of ear biopsy specimens. Hum Pathol 11:19–22, 1980.

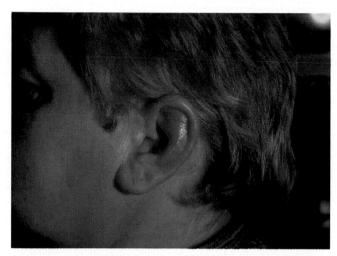

Figure 24-6. Relapsing polychondritis (RP), presenting with diffuse redness and swelling of the ear, which is warm to touch and is painful.

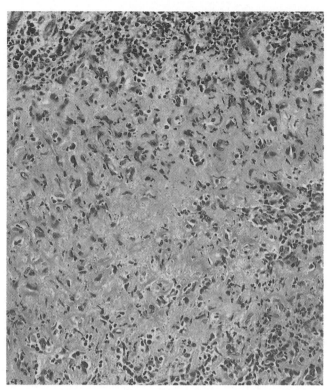

Figure 24-8. The inflammatory cell infiltrate in RP consists of a mixture of polymorphonuclear leukocytes, lymphocytes, plasma cells, and eosinophils, permeating throughout the auricular cartilage.

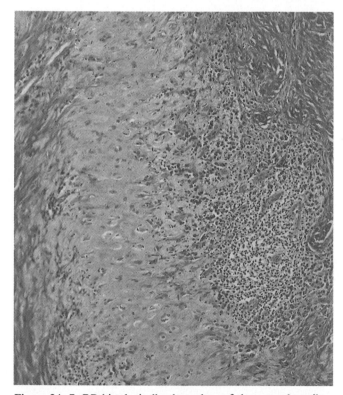

Figure 24-7. RP histologically shows loss of the normal cartilage basophilia, replaced by an acidophilic appearance with infiltration of peri- and intrachondrial areas by a severe mixed inflammatory cell infiltrate, resulting in a loss of the normally distinct perichondrial-cartilaginous interface.

4. Angiolymphoid Hyperplasia with Eosinophilia

Definition: Nodular, angiomatous, subcutaneous proliferation with predilection for the external ear and other head and neck sites.

Synonym: Histiocytoid hemangioma.

Clinical

- No sex predilection; may occur at any age, but most frequently seen in the third to fifth decades of life.
- Common locations include the external auricle, external auditory canal, scalp, and forehead.
- Symptoms include pruritus and bleeding after scratching.
- May be associated with regional lymphadenopathy and peripheral eosinophilia.
- The etiology is unknown.

Pathology

- Two types of lesions may be identified, including:
- Multiple, superficial, skin-colored to dull red-appearing nodules or papules, measuring from a few millimeters to 1.0 cm.
- The lesions may coalesce to form a large, subcutaneous plaque, measuring from 1 to 10 cm in diameter.

Histology

- Typical nodules are composed of a proliferation of vascular spaces and an inflammatory infiltrate rich in eosinophils.
- The vascular component varies in size, from the dimensions of a capillary to medium-sized arteries and veins; vascular spaces are lined by plump-appearing endothelial cells with pleomorphic changes and hyperchromatic nuclei.
- The inflammatory component is characterized by an admixture of lymphocytes, histiocytes, and eosinophils; however, on occasion eosinophils may be few in number or absent; a prominent diffuse lymphoid hyperplasia with germinal centers is seen.

Differential Diagnosis

- Lobular capillary hemangioma (pyogenic granuloma) (Chapter 4A, #2).
- Angiosarcoma (Chapter 4B, #9).

Treatment and Prognosis

- Local surgical excision or desiccation are the treatments of choice and are curative.
- Recurrence can occasionally occur.

Additional Facts

- *Kimura's disease* occurs in Asians, in whom clinical manifestations are different from those of non-Asians; these manifestations include:
  Purported male predominance.
  Larger lesions identified in locations other than in the head and neck.
  Commonly associated with regional lymphadenopathy and peripheral eosinophilia.
- Based on the difference in clinical presentations as well as the apparent absence of an enlarged, plump-appearing, endothelial cell, controversy exists whether Kimura's disease and angiolymphoid hyperplasia with eosinophilia represent two different disease processes; furthermore, it has been suggested that angiolymphoid hyperplasia with eosinophilia should be categorized under the group of lesions referred to as histiocytoid hemangioma, which includes epithelioid hemangioma, hemangioendothelioma of bone, and epithelioid hemangioendothelioma.

References

Barnes L, Koss W, Nieland: Angiolymphoid hyperplasia with eosinophilia: a disease that may be confused with malignancy. Head Neck Surg 2:425–434, 1980.

Castro C, Winkelmann RK: Angiolymphoid hyperplasia with eosinophilia in the skin. Cancer 34:1696–1705, 1974.

Googe PB, Harris NL, Mihm MC: Kimura's disease and angiolymphoid hyperplasia with eosinophilia: two distinct histopathological entities. J Cutan Pathol 14:263–271, 1987.

Kuo TT, Shih LY, Chan HL: Kimura's disease: involvement of regional lymph nodes and distinction from angiolymphoid hyperplasia with eosinophilia. Am J Surg Pathol 12:843–854, 1988.

Olsen TG, Helwig EB: Angiolymphoid hyperplasia with eosinophilia: a clinicopathologic study of 116 patients. J Am Acad Dermatol 12:781–796, 1985.

Razquin S, Mayayo E, Citores MA, Alvira R: Angiolymphoid hyperplasia with eosinophilia of the tongue: report of a case and review of the literature. Hum Pathol 22:837–839, 1991.

Rosai J, Gold J, Landy R: The histiocytoid hemangioma: a unifying concept embracing several previously described entities of skin, soft tissues, large vessels, bone and heart. Hum Pathol 10:707–730, 1979.

Thompson JW, Colman M, Williamson C, Ward PH: Angiolymphoid hyperplasia with eosinophilia of the external ear canal: treatment with laser excision. Arch Otolaryngol Head Neck Surg 107:316–319, 1981.

Urabe A, Tsuneyoshi M, Enjoji M: Epithelioid hemangioma versus Kimura's disease: a comparative clinicopathologic study. Am J Surg Pathol 11:758–766, 1987.

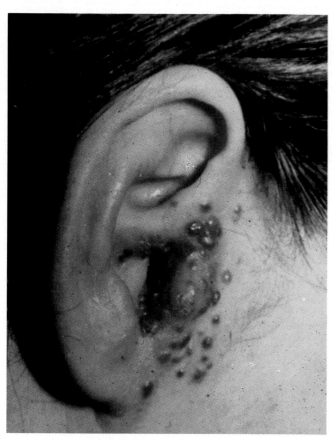

Figure 24–9. Angiolymphoid hyperplasia with eosinophilia (ALHE), seen as multiple, superficial, dull red–appearing papules; some of the papules appear to be coalescing into plaque-like lesions.

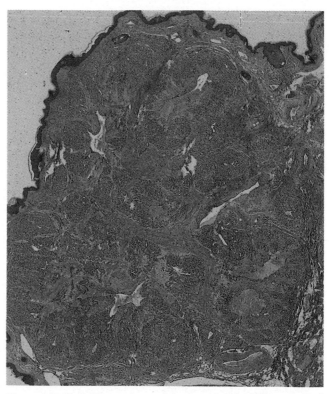

Figure 24–10. Subcutaneous nodular growth of ALHE composed of a proliferation of vascular spaces, varying in size from the dimensions of a capillary to medium-sized arteries and veins, and a mixed chronic inflammatory infiltrate.

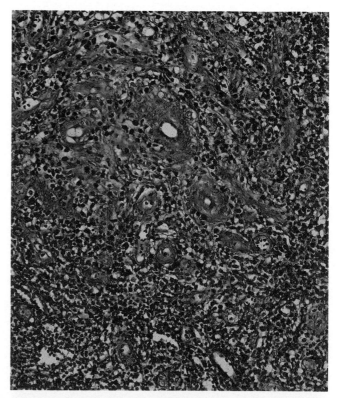

Figure 24–11. The vascular spaces of ALHE are lined by plump-appearing endothelial cells with pleomorphic changes with an associated inflammatory component, characterized by an admixture of numerous eosinophils, and lymphocytes and histiocytes.

5. Necrotizing "Malignant" External Otitis

Definition: Virulent and potentially fatal form of external otitis related to *Pseudomonas aeruginosa* infection.

Synonyms: Necrotizing granulomatous otitis.

Clinical

- No sex predilection; primarily affects older patients.
- Typical clinical setting is that of a diabetic patient or a patient who is chronically debilitated or immunologically deficient.
- Originates in the external auditory canal, with initial symptoms of an acute otitis externa.
- With progression of disease, pain, purulent otorrhea, and swelling occur.
- With time, the infectious process may extend into the surrounding soft tissue structures (cellulitis), cartilage (chondritis), bone (osteomyelitis), base of skull, and the middle ear space, leading to cranial nerve palsies, meningitis, intracranial venous thrombosis, and brain abscess.
- Pathogenesis is thought to be caused by tissue ischemia secondary to an underlying predisposing pathologic state (diabetic angiopathy), giving fertile ground for bacterial infection.

Pathology

Gross

- Swollen, draining ear with a hemorrhagic and necrotic appearance.

Histology

- Necrotizing inflammation with granulation tissue and an acute and chronic inflammatory cell infiltrate; epithelial ulceration is commonly seen.
- Thick, acellular collagen is seen replacing most of the tissue, extending from the cartilage to the overlying dermis.
- By tissue Gram stain, the organisms can be seen as numerous, gram-negative rods.
- The squamous epithelium is commonly ulcerated; intact epithelium may show marked reactive or atypical changes.

Differential Diagnosis

- Squamous cell carcinoma (Chapter 25C, #2).

Treatment and Prognosis

- Antibiotics, surgical debridement, and control of diabetes in patients suffering from that disease are the treatments of choice.
- Hyperbaric oxygen therapy may be used as an adjunctive modality.
- Mortality rates may exceed 50% if the diagnosis and treatment are delayed; cures can be achieved with early recognition and aggressive treatment.
- Deaths result from extensive spread of the infection to adjacent structures, including intracranial involvement.

References

Chandler JR: Malignant external otitis: further considerations. Ann Otol Rhinol Laryngol 86:417–428, 1977.

Damiani JM, Damiani DD, Kinney SE: Malignant external otitis with multiple cranial nerve involvement. Am J Otol 1:115–120, 1979.

Joachims HZ, Danino J, Raz R: Malignant external otitis: treatment with fluoroquinolones. Am J Otolaryngol 9:102–105, 1988.

Kohut RI, Lindsay JR: Necrotizing ("malignant") external otitis: histopathological processes. Ann Otol Rhinol Laryngol 88:714–720, 1979.

Ostfeld E, Segal M, Czernobilsky B: Malignant external otitis: early histopathologic changes and pathogenic mechanism. Laryngoscope 91:965–970, 1981.

Zaky DA, Bentley DW, Lowy K, Betts RF, Douglas RG: Malignant external otitis: a severe form of otitis in diabetic patients. Am J Med 61:298–302, 1976.

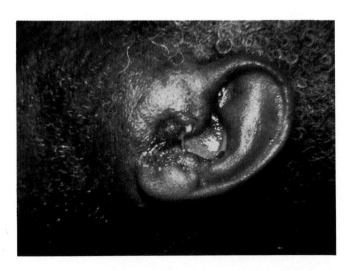

Figure 24–12. Necrotizing external otitis, characterized by a swollen, draining ear with a necrotic-appearing exudate.

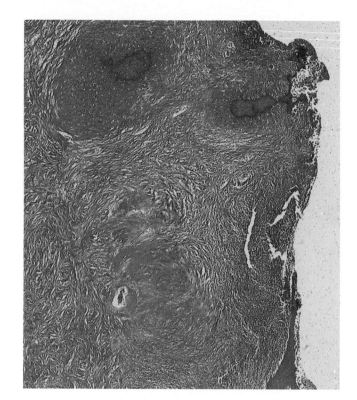

Figure 24-13. Histology of necrotizing external otitis with epithelial ulceration, an acute and chronic inflammatory cell infiltrate extending to bone, and thick, acellular collagenous bands.

B. MIDDLE EAR AND TEMPORAL BONE

1. Otitis Media

Definition: Acute or chronic infectious disease of the middle ear space.

Clinical

- Predominantly but not exclusively a childhood disease.
- Most common organisms implicated in causing disease are *Streptococcus pneumoniae* and *Hemophilus influenza.*
- No sex predilection; may occur at any age, but is particularly common in children under 3 years of age.
- Symptoms include fever, otalgia, and decreased hearing, typically preceded by several days of an upper respiratory tract infection.
- Otoscopic examination reveals a hyperemic, opaque, bulging tympanic membrane with limited mobility; purulent otorrhea may be present.
- Bilateral involvement is not uncommon.
- Middle ear infection is thought to result from infection via the eustachian tube at the time of or following a pharyngitis (bacterial or viral).
- In general, this is a medically treated illness; however, at times tissue is removed and secondary changes accompanying the infectious process may lead to incorrect pathologic diagnosis.

Pathology

Gross

- Multiple small fragments of soft to rubbery granulation-appearing tissue admixed with firm to hard calcific debris.

Histology

- Fragments of tissue, showing an acute or chronic inflammatory cell infiltrate composed of polymorphonuclear leukocytes, lymphocytes, plasma cells, and histiocytes.
- A low, cuboidal epithelium may or may not be seen.
- Multinucleated giant cells and foamy histiocytes may be seen.
- Typically, in cases of chronic otitis media, a metaplastic glandular proliferation, which is a response of the middle ear epithelium to the infectious process, may be present; these glands:
  Vary in size and shape.
  May or may not contain secretions (serous or mucus).

Are lined by a columnar to cuboidal epithelium, with or without cilia or goblet-cell metaplasia.

Are separated by abundant stromal tissue.

May be so striking as to suggest a neoplastic process (adenoma; middle ear adenomas are not ciliated and this is a helpful differentiating finding).

■ Additional findings that may accompany otitis media include:

Tympanosclerosis: dystrophic calcification of the tympanic membrane or middle ear, associated with recurrent otitis media; may cause scarring and ossicular fixation.

Cholesterol granulomas: represent a foreign body granulomatous response to cholesterol crystals; arise in the middle ear in any condition in which hemorrhage occurs (e.g., otitis media), combined with interference in drainage and ventilation of the middle ear space; otoscopic picture is referred to as "blue ear syndrome."

Reactive bone formation.

Differential Diagnosis

■ Cholesteatoma (Chapter 24B, #3).
■ Histiocytosis X (Chapter 24B, #4).
■ Middle ear adenoma (Chapter 25B, #1).
■ Rhabdomyosarcoma (Chapter 9B, #5).

Treatment and Prognosis

■ Antibiotic therapy directed at the specific pathogen is curative.
■ Recurrent infections of the middle ear are common, especially in the pediatric population.
■ With the use of antibiotics, complications associated with otitis media do not generally occur; however, if left unchecked, complications may be lethal and may include acute mastoiditis, suppurative labyrinthitis, meningitis, and brain abscess.

Additional Facts

■ In adults, an unresolving otitis media should warrant detailed examinaton of the nasopharynx in order to rule out the presence of a (malignant) neoplasm.
■ Squamous cell carcinomas of the middle ear typically arise in patients suffering from (long-standing) chronic otitis media.
■ In view of the fact that the inflammatory cell infiltrate seen in cases of otitis media may be extremely dense, the pathologist must be vigilant in evaluating these specimens; this is especially true in the pediatric age group, so as not to overlook the presence of a rhabdomyosarcoma or eosinophilic granuloma.
■ Tympanosclerosis and cholesterol granulomas may occur independently of otitis media.
■ Cholesteatomas may or may not be associated with otitis media.

References

Barnes L: Cholesterol granuloma. *In:* Barnes L, ed. Surgical pathology of the head and neck. New York: Marcel Dekker, 1985; pp 471–472.

Ferlito A: Histopathogenesis of tympanosclerosis. J Laryngol Otol 93:25–37, 1979.

Friedmann I: The pathology of acute and chronic infections of the middle ear cleft. Ann Otol Rhinol Laryngol 80:390–396, 1971.

Godolfsky E, Hoffman RA, Holliday RA, Cohen NL: Cholesterol cysts of the temporal bone: diagnosis and treatment. Ann Otol Rhinol Laryngol 100:181–187, 1991.

Sade J: Pathology and pathogenesis of serous otitis media. Arch Otolaryngol Head Neck Surg 84:297–305, 1966.

Schuknecht HF: Infections. *In:* Schuknecht HF, ed. Pathology of the ear. Cambridge, MA.: Harvard University Press, 1974; pp 215–271.

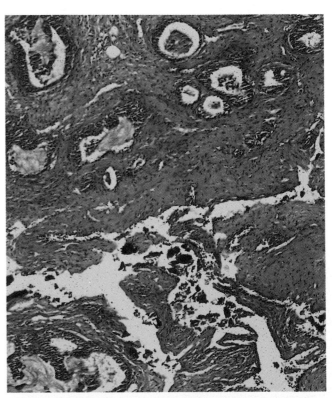

Figure 24–14. Histology of chronic otitis media, showing a glandular proliferation separated by a fibrous and focally inflamed stroma, and separate foci of calcifications; luminal secretions admixed with inflammatory cells can be seen within the glands.

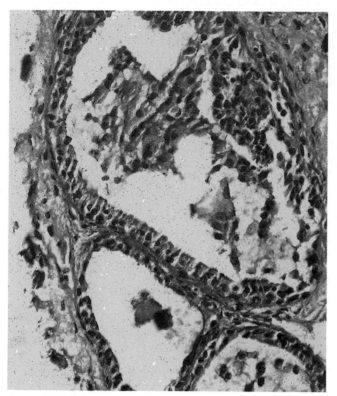

Figure 24–15. Metaplastic glands are lined by a respiratory-type epithelium, which is focally ciliated; luminal secretions are seen with desquamated epithelial cells and scattered inflammatory cells.

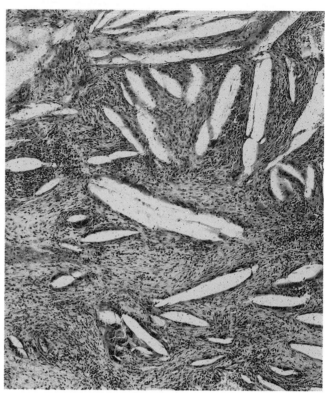

Figure 24–16. Focus of cholesterol granuloma formation, identified in association with an otitis media.

2. Otic or Aural Polyp

Definition: Inflammatory proliferation originating from the middle ear mucosa.

Clinical

- No sex predilection; may occur at any age.
- Symptoms include otorrhea, conductive hearing loss, or a mass protruding from the external auditory canal.
- Results secondary to chronic otitis media, with perforation of the tympanic membrane and extension from the middle ear into the external auditory canal.
- In large polyps completely obstructing the external ear, radiographic studies are an invaluable aid in identifying the origin of the polyp.

Pathology

Gross

- Polypoid, soft to rubbery, tan-white to pink-red–appearing tissue.

Histology

- When the epithelium is present, it appears as pseudostratified columnar or cuboidal cells with or without cilia and may demonstrate squamous metaplasia; a (metaplastic) glandular proliferation may be present.
- The cellular component consists of an acute or chronic inflammatory cell response, composed of polymorphonuclear leukocytes, lymphocytes, plasma cells, and histiocytes set in a stroma that is composed of granulation tissue that varies in appearance from edematous and richly vascularized to fibrous with a decreased vascular component.
- Giant cell granulomas may be seen.
- Tympanosclerosis and cholesterol granulomas may be present.
- Special stains for organisms (fungi, spirochetes, mycobacteriae, protozoa, and parasites) are indicated in order to rule out an infectious etiology.

Differential Diagnosis

- Histiocytosis X (Chapter 24B, #4).
- Middle ear adenoma (Chapter 25B, #1).

■ Rhabdomyosarcoma (Chapter 9B, #5).
■ Extramedullary plasmacytoma (Chapter 9B, #4).

Treatment and Prognosis

■ In the absence of an infectious etiology, local surgical excision is curative.

Additional Facts

■ The cellular component may be very dense, obscuring an underlying neoplastic process (rhabdomyosarcoma, eosinophilic granuloma, carcinoma).

References

Gaafar H, Maher A, Al-Ghazzawi E: Aural polypi: a histopathological and histochemical study. ORL J Otorhinolaryngol Relat Spec 44:108–115, 1982.
Hyams VJ, Batsakis JG, Michaels L: Inflammatory polyps of the middle ear. *In:* Hyams VJ, Batsakis JG, Michaels L, eds. Tumors of the upper respiratory tract and ear. Atlas of tumor pathology, Fascicle 25, 2nd series. Washington, D.C.: Armed Forces Institute of Pathology, 1988; p 301.

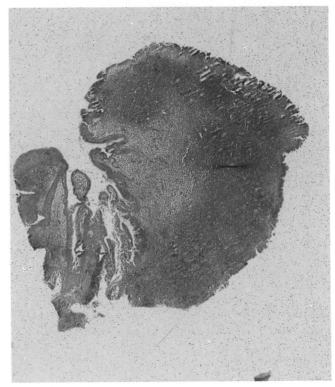

Figure 24–17. Otic polyp: the surface is composed of a pseudostratified columnar epithelium with squamous metaplasia overlying an intensely inflamed stroma.

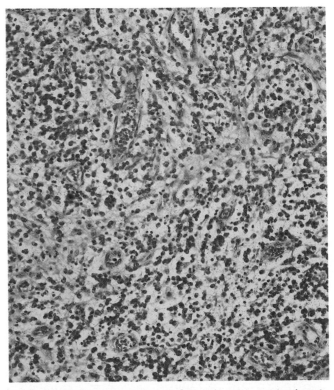

Figure 24–18. Edematous stroma of the otic polyp, predominantly composed of plasma cells and lymphocytes.

3. Cholesteatoma

Definition: Invasive, pseudoneoplastic disease characterized by the presence of stratified squamous epithelium that forms a saclike accumulation of keratin within the middle ear space.

Synonyms: Keratoma.

Clinical

- Affects males more than females; can occur at any age, but is most common in the third and fourth decades of life.
- The middle ear is the most common site of occurrence; infrequently, cholesteatoma may originate in the external auditory canal.
- Initially, cholesteatomas remain clinically silent until extensive invasion of the middle ear space and mastoid occurs.
- Symptoms include hearing loss, malodorous discharge, and pain, and may be associated with a polyp arising in the attic of the middle ear or a perforated tympanic membrane.
- Otoscopic examination may reveal the presence of white debris within the middle ear, which is considered diagnostic.
- After gaining access into the middle ear, cholesteatomas are invasive and destructive.
- The majority of cholesteatomas are acquired and either arise de novo without a prior history of middle ear disease or arise after a middle ear infection.
- A small percentage of cases are congenital.
- The pathogenesis is thought to occur via migration of squamous epithelium from the external auditory canal or from the external surface of the tympanic membrane into the middle ear; the mechanism by which the epithelium enters the middle ear probably occurs by a combination of:
  - Perforation of the tympanic membrane, particularly in its superior aspect, referred to as the pars flaccida or Shrapnell's membrane, following an infection.
  - Invagination or retraction of the tympanic membrane into the middle ear as a result of long-standing negative pressure on the membrane secondary to blockage or obstruction of the eustacian tube.
- Other theories by which cholesteatomas are thought to occur include:
  - Traumatic implantation.
  - Squamous metaplasia of the middle ear epithelium.
  - Congenital.

Pathology

Gross

- Cystic, white to pearly appearing mass of varying size, containing creamy or waxy granular material.

Histology

- The diagnosis of cholesteatoma is made in the presence of the following findings:
  1. Stratified keratinizing squamous epithelium.
  2. Subepithelial fibroconnective or granulation tissue.
  3. Keratin debris.
- **Note:** the presence of keratin debris alone is **not** diagnostic of a cholesteatoma.

Differential Diagnosis

- Keratosis obturans (see below).
- Squamous cell carcinoma (Chapter 25D, #1).

Treatment and Prognosis

- Complete surgical excision of all histologic components of the cholesteatoma is the treatment of choice.
- If incompletely excised, cholesteatomas, despite their bland histologic appearance, are progressive and destructive, and may be lethal.
- Complications arising from cholesteatomas include:
  Widespread bone destruction, which may lead to hearing loss, facial nerve paralysis, labrynthitis, meningitis, and epidural or brain abscess.

Additional Facts

- The destructive properties of cholesteatomas are caused by production of collagenase by **both** the squamous epithelial and the fibrous tissue components; collagenase has osteodestructive capabilities by its resorption of bony structures.
- The term cholesteatoma is a misnomer, in that it is not a neoplasm, nor does it contain cholesterol.
- Cholesteatomas do not transform into squamous cell carcinomas, but a squamous cell carcinoma may arise in the setting of long-standing chronic otitis media.
- Cholesterol granuloma is not synonymous with cholesteatoma.

Keratosis Obturans

- Results when the normal self-cleaning mechanism of keratin maturation and lateral extrusion from the external auditory canal is defective, causing accumulation of keratin debris deep within the bony aspect of the external auditory canal; etiology remains unclear.
- Occurs most commonly in the first two decades of life; symptoms generally relate to (conductive) hearing loss due to the keratin plug; associated pain is not uncommon.
- Keratin debris may exert pressure effects on the bony canal wall, resulting in widening of the external auditory canal, bone remodelling, and inflamed epithelium.

■ Histologic appearance is that of tightly packed keratin squames in a lamellar pattern.

■ Differential diagnosis is from external canal cholesteatoma, which generally occurs in older individuals, presents with otorrhea and unilateral chronic pain, does not produce a conductive hearing loss, and is composed histologically of loosely packed, irregularly arranged keratin squames.

■ Treatment for keratosis obturans is (repeated) debridement of the keratin debris.

References

Michaels L: Pathology of cholesteatomas: a review. J R Soc Med 72:366–369, 1979.

Palva T: Surgical treatment of cholesteatomatous ear disease. J Laryngol Otol 99:539–544, 1985.

Palva T, Makïnen: Why does middle ear cholesteatoma recur? Histopathologic observations. Arch Otolaryngol Head Neck Surg 109:513–518, 1983.

Ruedi L: Pathogenesis and surgical treatment of middle ear cholesteatoma. Acta Otolaryngol (Stockh) [Suppl] 361:6–45, 1979.

Schuknecht HF: Cholesteatoma (keratoma). *In:* Schuknecht HF, ed. Pathology of the ear. Cambridge, MA.: Harvard University Press, 1974; pp 225–228.

Swartz JD: Cholesteatomas of the middle ear: diagnosis, etiology, and complications. Radiol Clin North Am 22:15–35, 1984.

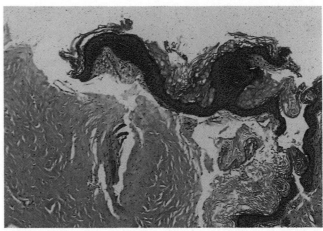

Figure 24–19. Cholesteatoma composed of stratified, keratinizing squamous epithelium, subepithelial fibroconnective tissue, and keratin debris; this histologic picture of a specimen from the middle ear is diagnostic for cholesteatoma.

4. Eosinophilic Granuloma

Definition: Idiopathic histiocytic proliferation, characterized by single or multiple bone lesions.

Synonyms: Idiopathic histiocytosis; nonlipid histiocytosis.

Clinical

■ Eosinophilic granuloma falls under the category of a group of lesions, collectively referred to as histiocytosis X, which additionally includes:

Letterer-Siwe syndrome—systemic disease with an acute, rapidly fatal course.

Multifocal eosinophilic granuloma or Hand-Schüller-Christian disease—chronic disease course that may be rapidly progressive in very young patients.

■ Affects males more than females; most commonly seen in the second and third decades of life.

■ The most frequent osseous sites involved occur in the skull (including the middle ear/temporal bone); other common sites of involvement are the femur, ribs, and pelvic bones.

■ In patients with middle ear/temporal bone involvement, symptoms include aural discharge, swelling of the temporal bone area, otitis media, bone pain, otalgia, loss of hearing, and vertigo.

Radiology

■ Single or multiple, sharply circumscribed, osteolytic lesions.

Pathology

Gross

■ Curetted material is soft, with a red-brown to slightly yellow appearance.

Histology

■ Proliferation of (histiocytic) cells in sheets, nests, or clusters composed of round, vesicular nuclei with lobation or indentation of the nuclear membrane and a moderate amount of eosinophilic cytoplasm; nucleoli are generally inconspicuous, but may be small and centrally located.

■ In addition to the histiocytes, admixtures of other inflammatory cells are seen, predominantly consisting of eosinophils; neutrophils, plasma cells, and lymphocytes also can be seen.

■ Multinucleated giant cells may be present.

■ The histiocytes may display evidence of emperipolesis.

■ Mitoses are uncommonly seen.

- Immunohistochemistry: the histiocytes are diffusely S-100 protein positive.
- Electronmicroscopy: elongated granules can be seen within the histiocyte cytoplasm, referred to as Langerhans' or Birbeck's granules.

Differential Diagnosis

- Infectious diseases.
- Otitis media (Chapter 24B, #1).
- Extranodal sinus histiocytosis with massive lymphadenopathy (Rosai-Dorfman disease) (Chapter 3, #7).

Treatment and Prognosis

- Surgical excision (curettage) and low-dose radiotherapy (500 to 1500 rads) are the treatments of choice.
- Prognosis is very good.
- Recurrence may be part of a systemic or multifocal process and generally occurs within 6 months of the diagnosis; failure of a new bone lesion to occur within 1 year of diagnosis is considered a cure.

Additional Facts

- The histologic appearance for all forms of histiocytosis X is the same, except for the relative absence of eosinophils in Letterer-Siwe syndrome.
- Chemotherapy is used for multifocal and systemic disease.
- Eosinophilic granuloma may involve nonosseous sites, including lung and larynx.
- In general, the younger the patient at onset of disease and the more extensive the involvement (multiple sites including bone and viscera), the worse the prognosis.

References

Appling D, Jenkins HA, Patton GA: Eosinophilic granuloma in the temporal bone and skull. Otolaryngol Head Neck Surg 91:358–365, 1983.

DiNardo LJ, Wetmore RF: Head and neck manifestations of histiocytosis-X in children. Laryngoscope 99:721–724, 1989.

Dombowski ML: Eosinophilic granuloma of bone manifesting mandibular involvement. Oral Surg Oral Med Oral Pathol 50:116–123, 1980.

Ide F, Iwase T, Saito I, et al: Immunohistochemical and ultrastructural analysis of the proliferating cells in histiocytosis X. Cancer 53:917–921, 1984.

Kapadia SB: Histiocytosis X. In: Barnes L, ed. Surgical pathology of the head and neck. New York: Marcel Dekker, 1985; pp 1149–1152.

McCaffrey TV, McDonald TJ: Histiocytosis X of the ear and temporal bone: a review of 22 cases. Laryngoscope 89:1735–1742, 1979.

Sweet RM, Kornblut AD, Hyams VJ: Eosinophilic granuloma in the temporal bone. Laryngoscope 89:1545–1552, 1979.

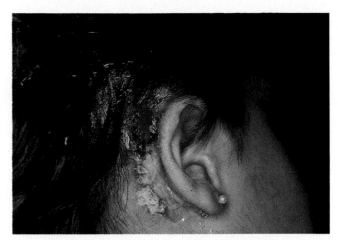

Figure 24–20. Young girl with temporal bone involvement by eosinophilic granuloma, presenting with swelling in this area and cutaneous extension.

Figure 24–21. Eosinophilic granuloma with sheet-like proliferation of histiocytic cells admixed with other inflammatory cells, predominantly consisting of eosinophils.

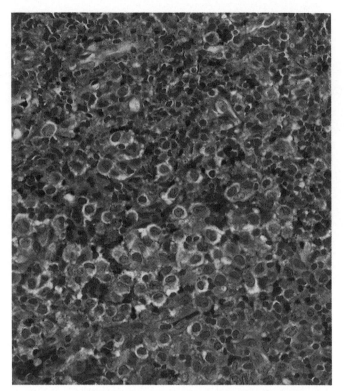

Figure 24–22. Clusters of the histiocytic cells of eosinophilic granuloma, composed of round, vesicular nuclei with lobation or indentation of the nuclear membrane and a moderate amount of eosinophilic cytoplasm; nucleoli are generally inconspicuous, but may be small and centrally located.

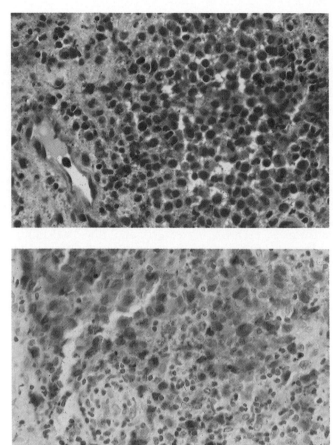

Figure 24–23. (*Top*) Typical cellular infiltrate of eosinophilic granuloma. (*Bottom*) Immunohistochemistry reveals the histiocytes to be diffusely S-100 protein positive.

CHAPTER 25

Neoplasms of the Ear

A. BENIGN NEOPLASMS OF THE EXTERNAL EAR

1. Keratoacanthoma

Definition: Benign, solitary squamous epithelial neoplasm, frequently arising on sun-exposed areas of the skin and characterized by rapid development followed by involution and regression.

Clinical

- Affects males more than females; most frequently seen in the sixth and seventh decades of life.
- The majority of cases occur on the face (most commonly on the cheek and nose); approximately 10% occur on the external ear (pinna).
- Initially, the lesion appears as an erythematous papule or may resemble a wart, but over a 1- to 2-month period undergoes rapid enlargement to appear as an exophytic or dome-shaped nodule measuring up to 2 cm in diameter and simulating a squamous cell carcinoma.
- The period of rapid proliferation is followed by a stationary period lasting up to several months, which in turn is followed by involution with spontaneous regression, ultimately leading to scar formation; the whole growth process may be seen over periods of several months up to a year.
- Etiology is unknown, but is probably the result of actinic damage.

Pathology

Gross

- The early lesion appears as an erythematous papule or a wart-like growth.
- The mature lesion is elevated and firm, with an exophytic or dome-shaped appearance characterized by skin-colored edges and a central cavity or crater filled with keratin debris; the lesion measures up to 2 cm and occasionally may reach sizes of up to 5 cm.

Histology

- The early lesion shows hyperkeratosis, parakeratosis, acanthosis with hypergranulosis, and papillomatosis with strands of atypical and dyskeratotic keratinocytes that form a central crater which extends into the epidermis.
- The mature lesion forms a crater that is filled with hyper- and orthokeratotic material, below which is the epithelial proliferation, composed of nests of large keratinocytes with a glassy-appearing or eosinophilic cytoplasm and prominent intercellular bridges.
- Dyskeratosis and squamous pearl formation are commonly seen.
- The transition area between the adjacent squamous epithelium and the hyperplastic epithelium that

forms the crater is noted by the formation of "shoulders," a characteristic low-power finding.

■ A variable, chronic, inflammatory infiltrate may be seen in the dermis surrounding the lesion that is composed of mature lymphocytes, histiocytes, eosinophils, and polymorphonuclear leukocytes; neutrophilic intraepithelial "microabscesses" are often seen.

■ Vascular and perineural invasion may be seen.

■ With time, the lesion involutes, characterized by regression of the epithelial proliferation, a shallower central crater, granulation tissue proliferation, and fibrosis of the dermis.

■ Involucrin immunoreactivity is uniformly present in the proliferating lobules.

Differential Diagnosis

■ Benign keratosis.
■ Squamous cell carcinoma (Chapter 25C, #2).

Treatment and Prognosis

■ Complete surgical excision is the treatment of choice and is curative.
■ In a small percentage of cases, keratoacanthomas may recur.

Additional Facts

■ Keratoacanthomas have been reported to metastasize; however, the metastases have been squamous cell carcinomas, suggesting that the primary tumors may have also been squamous cell carcinomas.

■ The presence of vascular or perineural invasion is not a finding indicative of malignancy.

■ Multiple keratoacanthomas can occur in association with immunosuppression, with adnexal and visceral neoplasms (Torre's syndrome), or with involvement of oral and laryngeal mucosae (eruptive keratoacanthoma).

■ Differentiating a keratoacanthoma from a squamous cell carcinoma is based on the overall architecture, rather than on cytologic examination; differentiation can be extremely difficult, especially if the biopsy specimen is taken from the central portion of the tumor.

■ Despite the end result of involution and regression, keratoacanthomas should be treated surgically for the following reasons:
  Cosmetic considerations.
  Allow for the best overall architectural evaluation to confirm the diagnosis and help differentiate from a squamous cell carcinoma.
  The treatment would be the same for a well-differentiated squamous cell carcinoma in this location.

References

Chalet MD, Connors RC, Ackerman AB: Squamous cell carcinoma vs keratoacanthoma: criteria for histologic differentiation. J Dermatol Oncol Surg 1:16–17, 1975.

Goodwin RE, Fisher GH: Keratoacanthoma of the head and neck. Ann Otol Rhinol Laryngol 89:72–74, 1980.

Janecka IP, Wolff M, Crikelair GF, Cosman B: Aggressive histologic features of keratoacanthoma. J Cutan Pathol 4:342–348, 1977.

Lapins NA, Helwig EB: Perineural invasion by keratoacanthoma. Arch Dermatol 116:791–793, 1980.

Murphy GF, Elder DE: Keratoacanthoma. In: Murphy GF, Elder DE, eds. Non-melanocytic tumors of the skin. Atlas of tumor pathology, Fascicle 1, 3rd series. Washington, D.C.: Armed Forces Institute of Pathology, 1991; pp 21–27.

Patterson HC: Facial keratoacanthoma. Otolaryngol Head Neck Surg 91:263–270, 1983.

Rook A, Whimster I: Keratoacanthoma: a thirty year perspective. Br J Dermatol 100:41–47, 1979.

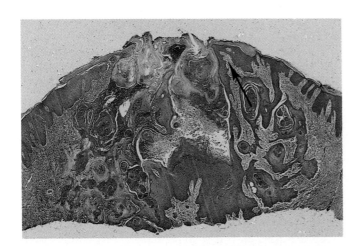

Figure 25–1. The mature lesion of keratoacanthoma forming a crater filled with hyper- and orthokeratotic material, below which is an epithelial proliferation; a characteristic low-power finding is the presence of "shoulders" representing the transition area between the adjacent squamous epithelium and the hyperplastic epithelium forming the crater *(arrow)*.

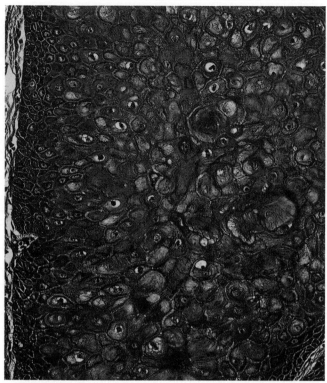

Figure 25–2. The epithelial component of keratoacanthoma is composed of nests of large keratinocytes with a "glassy" appearance or eosinophilic cytoplasm and prominent intercellular bridges.

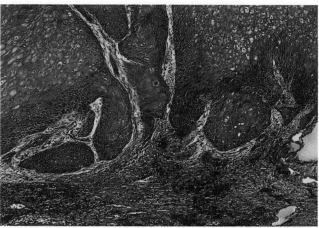

Figure 25–3. Deep portions of keratoacanthoma may demonstrate irregular epithelial nests with atypical and dyskeratotic keratinocytes and, if biopsied, may be mistakenly diagnosed as a squamous cell carcinoma.

2. Ceruminal Gland Adenoma

Definition: Benign tumor of cerumen-secreting, modified apocrine glands (ceruminal glands), located in the external auditory canal.

Synonym: Ceruminoma.

Clinical

■ In general, ceruminal gland neoplasms are uncommon, but represent one of the more common tumors of the external auditory canal.
■ Classification of ceruminal gland neoplasms include:
  Benign: ceruminoma, pleomorphic adenoma, and syringocystadenoma papilliferum.
  Malignant: adenocarcinoma and adenoid cystic carcinoma.
■ The present clinicopathologic description is limited to ceruminal gland adenoma.
■ Affects males more than females; occurs over a wide age range, but is most frequently seen in the fifth and sixth decades of life.
■ Ceruminal glands are located in the dermis of the cartilaginous portion of the external auditory canal.

■ Symptoms include a slow-growing, external auditory canal mass or blockage, hearing difficulty and, infrequently, otic discharge.

Pathology

Gross

■ Skin covered, circumscribed, polypoid, or rounded mass, ranging in size from 1 to 4 cm in diameter.
■ Ulceration is uncommon and may suggest a malignant neoplasm.

Histology

■ Unencapsulated but well-demarcated glandular proliferation.
■ The glands vary in size and may have various combinations of growth patterns, including solid, cystic, and papillary; a back-to-back glandular pattern is commonly seen.
■ The glands are composed of two cell layers: the inner or luminal epithelial cell is cuboidal or columnar-appearing, with an eosinophilic cytoplasm and a decapitation-type secretion (apical "snouts") characteristic of apocrine-derived cells;

the outer cellular layer is a spindle cell with a hyperchromatic nucleus and represents myoepithelial derivation.

■ A golden, yellow-brown, granular-appearing pigment can be seen in the inner lining cells and represents cerumen.

■ Cellular pleomorphism and mitoses can be seen, but are not prominent.

■ The intervening stroma shows a variable admixture of fibromyxomatous tissue.

■ Histochemistry: diastase-resistant, PAS-positive or mucicarmine-positive intracytoplasmic or intraluminal material may be seen.

Differential Diagnosis

■ Benign mixed tumor of ceruminal or parotid gland origin (Chapter 19A, #1).

■ Middle ear adenoma (Chapter 25B, #1).

■ Ceruminal gland adenocarcinoma (Chapter 25C, #3).

Treatment and Prognosis

■ Complete surgical excision is the treatment of choice and is curative.

■ Recurrence of the tumor can occur and relates to inadequate surgical excision.

Additional Facts

■ Mucoepidermoid carcinomas of ceruminal gland origin have been described but are considered extremely uncommon and may in fact represent a primary parotid gland tumor that presents in the external auditory canal or may be a mucin-producing ceruminal gland adenocarcinoma.

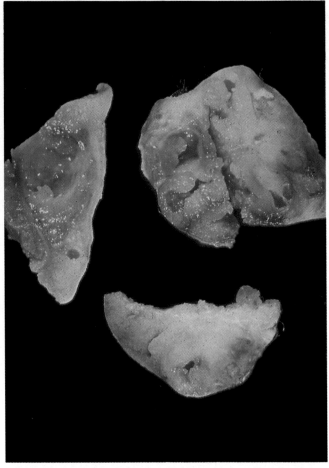

Figure 25–4. Skin covered, well-delineated ceruminal gland adenoma with a glistening, golden-yellow appearance.

References

Hyams VJ, Batsakis JG, Michaels L: Ceruminal gland neoplasms. *In*: Hyams VJ, Batsakis JG, Michaels L, eds. Tumors of the upper respiratory tract and ear. Atlas of tumor pathology, Fascicle 25, 2nd series. Washington, D.C.: Armed Forces Institute of Pathology, 1988; pp 285–291.

Dehner LP, Chen KTK: Primary tumors of the external and middle ear: benign and malignant glandular neoplasms. Arch Otolaryngol Head Neck Surg 106:13–19, 1980.

Peel RL: Ceruminous gland tumors. *In*: Barnes L, ed. Surgical pathology of the head and neck. New York: Marcel Dekker, 1985; pp 473–477.

Wetli CV, Pardo V, Millard M, Gerston K: Tumors of ceruminous glands. Cancer 29:1169–1178, 1972.

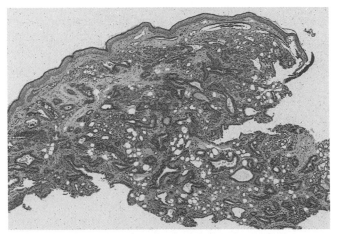

Figure 25–5. Ceruminal gland adenoma: subcutaneous unencapsulated glandular proliferation.

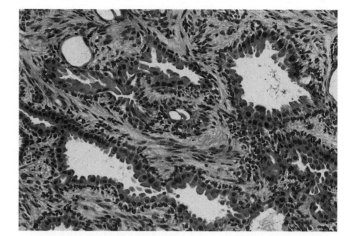

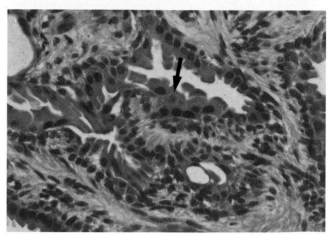

Figure 25–6. Ceruminal gland adenoma. *(Top)* Glands are composed of two cell layers: the inner or luminal epithelial cell is cuboidal or columnar-appearing, with an eosinophilic cytoplasm and a decapitation-type secretion (apical "snouts") characteristic for apocrine-derived cells; the outer cellular layer is a spindle cell with a hyperchromatic nucleus. *(Bottom)* Focally, golden yellow-brown granular-appearing pigment can be seen in the inner lining cells *(arrows)*.

B. BENIGN NEOPLASMS OF THE MIDDLE EAR

1. Middle Ear Adenoma

Definition: Benign glandular neoplasm arising from the middle ear mucosa.

Clinical

■ Generally considered a rare neoplasm.
■ No sex predilection; occurs over a wide age range, but is most common in the third to fifth decades of life.
■ Any portion of the middle ear may be affected, including the eustachian tube, mastoid air spaces, ossicles, and chorda tympani nerve.
■ The most common symptom is that of unilateral conductive hearing loss; fullness, tinnitus, and dizziness may also occur; however, pain, otic discharge, and facial nerve paralysis rarely occur, and these symptoms may be indicative of a malignant process.
■ Otoscopic examination in the majority of cases identifies an intact tympanic membrane with the tumor confined to the middle ear space, with possible extension to the mastoid; occasionally, the adenoma perforates through the tympanic membrane, with extension into and presentation as an external auditory canal mass.
■ Middle ear adenomas are not related to a prior history of chronic otitis media.
■ Concomitant cholesteatomas may occur and may be the cause of bone destruction or facial nerve abnormalities.

Radiology

■ In its more typical presentation, the middle ear adenoma appears as a relatively avascular soft-tissue density without evidence of destructive, invasive, or erosive properties.

Pathology

Gross

■ Gray-white to red-brown, rubbery to firm mass, free of significant bleeding on manipulation.

Histology

■ Unencapsulated glandular lesion with solid, cystic, sheetlike, trabecular, or papillary growth patterns; a back-to-back glandular pattern is commonly seen.
■ The glands are composed of a single layer of cuboidal to columnar cells, with a varying amount of eosinophilic cytoplasm and a round to oval nucleus, with chromatin ranging from densely packed (hyperchromatic) to a more dispersed "salt-and-pepper" pattern; nucleoli may be seen and are generally eccentrically located.
■ The cells may have a predominant plasmacytoid appearance, and this is particularly evident in the solid growth pattern.
■ Pleomorphism may be prominent, but mitoses are uncommon; perineural invasion may occur.
■ Some neoplasms demonstrate a marked papillary growth, which has been associated with a more aggressive behavior.
■ The stromal component is sparse and appears fibrous or myxoid.
■ Histochemistry: intraluminal mucin-positive material may be seen; intracytoplasmic mucin material is only rarely identified; neoplastic cells may be argyrophilic positive.
■ Immunohistochemistry: cytokeratin and epithelial membrane antigen are consistently positive; neuroendocrine differentiation may occur as identified by chromogranin, synaptophysin, neuron-specific enolase, S-100 protein, and Leu-7 reactivity.

Differential Diagnosis

■ Metaplastic glandular proliferation secondary to otitis media (Chapter 24B, #1).
■ Ceruminal gland adenoma (Chapter 25A, #2).
■ Jugulotympanic paraganglioma (Chapter 25C, #2).
■ Acoustic neuroma (Chapter 25C, #3).
■ Meningioma (Chapter 25C, #4).
■ Middle ear adenocarcinoma (Chapter 25D, #2).
■ Rhabdomyosarcoma (Chapter 9B, #5).

Treatment and Prognosis

■ Complete surgical excision is the treatment of choice, which may be conservative if the lesion is small and confined to the middle ear, or more radical in a larger lesion that is associated with more extensive structural involvement.
■ Recurrences may occur if the tumor is inadequately excised.
■ Some middle ear adenomas may be locally aggressive and rarely may invade vital structures, causing death; metastatic disease does not occur.

Additional Facts

■ In general, the clinical, radiologic, and pathologic findings indicate that the tumor is benign (absence of associated neural deficits, invasion or destruction of adjacent structures, or pleomorphism and increased mitotic activity); nevertheless, the histologic appearance is not always predictive of the clinical behavior.
■ Adenomas with neuroendocrine differentiation have been termed *carcinoid tumors of the middle ear;* rather than representing a separate, distinct neoplasm of the middle ear, these carcinoid tumors are closely related to the adenomas (cytoarchitecturally and biologically) and represent adenomas with neuroendocrine differentiation.

References

Batsakis JG: Adenomatous tumors of the middle ear. Ann Otol Rhinol Laryngol 98:749–752, 1989.

Benecke JE, Noel FL, Carberry JN, House JW, Patterson M: Adenomatous tumors of the middle ear and mastoid. Am J Otol 11:20–26, 1990.

Hyams VJ, Michaels L: Benign adenomatous neoplasm (adenoma) of the middle ear. Clin Otolaryngol 1:17–26, 1976.

Hyams VJ, Batsakis JG, Michaels L: Adenoma of the middle ear. *In*: Hyams VJ, Batsakis JG, Michaels L, eds. Atlas of tumor pathology: tumors of the upper respiratory tract and ear. Fascicle 25, 2nd series. Washington, D.C.: Armed Forces Institute of Pathology, 1988; pp 316–320.

Latif MA, Madders DJ, Shaw PAV: Carcinoid tumour of the middle ear associated with systemic symptoms. J Laryngol Otol 101:480–486, 1987.

McNutt MA, Bolen JW: Adenomatous tumor of the middle ear: an ultrastructural and immunocytochemical study. Am J Clin Pathol 84:541–547, 1985.

Mills SE, Fechner RE: Middle ear adenoma: a cytologically uniform neoplasm displaying a variety of architectural patterns. Am J Surg Pathol 8:677–685, 1984.

Riches WG, Johnston WH: Primary adenomatous neoplasms of the middle ear: light and electron microscopic features of a group distinct from the ceruminomas. Am J Clin Pathol 77:153–161, 1982.

Stanley MW, Horwitz CA, Levinson RM, Sibley RK: Carcinoid tumors of the middle ear. Am J Clin Pathol 87:592–600, 1987.

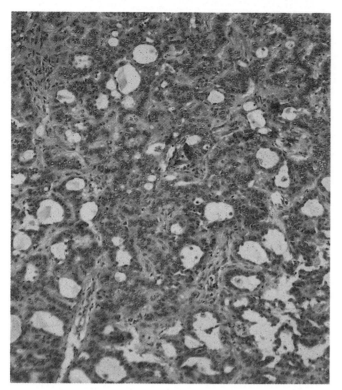

Figure 25–7. Middle ear adenoma consisting of unencapsulated glandular proliferation in cystic, solid, and back-to-back glandular growth patterns.

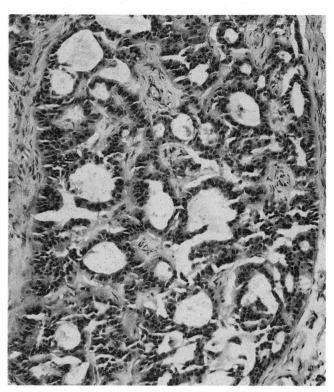

Figure 25–9. Middle ear adenoma: glands are composed of a single layer of cuboidal to columnar cells, with a varying amount of eosinophilic cytoplasm and round to oval nuclei.

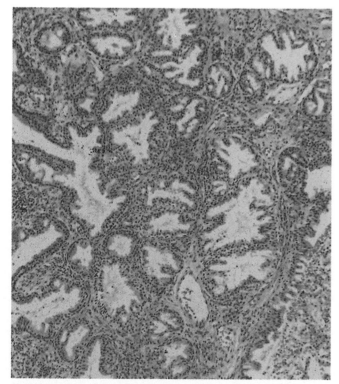

Figure 25–8. Middle ear adenoma with a papillary growth.

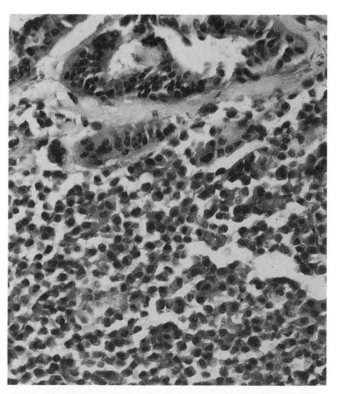

Figure 25–10. Middle ear adenomas may have a cellular component that is predominantly plasmacytoid in appearance, evident in this solid growth pattern.

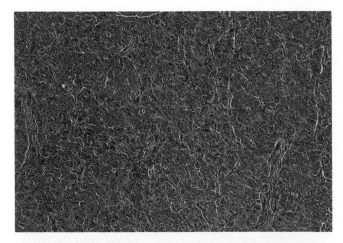

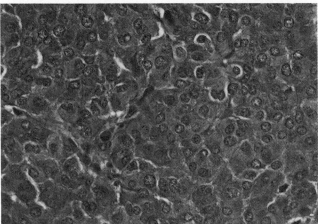

Figure 25-11. Some middle ear adenomas have neuroendocrine differentiation. *(Top)* Organoid growth. *(Bottom)* The presence of uniform cells with dispersed "salt and pepper" chromatin pattern.

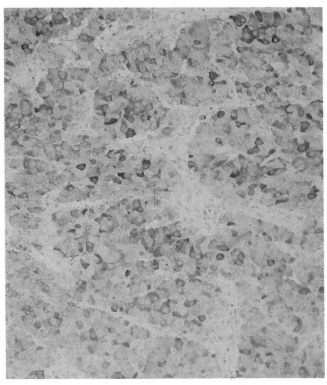

Figure 25-12. Immunohistochemistry of the middle ear adenomas with neuroendocrine features display cytokeratin and chromogranin reactivity; this illustration shows chromogranin immunoreactivity in the previously illustrated adenoma.

2. Jugulotympanic Paraganglioma

Definition: Benign neoplasm arising from the extra-adrenal, neural crest-derived paraganglia, specifically located in the middle ear or temporal bone region.

Synonyms: Glomus jugulare tumor; glomus tympanicum tumor.

Clinical

■ Considered the most common tumor of the middle ear.

■ Affects females more than males; most commonly seen in the fifth to seventh decades of life.

■ Jugulotympanic paragangliomas occur in one of three locations:

1. In the adventitia of the jugular vein *(glomus jugulare tumor).*

2. Associated with the posterior auricular branch of the vagus nerve, also known as Arnold's nerve *(glomus tympanicum tumor).*

3. Along the tympanic branch of the glossopharyngeal nerve, also known as Jacobson's nerve *(glomus tympanicum tumor).*

■ The majority of the jugulotympanic paragangliomas arise in the jugular bulb (85%), leading to a mass lesion in the middle ear or external auditory canal; approximately 12% take origin from Jacobson's nerve, presenting as a middle ear tumor, and approximately 3% arise from Arnold's nerve, originating in the external auditory canal.

■ The most common symptom is conductive hearing loss; other symptoms include tinnitus, fullness, otic discharge, pain, hemorrhage, facial nerve abnormalities, and vertigo.

■ Often are locally invasive neoplasms, with extension into and destruction of adjacent structures, including the temporal bone and mastoid.

Radiology

- CT scan: soft tissue mass, often with evidence of extensive destruction of adjacent structures.
- Carotid angiography: vascularized lesion fed by branches of nearby large arteries.

Pathology

Gross

- Polypoid, red, friable mass, identified behind an intact tympanic membrane or within the external auditory canal, measuring from a few millimeters to a large mass completely filling the middle ear space.
- Typically, paragangliomas bleed profusely on manipulation.

Histology

- Cell nest or "zellballen" pattern is characteristic of paragangliomas.
- The stroma surrounding and separating the nests is composed of a prominent fibrovascular tissue.
- The neoplasm is composed predominantly of chief cells, which are round or oval with uniform nuclei, dispersed chromatin pattern, and abundant eosinophilic, granular, or vacuolated cytoplasm.
- Sustentacular cells may be seen; these cells represent modified Schwann cells and are seen at the periphery of the cell nests as spindle-shaped, basophilic-appearing cells.
- No glandular or alveolar differentiation is seen.
- Cellular pleomorphism can be seen; mitoses and necrosis are infrequently identified.
- Spindling of the chief cells may be seen and infrequently may predominate.
- The tumor cells are argyrophilic, and the presence of reticulin staining delineates the cell nests; argentaffin, mucicarmine, and periodic acid-Schiff (PAS) stains are negative.
- Immunohistochemical profile:
  Chief cells: chromogranin, synaptophysin, neuron-specific enolase, neurofilaments, and a variety of peptides are positive.
  Sustentacular cells: S-100 protein positive.
- Electronmicroscopic: the hallmark of the electron-microscopic findings is the presence of neurosecretory granules.
- Note: biopsy specimens of middle ear paragangliomas are often small and display artifactual distortion, excluding identification of the classic histologic features.

Differential Diagnosis

- Middle ear adenoma, with or without neuroendocrine differentiation (Chapter 25B, #1).
- Acoustic neuroma (Chapter 25B, #3).
- Meningioma (Chapter 25B, #4).

Treatment and Prognosis

- Complete surgical excision is the treatment of choice; however, the location and invasive nature of these lesions often preclude the capability of complete surgical eradication; in such cases, radiotherapy is a useful adjunct to surgery, because radiotherapy results in a decrease or ablation of vascularity and promotes fibrosis.
- Preoperative embolization has been advocated as useful to decrease the vascularity of the tumor and allow for safer surgery.
- Local recurrence of the tumor can be seen in as high as 50% of the cases.
- Although these are slow-growing neoplasms, prognosis is guarded, because they often infiltrate and invade adjacent structures.
- Although malignancy is rare, these neoplasms may result in increased morbidity and mortality as a result of invasion of vital structures (cranial cavity).

Additional Facts

- The histologic appearance does not correlate to the biologic behavior of the tumor.
- Neurologic abnormalities, including cranial nerve palsies, cerebellar dysfunction, dysphagia, and hoarseness, may be seen and correlate to the invasive capabilities of this neoplasm.
- Functioning jugulotympanic paragangliomas, as evidenced by endocrinopathic manifestations, occur but are extremely uncommon.
- Malignant jugulotympanic paragangliomas occur, are associated with histologic criteria of malignancy (increased mitotic activity, necrosis usually seen within the center of the cell nests, vascular invasion) and metastasize to cervical lymph nodes, lungs, and liver.

References

Glassock CG, Welling B, Chironis P, Glassock ME, Woods CI: Glomus tympanicum tumors: contemporary concepts in conservation surgery. Laryngoscope 99:875–884, 1989.

Hyams VJ, Batsakis JG, Michaels L: Jugulotympanic paraganglioma. In: Hyams VJ, Batsakis JG, Michaels L, eds. Tumors of the upper respiratory tract and ear. Atlas of tumor pathology, Fascicle 25, 2nd series. Washington, D.C.: Armed Forces Institute of Pathology, 1988; pp 306–311.

Johnstone PAS, Foss RD, Desilets DJ: Malignant jugulotympanic paraganglioma. Arch Pathol Lab Med 114:976–979, 1990.

Konefal JB, Pilepich MV, Spector GJ, Perez CA: Radiation therapy in the treatment of chemodectomas. Laryngoscope 97:1331–1335, 1987.

Larson TC, Reese DF, Baker HL, McDonald TJ: Glomus tympanicum chemodectomas: radiographic and clinical characteristics. 97:1331–1335, 1987.

Peel RL: Tumors of the paraganglionic nervous system. In: Barnes L, ed. Surgical pathology of the head and neck. New York: Marcel Dekker, 1985; pp 684–695.

Schuknecht HF: Glomus body tumor. In: Schuknecht HF, ed. Pathology of the ear. Cambridge, MA: Harvard University Press, 1974; pp 420–424.

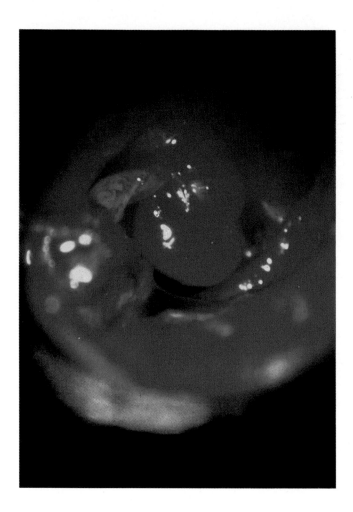

Figure 25–13. Jugulotympanic paraganglioma, characterized by a bright red polypoid mass originating in the middle ear space.

Figure 25–14. The histologic appearance of middle ear paragangliomas is often distorted or masked secondary to artifactual changes, but the characteristic cell nest appearance is usually focally maintained.

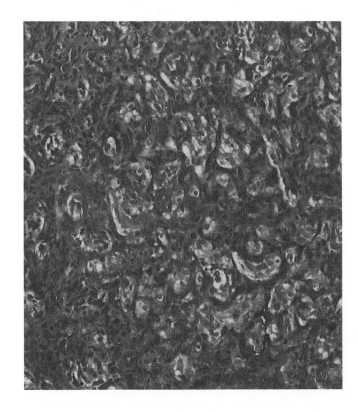

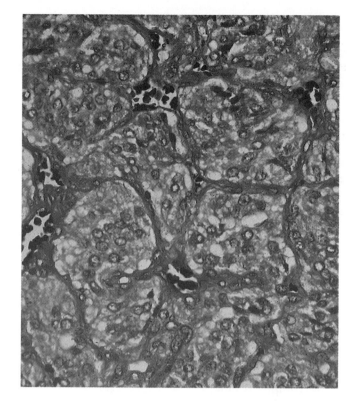

Figure 25–15. Characteristic appearance of all paragangliomas is that of a cell nest pattern separated by fibrovascular stroma and composed predominantly of chief cells, which are round or oval with uniform nuclei, dispersed chromatin pattern, and abundant eosinophilic, granular, or vacuolated cytoplasm; the peripherally located sustentacular cells are difficult to identify by light microscopy and appear as spindle-shaped cells with a basophilic appearance.

3. Acoustic Neuroma

Definition: Benign neoplasm arising from Schwann cells, specifically originating from the VIIIth cranial nerve.

Synonyms: Acoustic schwannoma or neurilemmoma.

Clinical

■ Account for up to 10% of all intracranial neoplasms and up to 90% of all tumors of the cerebellopontine angle.

■ Affects females more than males; may affect any age, but are most common in the fourth to seventh decades of life.

■ Neurilemmomas may take origin from any cranial nerve; however, aside from the VIIIth nerve and much less frequently the Vth nerve, involvement of cranial nerves is uncommon.

■ Acoustic neuromas typically develop at the neuroglial-neurolemmal junction, termed the Rednik-Obersteiner line, identified immediately inside the meatus of the internal auditory canal; however, the site of this junction varies and so too does the site of acoustic neuromas.

■ The majority of acoustic neuromas involve the superior or vestibular portion of the VIIIth nerve, as compared to involvement of the cochlear portion of the VIIIth nerve.

■ Symptoms include progressive (sensorineural) hearing loss, tinnitus, and loss of equilibrium; with progression, the tumor enlarges and may compress adjacent cranial nerves (V, VII, IX, X, XI), the cerebellum, and the brainstem, leading to facial paresthesia and numbness, headaches, nausea, vomiting, diplopia, and ataxia.

■ Symptoms of neurofibromatosis may be seen in up to 16% of patients, and those with neurofibromatosis who develop acoustic neuromas generally are symptomatic at an earlier age (second decade) and have a higher incidence of bilateral acoustic neuromas.

Radiology

■ CT and MRI: flaring, asymmetrical widening or erosion of the internal auditory canal; these techniques are capable of detecting tumors with dimensions of 1 cm and less.

Pathology

Gross

■ Unilateral, circumscribed, tan-white, rubbery to firm mass, which may appear yellow and have cystic change.

■ Sizes range from a few millimeters up to 4 to 5 cm in greatest diameter.

Histology

■ Tumors are composed of alternating regions, which are composed of compact spindle cells called Antoni A areas, and loose, hypocellular zones called Antoni B areas; in a given tumor, the proportion of these components varies.
■ Nuclei are vesicular to hyperchromatic, elongated and twisted, with indistinct cytoplasmic borders.
■ Cells are arranged in short, interlacing fascicles, and whorling or palisading of nuclei may be seen; nuclear palisading with nuclear alignment in rows is called Verocay bodies.
■ Antoni B areas display a disorderly cellular arrangement, myxoid stroma, and a chronic inflammatory cell infiltrate.
■ Increased vascularity is prominent, composed of large vessels with thickened (hyalinized) walls.
■ Mitoses, usually sparse in number, and cellular pleomorphism with hyperchromasia can be identified but are not evidence of malignancy.
■ Cellularity may vary, and some benign schwannomas can be very cellular, conferring the name cellular schwannoma.
■ Retrogressive changes, including cystic degeneration, necrosis, hyalinization, calcification, and hemorrhage, may be seen.
■ Immunohistochemistry: S-100 protein is uniformly and intensely positive.

Differential Diagnosis

■ Middle ear adenoma (Chapter 25B, #1).
■ Jugulotympanic paraganglioma (Chapter 25B, #2).
■ Meningioma (Chapter 25B, #4).

Treatment and Prognosis

■ Complete surgical excision is the treatment of choice and is curative.
■ Death may occur secondary to herniation of the brainstem in untreated or large neoplasms.

Additional Facts

■ Malignant (acoustic) schwannomas are exceedingly rare and, if present, neurofibromatosis should be suspected.

References

Erickson LS, Sorenson GD, McGavaran MH: A review of 140 acoustic neurinomas (neurilemmoma). Laryngoscope 75:601–626, 1965.
Kasantikul V, Netsky MG, Glassock ME, Hays JW: Acoustic neurilemmoma: clinico-anatomical study of 103 patients. J Neurosurg 52:28–35, 1980.
Peel RL: Acoustic neuroma. In: Barnes L, ed. Surgical pathology of the head and neck. New York: Marcel Dekker, 1985; pp 700–704.
Schuknecht HF: Vestibular schwannoma. In: Schuknecht HF, ed. Pathology of the ear. Cambridge, MA: Harvard University Press, 1974; pp 425–438.
Tos M, Thomsen J: Management of acoustic neuroma: a review. Acta Otolaryngol (Stockh) 111:616–632, 1991.

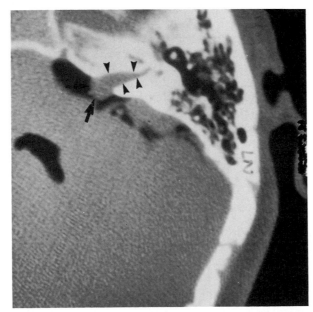

Figure 25–16. Axial CT air cisternogram of acoustic neuroma: intrathecally injected air outlines a left intracanalicular tumor *(arrows)*, which extends into the cerebellopontine angle. The left internal auditory canal *(arrowheads)* is slightly enlarged, a typical feature of VIIIth nerve schwannomas. MR imaging has virtually replaced invasive diagnostic techniques. (Courtesy of Franz J. Wippold II, M.D., Mallinckrodt Institute of Radiology, St. Louis, MO.)

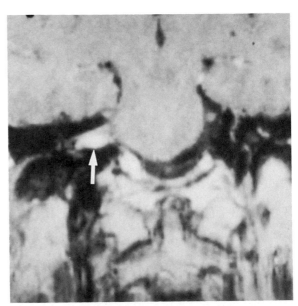

Figure 25–17. Coronal MR T1-weighted image, enhanced, of an acoustic neuroma: contrast enhanced tumor *(arrow)*, largely confined by the right internal auditory canal. Contrast-enhanced MR is now the preferred imaging modality for evaluation of neurosensory hearing loss and suspected cerebellopontine angle masses. (Courtesy of Franz J. Wippold II, M.D., Mallinckrodt Institute of Radiology, St. Louis, MO.)

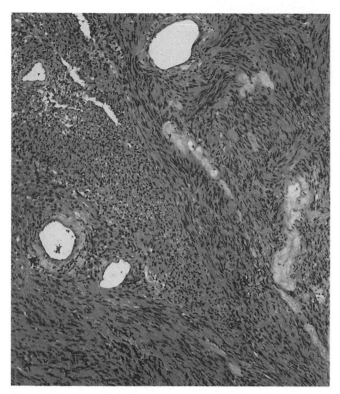

Figure 25-18. Acoustic neuroma, composed of a spindle-cell proliferation with cells arranged in short, interlacing fascicles, whorling or palisading of nuclei, and an associated increased vascularity marked by thickened (hyalinized) vascular walls.

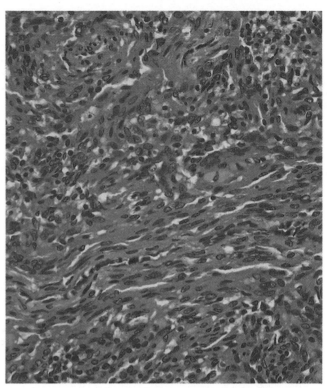

Figure 25-19. Acoustic neuroma: nuclei are vesicular to hyperchromatic, elongated, and twisted with indistinct cytoplasmic borders; scattered chronic inflammatory cells can be seen.

4. Meningioma

Definition: Benign neoplasms arising from arachnoid cells that form the arachnoid villi, seen in relation to the dural sinuses.

Clinical

■ Represent from 13% to 18% of all intracranial tumors.
■ Represent the second most common tumor of the cerebellopontine angle.
■ Affect females more than males; occur over a wide age range, but are most commonly seen in the fifth decade of life and infrequently in children.
■ Occurrence outside the central nervous system (CNS) is considered ectopic; are divided into those meningiomas with no identifiable CNS connection (primary) and those with CNS connection (secondary).
■ The most common site of occurrence of the ectopically located meningiomas is the head and neck region and includes middle ear and temporal bone (internal auditory canal, jugular foramen, geniculate ganglion, roof of the eustachian tube, sulcus of the greater petrosal nerve), sinonasal cavity, orbit, oral cavity, and parotid gland.
■ Symptoms vary according to site, and in the middle ear and temporal bone area clinically simulate an acoustic neuroma with symptoms including progressive loss of hearing, loss of equilibrium, headaches, cerebellar dysfunction, and cranial nerve abnormalities.

Radiology

■ A feature that correlates to the histology and is considered a pathognomonic feature for meningioma in this location is the presence of speckled calcification in a soft tissue mass.

Pathology

Gross

■ Lobular-appearing, tan-white to gray, rubbery to firm mass with a gritty consistency.
■ In contrast to their intracranial counterparts, which are well-delineated and circumscribed lesions, meningiomas of the middle ear tend to be infiltra-

tive with extension and invasion of adjacent structures.

Histology

Four histologic variants have been described and include syncytial or meningothelial, fibroblastic, transitional (combination of syncytial and fibroblastic), and angioblastic; in the middle ear, the most common histologic subtype is the meningothelial type, which has the following features:

■ Lobular growth, with tumor nests separated by a variable amount of fibrous tissue.
■ The cells have a whorled appearance and are composed of round to oval or spindle-shaped nuclei with pale-staining cytoplasm and indistinct cell borders.
■ Characteristically, the nuclei have a punched-out or empty appearance, resulting from intranuclear cytoplasmic inclusions.
■ Psammoma bodies, typical and numerous in intracranial meningothelial meningiomas, may be seen but are not found as often in meningiomas occurring in the middle ear region.
■ Mild cellular pleomorphism may be seen; mitoses are uncommon.
■ Immunohistochemistry: immunoreactivity with vimentin and epithelial membrane antigen (EMA).

Differential Diagnosis

■ Middle ear adenoma (Chapter 25B, #1).
■ Jugulotympanic paraganglioma (Chapter 25B, #2).
■ Acoustic neuroma (Chapter 25B, #3).
■ "Juvenile" active ossifying fibroma when meningiomas occur in association with the sinonasal cavities or orbit (Chapter 4A, #7).

Treatment and Prognosis

■ Complete surgical excision is the treatment of choice and is curative.
■ Local recurrence relates to inadequate excision.
■ Malignant change rarely, if ever, occurs.

Additional Facts

■ There is no correlation between the histologic subtype and clinical behavior, except for the angioblastic variant, which has been associated with a more aggressive behavior.
■ Patients with neurofibromatosis have an increased incidence of developing a meningioma.
■ Aside from bilateral meningiomas, patients with neurofibromatosis also experience increased incidence of multiple, separately occurring meningiomas in intra- and extracranial locations.
■ Development of meningiomas in the middle ear and temporal bone results either from direct extension of an intracranial meningioma or independent of intracranial origin from ectopically located arachnoid cells.

References

Friedman CD, Costantino PD, Teitelbaum B, Berktold RE, Sisson GA: Primary extracranial meningioma of the head and neck. Laryngoscope 100:41–48, 1990.

Granich MS, Pilch BZ, Goodman ML: Meningiomas presenting in the paranasal sinuses and temporal bone. Head Neck Surg 5:319–328, 1983.

Hyams VJ, Batsakis JG, Michaels L: Meningioma of the temporal bone. In: Hyams VJ, Batsakis JG, Michaels L, eds. Tumors of the upper respiratory tract and ear. Atlas of tumor pathology, Fascicle 25, 2nd series. Washington, D.C.: Armed Forces Institute of Pathology, 1988; pp 312–316.

Perzin KH, Pushparaj N: Nonepithelial tumors of the nasal cavity, paranasal sinuses and nasopharynx: a clinicopathologic study XIII: meningiomas. Cancer 54:1860–1869, 1984.

Rietz DH, Ford CN, Kurtycz DF, Brandenburg JH, Hafez GH: Significance of apparent intratympanic meningiomas. Laryngoscope 93:1397–1404, 1983.

Salama N, Stafford N: Meningiomas presenting in the middle ear. Laryngoscope 92:92–97, 1982.

Schnitt SJ, Vogel H: Meningiomas: diagnostic value of immunoperoxidase staining for epithelial membrane antigen. Am J Surg Pathol 10:640–649, 1986.

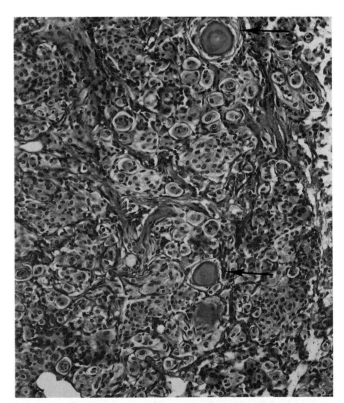

Figure 25–20. Middle ear meningioma displaying a lobular growth with tumor nests separated by a variable amount of fibrous tissue; psammomatoid bodies are seen (arrows).

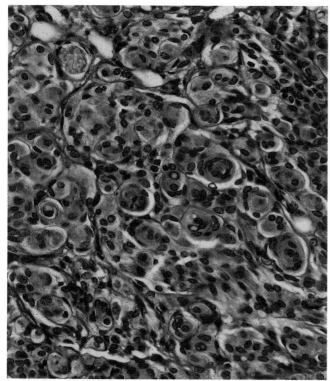

Figure 25–21. Middle ear meningioma: cells have a whorled appearance and are composed of round to oval or spindle-shaped nuclei with pale-staining cytoplasm and indistinct cell borders; characteristically, the nuclei have a punched-out or empty appearance, resulting from intranuclear cytoplasmic inclusions.

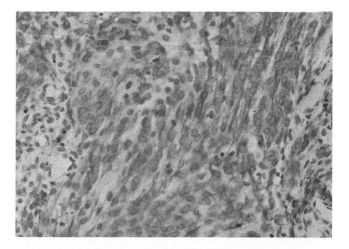

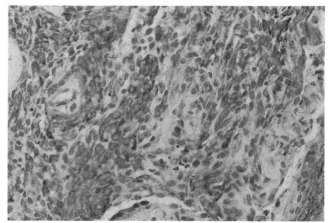

Figure 25–22. Immunohistochemistry of meningioma. *(Top)* Epithelial membrane antigen (EMA). *(Bottom)* Vimentin.

C. MALIGNANT NEOPLASMS OF THE EXTERNAL EAR

1. Basal Cell Carcinoma

Definition: Slow-growing, locally infiltrative malignant neoplasm of the skin and subcutaneous adnexal tissue.
Synonym: Basal cell epithelioma.

Clinical

■ Represents the most common cutaneous malignancy.
■ Affects males more than females; generally is a tumor affecting adults and is most commonly seen in the seventh decade of life.
■ The sun-exposed areas of the head and neck are the most frequent sites of occurrence and, therefore, may occur in virtually all cutaneous sites of this region; the more common locations include the nose, eyelids, nasolabial area, and the auricular area (pinna).
■ In general, basal cell carcinomas are asymptomatic; presentation usually occurs because the patient notices a growth.
■ Basal cell carcinomas of the external auditory canal are uncommon; however, when this area is involved, it typically has extensive subcutaneous involvement, which may not be clinically appreciated.
■ Basal cell carcinomas take origin from a pluripotential cell in either the basal cell layer of the surface epithelium or in the epithelium of the subcutaneous adnexae.
■ Etiology is related to prolonged sun exposure with resulting actinic damage.
■ Basal cell carcinomas may be inherited in the au-

tosomal dominant disorder called *nevoid basal cell carcinoma syndrome,* which includes:

Multiple basal cell carcinomas, most commonly involving the nose, mouth, eyes, and ear regions.

Occurrence in childhood.

Association with palmar and plantar pitting, odontogenic keratocysts of the jaws, skeletal developmental abnormalities (bifid ribs, brachymetacarpalism, and vertebral anomalies), ectopic calcification in dermal and soft tissue sites, and neurologic abnormalities (mental retardation).

Pathology

Gross

■ Initially, the lesion is a raised papule or nodule with a waxy or translucent appearance covered by a fine capillary network (telangiectasia).

■ With time, the central portion ulcerates and is surrounded by raised, pearly appearing borders, creating the typical papulonodular ulcerative lesion which is referred to as so-called "rodent ulcer."

Histology

■ Although a variety of histologic growth patterns are identified, all basal cell carcinomas arise in continuity with the basal cell layer of the epithelium or from the adnexae and are composed of fairly uniform cells with hyperchromatic, oval, or elongated nuclei, scant cytoplasm, and palisading appearance of the nuclei at the periphery of the tumor nests; a characteristic retraction (separation) of the surrounding stroma from the peripheral portions of the tumor nests is commonly seen.

■ The various growth patterns include:

Solid type, made up of islands or sheets of tumor cells; this is the most common histologic subtype.

Adenoid type, in which the tumor islands are arranged in anastamosing cords, creating a lace-like or adenoid pattern.

Morphea or sclerosing type, in which strands of tumor cells are embedded in a dense, sclerotic stroma.

■ Additional histologic variants of basal cell carcinoma include:

Keratotic basal cell carcinoma, composed of keratin microcysts or horn cysts lined by flattened, parakeratotic cells identified within the tumor islands.

Metatypical or basosquamous carcinoma, composed of a basal cell carcinoma with squamous cell differentiation.

■ In any one lesion, multiple growth patterns may be identified.

■ Cellular pleomorphism, increased mitoses, and necrosis may be seen and vary from case to case.

■ Melanin pigmentation may be seen in tumor islands.

Differential Diagnosis

■ Adnexal neoplasms (trichoepithelioma).
■ Merkel cell carcinoma (see below).
■ Squamous cell carcinoma (Chapter 25C, #2).

Treatment and Prognosis

■ Complete surgical excision is the treatment of choice; electrodessication and irradiation may be used; irradiation is used particularly in cases that cannot be completely excised.

■ Prognosis is excellent after complete excision.

■ Local recurrences are not uncommon and are especially high in the morphea or sclerosing type of basal cell carcinoma.

■ Metastases are rare, except for:

Neglected or long-standing tumors that attain large sizes and become deeply and extensively infiltrative.

The basosquamous carcinoma which, for all intents and purposes, behaves as a squamous cell carcinoma, with metastatic rates seen in approximately 6% of patients; this form of basal cell carcinoma requires a more aggressive surgical approach and a closer follow-up than other types of basal cell carcinomas.

■ When metastases occur, spread is usually to regional lymph nodes and to the lungs; metastatic disease is associated with poor prognosis, irrespective of any therapeutic intervention.

■ Basal cell carcinomas of the external auditory canal are notorious for extensive local invasion and extension to the middle ear, mastoid region, temporal bone, and potentially into the cranial cavity; radical surgical excision may be necessary in order to eradicate tumors in this location.

Additional Facts

■ Unlike squamous cell carcinoma, basal cell carcinomas do not have a premalignant counterpart.

■ Aside from the metatypical and sclerosing types, histology does not correlate with the biologic behavior.

Merkel Cell Carcinoma

■ Neuroendocrine carcinoma of the skin, primarily arising from Merkel cells, which may be clinically mistaken for a basal cell carcinoma when it occurs on the face of elderly patients.

■ No sex predilection; most common in the seventh and eighth decades of life.

■ Slow-growing tumor with predilection for cutaneous sites of the head and neck (face), extremities, and buttocks.

■ Characterized histologically by an undifferentiated,

malignant small-cell infiltrate, primarily seen in the dermis and subcutaneous tissues and, generally, not involving the epidermis, from which the cellular infiltrate is separated by a narrow rim of papillary dermis; epithelial involvement may occur and results in ulceration.

■ Growth patterns include diffuse, densely packed, cellular infiltrate, trabeculae, cords, and cell nests; nuclei are round with dispersed (stippled) chromatin, contain multiple small nucleoli, and the cytoplasm is scanty, poorly defined, and acidophilic; numerous mitotic figures and necrosis are seen.

■ Histochemistry: argyrophilia may be seen.

■ Immunohistochemistry: keratin (paranuclear stippled pattern), chromogranin, and neuron specific enolase positive.

■ Wide local surgical excision is the treatment of choice, with lymph node dissection when palpable nodes are present; radiotherapy may be beneficial in conjunction with surgery.

■ Aggressive tumor that has a tendency to recur; regional lymph node metastases commonly occur, as do distant (visceral) metastases (lung, liver, bone).

References

Silverman AR, Nieland ML: Basal cell carcinoma. *In*: Barnes L, ed. Surgical pathology of the head and neck. New York: Marcel Dekker, 1985; pp 1583–1591.

Murphy GF, Elder DE: Basal cell carcinoma. *In*: Murphy GF, Elder DE, eds. Non-melanocytic tumors of the skin. Atlas of tumor pathology, Fascicle 1, 3rd series. Washington, D.C.: Armed Forces Institute of Pathology, 1991; pp 47–58.

Murphy GF, Elder DE: Neuroendocrine carcinoma. *In*: Murphy GF, Elder DE, eds. Non-melanocytic tumors of the skin. Atlas of tumor pathology, Fascicle 1, 3rd series. Washington, D.C.: Armed Forces Institute of Pathology, 1991; pp 248–251.

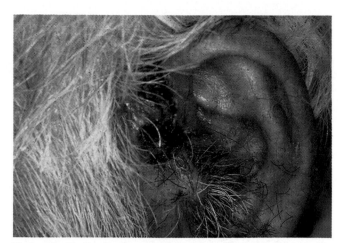

Figure 25–23. Basal cell carcinoma arising anterior to the ear with central ulceration surrounded by raised, pearly appearing borders.

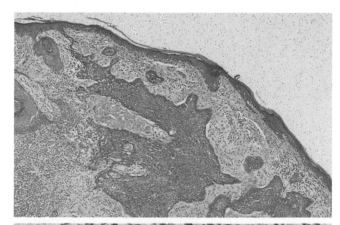

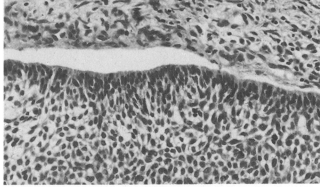

Figure 25–24. Basal cell carcinoma of the external ear. *(Top)* Infiltrating tumor focally connected and arising in continuity with the overlying keratinizing squamous epithelium. *(Bottom)* Portion of tumor nodule composed of uniform cells with round to oval hyperchromatic nuclei. Characteristic histologic features of basal cell carcinoma include peripheral nuclear palisading represented as the parallel alignment of basal cells at the periphery of the tumor nodule, and the epithelial–stromal separation artifact.

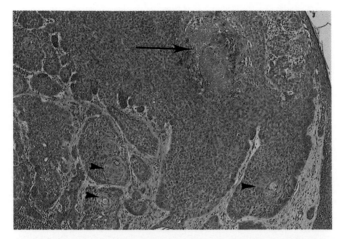

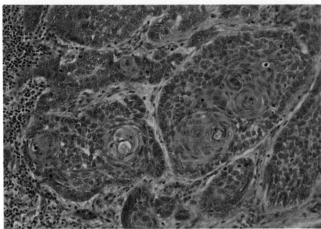

Figure 25–25. Basosquamous (metatypical) carcinoma of the external ear. *(Top)* The tumor arises from the surface *(upper right)* and infiltrates as solid nests and nodules composed of basaloid cells with peripheral nuclear palisading admixed with areas of squamous differentiation, including horn pearl formation with individual cell keratinization *(arrowheads)* and a large focus of keratinization *(arrow).* *(Bottom)* Higher magnification of the infiltrating tumor nodules seen above showing the foci of squamous differentiation admixed with the basaloid cells.

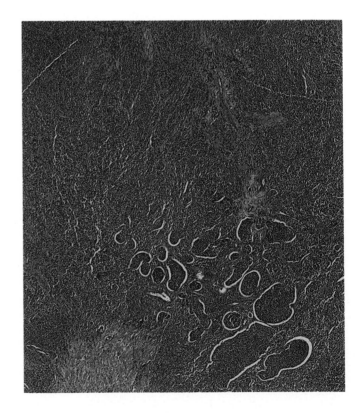

Figure 25–26. Merkel cell carcinoma: subcutaneous, diffuse, densely packed cellular infiltrate with trabecular, cord-like, and cell nest growth patterns.

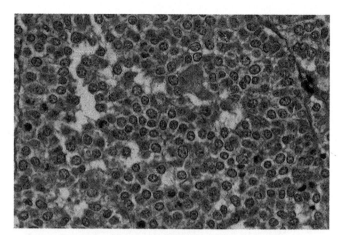

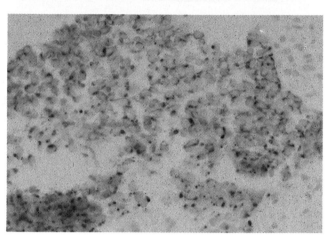

Figure 25–27. Merkel cell carcinoma. *(Top)* Cellular infiltrate is composed of cells with round nuclei, dispersed (stippled) chromatin pattern, small eosinophilic nucleoli, and scanty, poorly defined, acidophilic cytoplasm; numerous mitotic figures and necrosis are seen. *(Bottom)* Immunohistochemistry of Merkel cell carcinoma includes a characteristic, paranuclear stippled reactive pattern with cytokeratin.

2. Squamous Cell Carcinoma of the External Ear and External Auditory Canal

Definition: Malignant epithelial tumor arising from the surface epithelium.

Synonym: Epidermoid carcinoma.

Clinical

- Accounts for approximately 25% of all squamous cell carcinomas of the head and neck.
- Squamous cell carcinoma of the external ear:
  Affects males more than females; most frequently seen in the seventh and eighth decades of life.
  Presents with a nonhealing sore.
- Squamous cell carcinoma of the external auditory canal:
  Affects females more than males; most frequently seen in the sixth and seventh decades of life.
  Symptoms mimic those of a chronic otitis media, with pain, hearing deficits, and otorrhea (bloody or purulent).

Pathology

Gross

- External ear—polypoid, rubbery to firm nodules, frequently with ulceration.
- External auditory canal—visualization is difficult, given the location and concealment by a purulent or hemorrhagic exudate.

Histology

- In general, squamous cell carcinomas in this region tend to be well differentiated, composed of infiltrating nests of cells with keratinization and intercellular bridges.
- An adenoid or glandular appearance (adenoid squamous cell carcinoma or adenoacanthoma) may be identified.
- A spindle cell morphology may be seen in those squamous carcinomas arising on the external ear, with little evidence of squamous differentiation;

they are characterized by:

Surface ulceration; continuity of the tumor with the overlying epithelium may be seen in those cases not associated with ulceration.

Infiltrating but demarcated tumor composed of interlacing bundles or fascicular growth pattern.

Cells with elongated hyperchromatic nuclei, cellular pleomorphism with giant cells, and increased mitotic activity including atypical mitoses and a variable amount of amphophilic to eosinophilic cytoplasm.

Immunoreactivity: cytokeratin positive but S-100 protein and HMB-45 negative.

Differential Diagnosis

■ Pseudoepitheliomatous hyperplasia and other reactive hyperplasias (Chapter 13, #6; and Chapter 14A, #2).

■ Cholesteatoma of the external auditory canal (Chapter 24B, #3).

■ Atypical fibroxanthoma (Chapter 25C, #4).

■ Spindle cell malignant melanoma (Chapter 4B, #3).

Treatment and Prognosis

External Ear

■ Complete surgical excision is the treatment of choice.

■ In general, early detection and complete removal result in good prognosis; however, prognosis is dependent on the extent of disease and the presence or absence of metastasis.

■ Local recurrence may occur in up to 25% of patients and may correlate to tumor size.

■ Fatal outcomes are seen when tumor has spread beyond the auricle.

External Auditory Canal

■ Complete surgical excision is the treatment of choice; this often requires a radical procedure (mastoidectomy or temporal bone resection).

■ Radiotherapy may be indicated, depending on the extent of disease.

■ Prognosis is considered poor, with approximately 25% 5-year survival rate.

■ Histologic differentiation does not correlate with prognosis; squamous cell carcinomas in this location often go undetected for long periods of time, and presentation is with advanced disease involving the mastoid or middle ear.

■ Regional lymph node metastases are seen infrequently, and death is generally attributed to invasion of regional structures, particularly intracranial extension.

Additional Facts

■ Suspicion for the presence of a malignancy should be considered in patients with chronic ear infections who suddenly have a change in symptoms, including pain, bleeding, or facial paralysis.

References

Avila J, Bosch A, Aristizabel S, Frias Z, Marcial V: Carcinoma of the pinna. Cancer 40:2891–2895, 1977.

Bailin PL, Levins HL, Wood BG, Tucker HM: Cutaneous carcinoma of the auricular and preauricular region. Arch Otolaryngol 106:692–696, 1980.

Barnes L, Johnson JT: Clinical and pathological considerations in the evaluation of major head and neck specimens resected for cancer. Pathol Ann (pt 2) 21:83–110, 1986.

Conley J, Schuller DE: Malignancies of the ear. Laryngoscope 86:1147–1163, 1976.

Goodwin WJ, Jesse RH: Malignant neoplasms of the external auditory canal and temporal bone. Arch Otolaryngol Head Neck Surg 106:675–679, 1980.

Paaske PB, Witten J, Schwer S, Hansen HS: Results in treatment of carcinoma of the external auditory canal and middle ear. Cancer 59:156–160, 1987.

Shiffman NJ: Squamous cell carcinoma of the skin and pinna. Can J Surg 18:279–283, 1975.

Shih L, Crabtree JA: Carcinoma of the external auditory canal: an update. Laryngoscope 100:1215–1218, 1990.

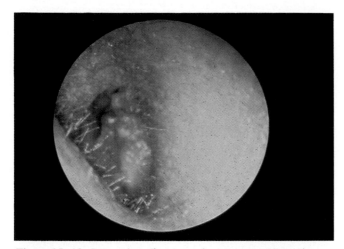

Figure 25–28. External auditory canal squamous cell carcinoma, consisting of a gray-white, pearly appearing polypoid lesion that fills the canal.

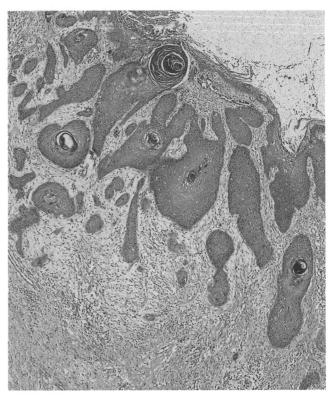

Figure 25–29. Infiltrating, well-differentiated squamous cell carcinoma of the external auditory canal.

3. Ceruminal Gland Adenocarcinoma

Definition: Malignant neoplasm of cerumen-secreting modified apocrine glands (ceruminal glands), located in the external auditory canal.

Clinical

- Affects males more than females; occurs over a wide age range, but is most frequently seen in the fifth and sixth decades of life.
- In addition and in contrast to the symptoms of ceruminal gland adenomas, which include a mass in the external auditory canal, hearing difficulty, and otic discharge, the adenocarcinomas are associated with pain as a more characteristic feature.

Pathology

Gross

- Ulcerated, polypoid, or rounded mass, ranging in size from 1 to 4 cm in diameter.

Histology

- Histologic similarity to ceruminomas.
- Features of adenocarcinoma that differ from the adenomas include:
  Loss of the glandular, double-cell layer, with identification of only the inner or luminal epithelial cell.
  The cells vary in appearance from those with minimal pleomorphism and atypia to cells with pleomorphism, nuclear anaplasia, and mitoses; the decapitation-type secretion (apical "snouts") may or may not be apparent.
  Tissue invasion and destruction.

Differential Diagnosis

- Ceruminal gland adenoma (Chapter 25A, #2).

Treatment and Prognosis

- Complete surgical excision is the treatment of choice and may be supplemented with radiotherapy.

- Recurrence of the tumor can occur and relates to inadequate surgical excision.
- Metastases rarely, if ever, occur.

References

Dehner LP, Chen KTK: Primary tumors of the external and middle ear: benign and malignant glandular neoplasms. Arch Otolaryngol Head Neck Surg 106:13–19, 1980.

Hageman MEJ, Becker AE: Intracranial invasion of a ceruminous gland tumor; a follow-up of 12 years. Arch Otolaryngol Head Neck Surg 100:395–397, 1974.

Hyams VJ, Batsakis JG, Michaels L: Ceruminal gland neoplasms. In: Hyams VJ, Batsakis JG, Michaels L, eds. Tumors of the upper respiratory tract and ear. Atlas of tumor pathology, Fascicle 25, 2nd series. Washington, D.C.: Armed Forces Institute of Pathology, 1988; pp 285–291.

Peel RL: Ceruminous gland tumors. In: Barnes L, ed. Surgical pathology of the head and neck. New York: Marcel Dekker, 1985; pp 473–477.

Wetli CV, Pardo V, Millard M, Gerston K: Tumors of ceruminous glands. Cancer 29:1169–1178, 1972.

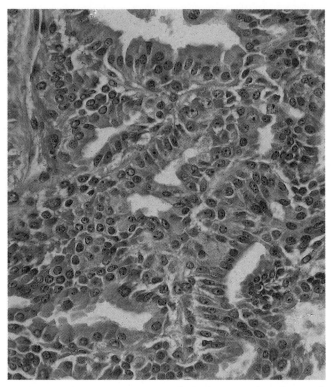

Figure 25–31. In contrast to ceruminal adenomas, the adenocarcinomas display loss of nuclear polarity, loss of the glandular double cell layer with identification of only the inner or luminal epithelial cell, cellular pleomorphism, anaplasia, and mitoses; the decapitation-type secretion (apical "snouts") is focally seen but may not be apparent.

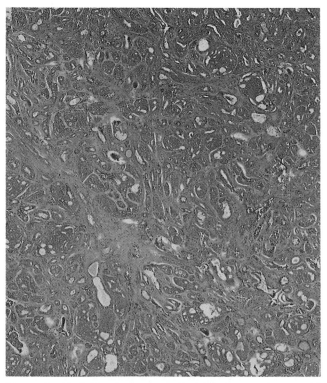

Figure 25–30. Infiltrating, ceruminal gland adenocarcinoma with glandular, cribriform, and solid growth patterns.

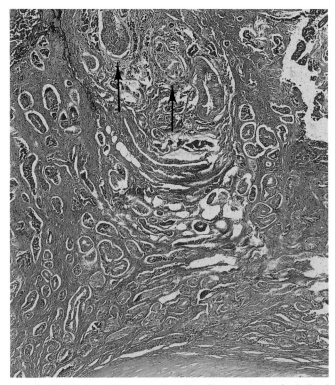

Figure 25–32. In addition to the other features, ceruminal gland adenocarcinomas may demonstrate neural invasion (arrows) as well as invasion of the auricular cartilage seen along the lower portion of the illustration.

4. Atypical Fibroxanthoma

Definition: Malignant fibrohistiocytic neoplasm identified on actinic-damaged cutaneous sites, composed of a pleomorphic cell population, with a locally aggressive clinical course.

Synonym: Superficial (low-grade) malignant fibrous histiocytoma.

Clinical

- Seen in two clinical forms, neither having a specific sex predilection:
  Common form, accounting for approximately 75% of cases affecting elderly patients, commonly involving the head and neck (nose, cheek, and ear).
  Less common form, accounting for approximately 25% of cases affecting younger patients, commonly involving superficial sites on the limbs and trunk.
- Both forms present with a generally asymptomatic solitary growth on the affected body site.
- Etiology is related to actinic damage.

Pathology

Gross

- Solitary, firm nodules, frequently associated with ulceration, measuring from 1 to 2 cm in diameter.

Histology

- Unencapsulated but circumscribed neoplasm, characterized by a bizarre cellular component arranged in a vague fascicular pattern; a storiform growth pattern is infrequently seen.
- Junctional activity between the neoplasm and the overlying epidermis is absent; surface atrophy or ulceration may be present.
- The cells are strikingly pleomorphic and bizarre, varying from spindle-shaped, plump, or rounded with hyperchromatic nuclei, often with multiple nuclei, prominent foamy cytoplasm, large acidophilic nucleoli, and the presence of multiple, atypical, multipolar mitotic figures.
- A mild, chronic inflammatory cell infiltrate may be seen.
- Necrosis is rarely seen.
- Superficial areas adjacent to the tumor show solar elastosis and vascular proliferation.

- Histochemistry: intracytoplasmic diastase-resistant, PAS-positive granular material may be seen.
- Immunohistochemistry: cytokeratin, S-100 protein, and HMB-45 are all negative.

Differential Diagnosis

- Spindle cell carcinoma (Chapter 14B, #2).
- Spindle cell malignant melanoma (Chapter 4B, #3).
- Dermatofibrosarcoma protuberans (Chapter 4A, #4).
- Leiomyosarcoma (Chapter 4B, #8).

Treatment and Prognosis

- Complete surgical excision is the treatment of choice and is curative.
- Prognosis is excellent.
- Local recurrence is uncommon, and although metastases have occurred, this event is exceptional.

Additional Facts

- The diagnosis of atypical fibroxanthoma is one of exclusion.
- Recurrent tumors may present as a large mass in the deep soft tissue, and these neoplasms should be considered and treated as a malignant fibrous histiocytoma.
- These tumors display ultrastructural variability, with evidence of fibrohistiocytic and myofibroblastic features and, to a lesser extent, features of Langerhans' cells.

References

Enzinger FM, Weiss SW: Atypical fibroxanthoma. *In*: Enzinger FM, Weiss SW, eds. Soft tissue tumors, 2nd ed. St. Louis: C.V. Mosby, 1988; pp 269–273.

Evans HL, Smith JL: Spindle cell squamous carcinoma and sarcoma-like tumors of the skin: a comparative study of 38 cases. Cancer 45:2687–2697, 1980.

Helwig EB, May D: Atypical fibroxanthoma of the skin with metastasis. Cancer 57:368–376, 1986.

Kuwano H, Hashimoto H, Enjoji M: Atypical fibroxanthoma distinguishable from spindle cell carcinoma in sarcoma-like skin lesions: a clinicopathologic and immunohistochemical study of 21 cases. Cancer 55:172–180, 1985.

Leong ASY, Milios J: Atypical fibroxanthoma of the skin: a clinicopathological and immunohistochemical study and a discussion of its histogenesis. Histopathology 11:463–475, 1987.

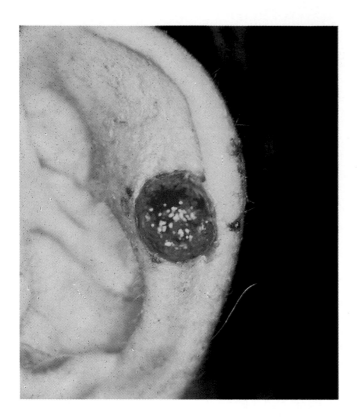

Figure 25–33. Atypical fibroxanthoma (AFX), presenting as a solitary, firm auricular nodule.

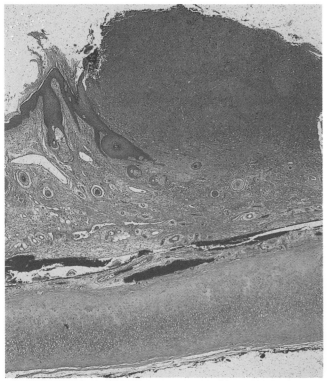

Figure 25–34. Histologic appearance of AFX is that of an unencapsulated but circumscribed neoplasm, characterized by a bizarre cellular component arranged in a vague fascicular pattern; this example depicts a raised lesion with surface ulceration.

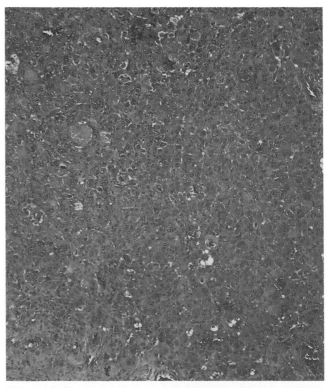

Figure 25–35. The cellular components of AFX are strikingly pleomorphic and bizarre, varying from spindle-shaped, plump, or rounded with hyperchromatic nuclei, often with multiple nuclei, prominent foamy cytoplasm, large acidophilic nucleoli, and the presence of multiple, atypical, multipolar mitotic figures.

D. MALIGNANT NEOPLASMS OF THE MIDDLE EAR

1. Squamous Cell Carcinoma

Definition: Malignant epithelial tumor of epidermoid cells arising as a primary neoplasm from the middle ear mucosal epithelium.

Clinical

- No sex predilection; most commonly seen in the sixth and seventh decades of life.
- Majority of patients have a long history of chronic otitis media, usually of greater than 20 years in duration.
- Early symptoms include pain with radiation to the scalp and face and hearing impairment; late symptoms include facial palsies and vertigo.
- Etiology also linked to radiation treatment for intracranial neoplasms and, although no longer used, radiotherapy for middle ear inflammatory conditions.
- Although concomitant cholesteatomas can be seen in up to 25% of cases, there is no correlation between cholesteatomas and the development of a middle ear squamous cell carcinoma.

Pathology

Histology

- The tumor varies from well to poorly differentiated, and may or may not be seen arising from the middle ear mucosa.
- Often, evidence of chronic otitis media is seen in association with the infiltrating carcinoma, as demonstrated by the presence of a chronic inflammatory cell infiltrate, calcifications (tympanosclerosis) and glandular proliferation.
- Evidence of a cholesteatoma may be present.

Differential Diagnosis

- Cholesteatoma (Chapter 24B, #3).
- Metastatic squamous cell carcinoma from a distant site or extension from a squamous carcinoma from an adjacent site (external ear, nasopharynx, parotid gland, or skin).

Treatment and Prognosis

- Radical surgery with radiotherapy is the treatment of choice; in advanced disease, chemotherapy may be of benefit.
- Prognosis is poor, with 5- and 10-year survival rates of 39% and 21%, respectively.
- Neoplasms often present in advanced stages with extensive bone destruction and spread to the eustachian tube, external auditory canal, mastoid, jugular fossa, internal auditory canal, and brain.
- Metastases may occur but are considered uncommon.

Additional Facts

- The development of a middle ear squamous cell carcinoma should be suspected in patients with a long history of chronic otitis media with the following clinical manifestations:
  Sudden onset of pain out of proportion to the clinical extent of disease.
  Onset or increase of otorrhea that is often hemorrhagic.
  Lack of clinical resolution after therapeutic doses of antibiotics.
- The bony capsule of the labyrinth is resistant to the spread of tumor.

References

Hyams VJ, Batsakis JG, Michaels L: Squamous cell carcinoma of the middle ear. *In*: Hyams VJ, Batsakis JG, Michaels L, eds. Tumors of the upper respiratory tract and ear. Atlas of tumor pathology, Fascicle 25, 2nd series. Washington, D.C.: Armed Forces Institute of Pathology, 1988; pp 326–327.

Kenyon GS, Marks PV, Scholtz CL, Dhillon R: Squamous cell carcinoma of the middle ear; a 25-year retrospective study. Ann Otol Rhinol Laryngol 94:273–277, 1985.

Michaels L, Wells M: Squamous cell carcinoma of the middle ear. Clin Otolaryngol 5:235–248, 1980.

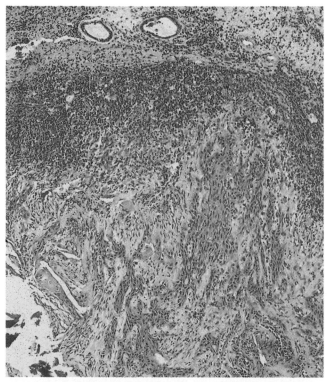

Figure 25–36. Middle ear squamous cell carcinoma arising in a setting of chronic otitis media; the latter consists of an inflamed stroma, glandular metaplasia *(top)*, and tympanosclerosis *(lower left)*; the carcinomatous component is seen throughout the center portion of the illustration.

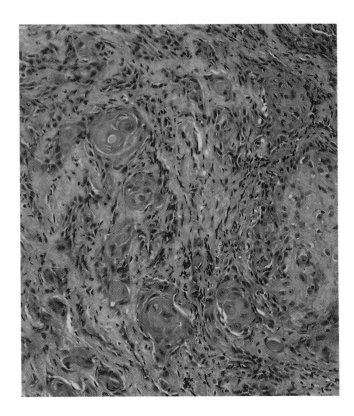

Figure 25–37. Squamous cell carcinoma of the middle ear: well-differentiated neoplasm composed of infiltrating nests of tumor with minimal pleomorphism and with keratinization.

2. Middle Ear Adenocarcinoma

Definition: Malignant glandular neoplasm arising from the middle ear mucosa.

Clinical

- Rare neoplasm, and metastases to the middle ear from adenocarcinomas of other (distant) sites must be considered.
- No sex predilection; occurs over a wide age range, between the second and sixth decades of life.
- Symptoms are typically present for many years and include progressive hearing loss and a unilateral draining ear; pain and vestibular manifestations are uncommon.
- Otoscopic examination in the majority of cases will identify an intact tympanic membrane with tumor confined to the middle ear space, with possible extension to the mastoid; occasionally, and similar to the middle ear adenoma, the adenocarcinoma will perforate through the tympanic membrane with extension into and presentation as an external auditory canal mass.
- There is no association between chronic otitis media and the development of these adenocarcinomas.

Pathology

Gross

- Variation in appearance from gray-white to red-brown, rubbery to firm mass, to spongy and cystic appearing.
- The neoplasm may attain large sizes, filling the middle ear space and encasing the ossicles.

Histology

- Unencapsulated, glandular lesion with variations in the histologic appearance, including:

  Similarity to adenomas, but with prominent pleomorphism, increased mitotic activity, extensive infiltration of surrounding soft tissue structures, including perineural and perivascular invasion and invasion of bone.

  A papillary and cystic variant (papillary cystadenocarcinoma), lined by cells with hyperchromatic nuclei and vacuolated cytoplasm that contain luminal eosinophilic secretions with scalloped edges.
- Histochemistry: intraluminal but not intracytoplasmic mucin-positive material may be seen.
- Immunohistochemistry: cytokeratin and epithelial

membrane antigen are consistently positive; thyroglobulin immunoreactivity is not seen.

Differential Diagnosis

■ Middle ear adenoma (Chapter 25B, #1).
■ Metastatic papillary carcinoma of thyroid gland origin.

Treatment and Prognosis

■ Complete surgical excision is the treatment of choice.
■ In general, these are slow-growing neoplasms that are locally aggressive but do not metastasize.
■ The papillary cystadenocarcinomas are considered low-grade malignant tumors.
■ Deaths may occur as a result of direct intracranial extension.

Additional Facts

■ Confinement to the middle ear space and association with the middle ear mucosa are supportive evidence of origin from the middle ear; nevertheless, metastatic adenocarcinoma from a separate site must be excluded prior to treatment.
■ Metastases to the middle ear and temporal bone can be seen from all sites, but are most common from the breast, lung, kidney, gastrointestinal tract, larynx, skin (melanoma), and prostate.

References

Glassock ME, McKennan KX, Levine SC, Jackson CG: Primary adenocarcinoma of the middle ear and temporal bone. Arch Otolaryngol Head Neck Surg 113:822–824, 1987.

Gulya AJ, Glassock ME, Pensack ML: Primary adenocarcinoma of the temporal bone with middle cranial fossa extension: case report. Laryngoscope 96:675–677, 1986.

Hyams VJ, Batsakis JG, Michaels L: Adenocarcinoma of the middle ear. In: Hyams VJ, Batsakis JG, Michaels L, eds. Tumors of the upper respiratory tract and ear. Atlas of tumor pathology, Fascicle 25, 2nd series. Washington, D.C.: Armed Forces Institute of Pathology, 1988; pp 320–323.

Pallanch JF, McDonald TJ, Weiland LH, Facer GW, Harner SG: Adenocarcinoma and adenoma of the middle ear. Laryngoscope 92:47–53, 1982.

Schuller DE, Conley JJ, Goodman JH, Clausen KP, Miller WJ: Primary adenocarcinoma of the middle ear. Otolaryngol Head Neck Surg 91:280–283, 1983.

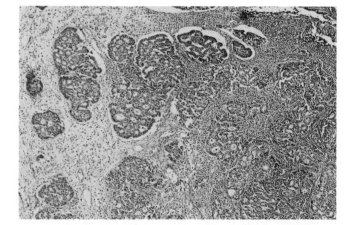

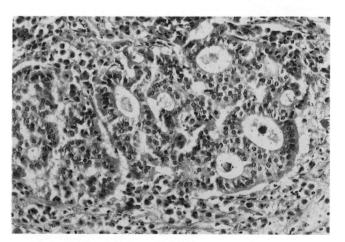

Figure 25–38. Middle ear adenocarcinoma. *(Top)* Unencapsulated, infiltrating glandular neoplasm. *(Bottom)* Complexity of growth, including a cribriform or back-to-back pattern with cellular pleomorphism, helps in distinguishing an adenoma from an adenocarcinoma.

3. Temporal Bone Adenocarcinoma of Endolymphatic Sac Origin

Definition: Low-grade malignant neoplasm of probable origination from the endolymphatic sac epithelium.

Clinical

- Rare neoplasm, with less than 25 reported cases.
- No sex predilection; occurs over a wide age range, from the second to eighth decades of life.
- The most common symptom is unilateral hearing loss, ranging from 6 months to 18 years in duration; the hearing loss is most frequently sensorineural, rather than conductive, but mixed types of hearing loss also occur.
- Other symptoms include tinnitus, vertigo, ataxia, and cranial nerve deficits.
- Etiology is unknown.

Radiology

- CT scan and MRI:
  Lytic temporal bone lesion measuring from 4 to 6 cm.
  The center of the lesions is most often seen at or near the posteriomedial face of the petrous bone.
  Extension of tumor to the posterior cranial cavity lead to suggestions that the tumor took origin from the cerebellopontine angle; extension results in cerebellar involvement and evidence of compression or shifting of the fourth ventricle, brain stem, or pineal gland.
- Angiographic studies show a vascular or hypervascular lesion.

Pathology

Histology

- Papillary and cystic neoplasm, lined by a single row of cells ranging from a flattened or attenuated appearance to columnar with uniform nuclei, situated either in the center of the cells or toward the luminal aspect, and pale eosinophilic to clear-appearing cytoplasm.
- The epithelium, particularly when attenuated, may be poorly demarcated from the underlying stroma, which is noted for the presence of numerous capillary-sized vascular spaces.
- Hypercellular areas can be seen, with crowded cystic glands that contain eosinophilic, colloid-like material, which may be scalloped at the edges.
- Areas of hypocellularity with fibrosis, hemorrhage, and chronic inflammatory cells can be seen.

- Histochemistry: colloid-like glandular material stains strongly with PAS; intracytoplasmic and intraluminal mucin staining is rarely positive; epithelial cells may occasionally stain positive for iron.
- Immunohistochemistry: cytokeratin positive; S-100 protein, glial fibrillary acidic protein (GFAP), synaptophysin, and Leu-7 may be positive; thyroglobulin immunoreactivity is not seen.

Differential Diagnosis

- Non-neoplastic reactive or inflammatory processes (Chapter 24B, #1).
- Choroid plexus papilloma.
- Middle ear adenoma/adenocarcinoma (Chapter 25B, #1; Chapter 25D, #2).
- Ceruminal gland adenocarcinoma (Chapter 25C, #3).
- Metastatic adenocarcinoma, particularly papillary carcinoma of the thyroid and renal cell carcinoma.

Treatment and Prognosis

- Radical surgery, including mastoidectomy and temporal bone resection, which may necessitate sacrifice of cranial nerves, is the treatment of choice and is potentially curative.
- Local recurrence results after inadequate surgical removal; operative morbidity may be high.
- Despite being low-grade and slow-growing, these neoplasms are capable of widespread infiltration and destruction, and may be lethal.
- Prognosis is dependent on the extent of disease and the adequacy of resection; earlier detection, when the tumors are relatively small and confined, may decrease the operative-associated morbidity and be curative.

Additional Facts

- The clinicopathologic and especially the radiologic findings may be highly suggestive of this neoplasm.
- Endolymphatic sac origin is supported by:
  The growth of this tumor from the region of the posteromedial petrous ridge, a site where the endolymphatic sac is located.
  Resemblance of normal endolymphatic sac epithelium to the tumor.

References

Carroll WR, Niparko JK, Zappia JJ, McClatchey KD: Primary adenocarcinoma of the temporal bone: a case with 40-year follow-up. Arch Otolaryngol Head Neck Surg 117:439–441, 1991.

Heffner DK: Low-grade adenocarcinoma of probable endolymphatic sac origin: a clinicopathologic study of 20 cases. Cancer 64:2292–2302, 1989.

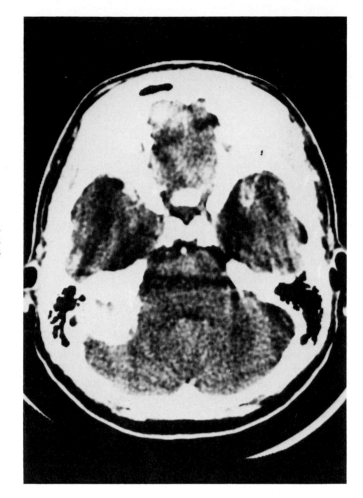

Figure 25–39. Cranial CT scan of temporal bone adenocarcinoma of (probable) endolymphatic sac origin (TBAES), as seen by a large, lytic expansile mass of the right mastoid and petrous bones with involvement of the cerebellopontine angle.

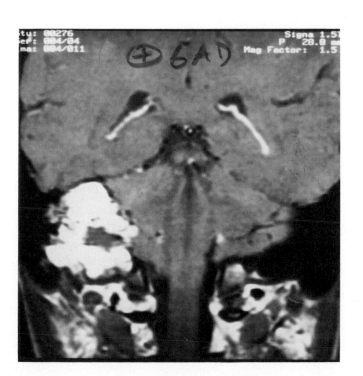

Figure 25–40. Coronal MR, T1-weighted image of TBAES showing a 4.0-cm mass involving the right temporal bone and cerebellopontine angle with involvement of the posteromedial portion of the petrous bone and extension into the posterior cranial fossa; multiple cystic areas can be seen.

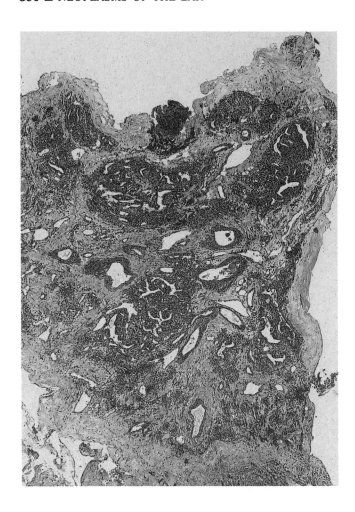

Figure 25–41. Histologic appearance of TBAES: lobules of tumor at low magnification may appear as granulation tissue in a setting of chronic otitis media.

Figure 25–42. Another pattern of TBAES is that of papillary proliferation; this neoplasm extensively invades bone.

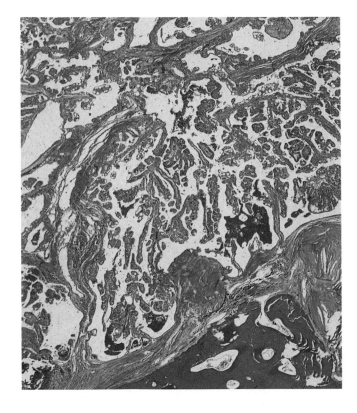

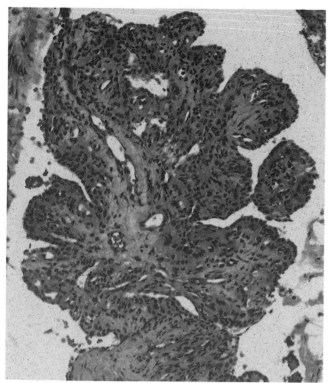

Figure 25-43. Morphologic appearance of TBAES includes a single row of cells ranging from flattened or attenuated-appearing, poorly demarcated from the underlying stroma, and merging with this stromal component, which is composed of numerous capillary-sized vascular spaces. The continuity and merging of the epithelial and stromal components is easily overlooked as part of a granulation tissue reaction.

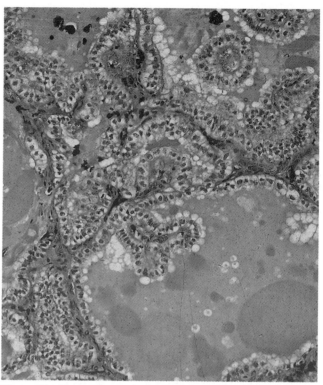

Figure 25-44. Another growth pattern of TBAES is that of a papillary and cystic neoplasm composed of columnar cells with uniform nuclei situated either in the center of the cells or toward the luminal aspect and pale eosinophilic to clear-appearing cytoplasm; the cystic spaces contain colloid-like material and, coupled with the scalloped appearance along the cellular aspect, are histologically similar to papillary carcinoma of thyroid gland origin. Given this histologic appearance, differentiation from a metastatic papillary carcinoma of the thyroid gland is required; TBAES cells are thyroglobulin negative.

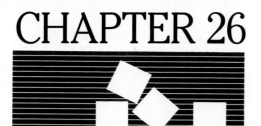

CHAPTER 26

Immunohistochemistry of Middle Ear Neoplasms

MIDDLE EAR NEOPLASMS

Table 26–1
IMMUNOHISTOCHEMISTRY OF MIDDLE EAR NEOPLASMS

	CK	CG	Syn	S-100	NSE	GFAP	Leu-7	Vim	EMA	Des	Myo
MEA	+	0	0	0	0	0	0	0	+	0	0
MEA with neuroen-docrine features	+	+	+	+/0	+	0	+	0	+	0	0
Paraganglioma	0	+	+	+*	+	0	+	0	0	0	0
Meningioma	0	0	0	0	0	0	0	+	+	0	0
Acoustic neuroma	0	0	0	+	+	0	0	0	0	0	0
Rhabdomyosarcoma	0	0	0	0	0	0	0	+/0	0	+	+

* Positive only in the peripherally located sustentacular cells.
MEA—middle ear adenoma; CK—cytokeratin; CG—chromogranin; Syn—synaptophysin; NSE—neuron-specific enolase; GFAP—glial fibrillary acidic protein; Vim—vimentin; EMA—epithelial membrane antigen; Des—desmin; Myo—myoglobin.
See individual chapters for references pertaining to specific tumors.

APPENDICES

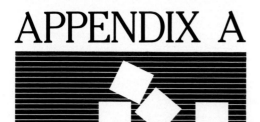

APPENDIX A

Nasal Cavity and Paranasal Sinuses — Embryology and Anatomy

NASAL CAVITY

Embryology

- The facial prominences (frontonasal, maxillary, and mandibular) appear around the fourth week of gestation and give rise to the boundaries and structures of the face.
- The nasal placodes, representing bilateral thickening of the surface ectoderm along the frontonasal prominence, form the nasal pits which, by growth of the surrounding mesenchyme, become progressively depressed along their length and give rise to the primitive nasal sacs, the forerunners of the nasal cavities.
- The anterior portion of the nasal cavity is the vestibule, the epithelium of which is ectodermally derived and represents the internal extension of the integument of the external nose; similarly, the epithelium lining the nasal cavities proper (Schneiderian membrane) is of ectoderm origin.
- The nasal septum develops from the merged medial nasal prominences.
- The regions of continuity between the nasal and oral cavities develop into the choanae after rupture of the oronasal membrane.
- The conchae (turbinates) develop as elevations along the lateral wall of each nasal cavity.
- The olfactory epithelia develop in the superoposterior portion of each nasal cavity and differentiate from cells in the ectodermally derived nasal cavity epithelium.

Innervation

- Innervation of the mucous membranes of the nose is supplied by the ophthalmic and maxillary branches of V (trigeminal) nerve via the pterygopalatine (sphenopalatine) ganglion.
- Olfactory mucous membranes contain the cells of origin of the olfactory nerve fibers, which collect into bundles that traverse the cribriform plate and end in the olfactory bulb.

Vascular Supply and Lymphatic Drainage

Arteries and Veins

- Arterial supply to the nasal cavity comes from several sources, including the sphenopalatine branch of the internal maxillary artery (a branch of the external carotid artery), the anterior and posterior ethmoidal arteries, branches of the ophthalmic artery (a branch of the internal carotid artery), and the facial artery (a branch of the external carotid artery).
- The veins of the nose parallel the arteries with drainage via the sphenopalatine foramen into the pterygoid plexus and then into the internal jugular vein, via the ophthalmic veins into the cavernous sinus and then into the dural venous sinuses, and via the facial vein into either the internal or external jugular vein.

Lymphatics

- Anterior portion of nose drains to the lymphatics draining the skin covering the external nose, and passes to the submandibular nodes.
- Majority of the lymphatics of the nasal cavity drain via the retropharyngeal lymph nodes to the deep cervical lymph nodes.

PARANASAL SINUSES

Embryology

- The paranasal sinuses (maxillary, ethmoid, sphenoid, and frontal) develop as outgrowths of the walls of the nasal cavities and become air-filled extensions of the nasal cavities.
- Some of the paranasal sinuses (the maxillary and portions of the ethmoidal cells) develop during late

fetal life, and others (frontal and sphenoid sinuses) are not present at birth but develop during the early years of life.

Innervation

Maxillary Sinuses

■ Innervation supplied by the maxillary branches of V (trigeminal) nerve, including the anterior, middle, and posterior superior alveolar nerves and the infraorbital nerve.

Ethmoid Sinuses

■ Innervation supplied by the ophthalmic and maxillary branches of V (trigeminal) nerve, including the nasociliary, anterior ethmoid, posterior ethmoid nerves and the orbital branches of the pterygopalatine (sphenopalatine) ganglion.

Frontal Sinuses

■ Innervation supplied by the supraorbital and supratrochlear branches of the frontal nerve, a derivative of the ophthalmic branch of V (trigeminal) nerve.

Sphenoid Sinuses

■ Innervation supplied by the ophthalmic and maxillary branches of V (trigeminal), including the posterior ethmoid nerve and the orbital branches of the pterygopalatine (sphenopalatine) ganglion.

Vascular Supply and Lymphatic Drainage

Arteries and Veins

Maxillary Sinuses

■ Major blood supply comes from branches of the maxillary artery (infraorbital, greater palatine, postero- and anterosuperior alveolar arteries, and sphenopalatine artery), with smaller contribution from the facial artery; both the maxillary and facial arteries are branches of the external carotid artery.
■ Venous drainage occurs anteriorly via the anterior facial vein to the jugular vein and posteriorly via the maxillary vein to the jugular system by way of the retromandibular vein; in addition, in the region of the infratemporal fossa, the maxillary vein communicates with the pterygoid venous plexus, which

anastomose with the dural sinuses through the base of the skull.

Ethmoid Sinuses

■ Receive their blood supply from both the internal and external carotid arteries via branches of the ophthalmic (anterior and posterior ethmoidal arteries) and maxillary (nasal branch of sphenopalatine artery) arteries, respectively.
■ Venous drainage occurs by two routes:
  1. Into the nose via the nasal veins, which flow to the maxillary vein, and then retromandibular vein and ultimately into the external jugular vein.
  2. Via the ethmoidal veins to the ophthalmic veins to the cavernous sinus.

Frontal Sinuses

■ Receive their blood supply from branches of the ophthalmic artery (supraorbital and supratrochlear arteries), a branch of the internal carotid artery.
■ Venous drainage is to the cavernous sinus by way of the superior ophthalmic vein.

Sphenoid Sinuses

■ Receives their blood supply from both the internal and external carotid arteries via branches of the ophthalmic (posterior ethmoidal artery) and maxillary (sphenopalatine artery) arteries, respectively.
■ Venous drainage occurs to the maxillary vein, which flows to the external jugular vein by way of the retropharyngeal vein and to the pterygoid plexus, which flows to the facial vein, which empties into the internal jugular vein.

Lymphatics

■ Maxillary sinuses: lymphatic drainage is to the submandibular lymph nodes.
■ Ethmoid sinuses: lymphatic drainage occurs to the submandibular (from the anterior and middle ethmoid groups) and the retropharyngeal (from posterior ethmoid group) lymph nodes.
■ Frontal sinuses: lymphatic drainage occurs to the submandibular lymph nodes.
■ Sphenoid sinuses: lymphatic drainage occurs to the retropharyngeal lymph nodes.

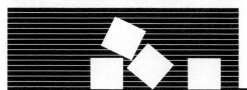

Oral Cavity, Nasopharynx, and Neck — Embryology and Anatomy

ORAL CAVITY

Embryology

- The primitive mouth or stomodeum partly develops from the surface ectoderm and partly from the endoderm of the cranial end of the foregut (the future site of the pharynx); initially, the oropharyngeal membrane separates these structures, but at the end of the fourth week of gestation, the oropharyngeal membrane disappears, allowing for direct communication of the mouth with the pharynx.
- Most of the epithelium of the oral cavity (lips, gums, palate) is of ectodermal origin.
- The epithelium of the tongue varies in its development:

  The anterior two thirds or oral tongue is of ectodermal origin, developing from the tuberculum impair, and is of first branchial arch derivation.

  The posterior or pharyngeal portion of the tongue is of endodermal origin, developing from the hypobranchial eminence, and is of third branchial arch derivation.
- Muscles of mastication (temporalis, masseter, medial and lateral pterygoids) are derived from the first branchial arch (mandibular arch).
- The mandible is formed from the mandibular prominence of the first branchial arch; the maxilla, zygomatic bone, and squamous part of the temporal bone derive from the maxillary prominence of the first branchial arch.
- Trigeminal nerve (V) (maxillary and mandibular branches) arises from the first branchial arch; facial nerve (VII) arises from the second branchial arch; glossopharyngeal nerve (IX) arises from the third branchial arch; vagus nerve (X) arises from the fourth branchial arch.

Innervation

- Innervation of the oral cavity structures are from cranial nerves V and VII:

  V nerve branches to the oral cavity include the maxillary nerve (entirely sensory) and the mandibular nerve (sensory and motor); each of these nerves is further divided into various nerve groups that innervate specific oral cavity structures (for more details, the reader is referred to specific anatomy texts).

  VII nerve: motor root supplies the muscles of the face; sensory root supplies the taste fibers via the chorda tympani for the presulcal area of the tongue, and via the palatine and greater petrosal nerves for the soft palate.
- Of special note is the innervation of the tongue:

  Motor innervation to the intrinsic muscles of the tongue is supplied by the hypoglossal (XII) nerve.

  Sensory nerves include lingual branch of the mandibular nerve for ordinary sensibility to the anterior tongue; the chorda tympani branch of the facial nerve for taste to the anterior tongue (excluding the circumvallate papillae); lingual branch of the glossopharyngeal (IX) nerve for taste and general sensibility to the mucous membranes at the base and lateral aspects of the tongue and to the circumvallate papillae; superior laryngeal nerve to the vallecular area (in front of the epiglottis).

Vascular Supply and Lymphatic Drainage

Arteries and Veins

- Arterial supply to the oral cavity structures comes via branches of the internal carotid artery (facial artery and its branches) and the external carotid artery (lingual and maxillary arteries and their branches).

■ Venous drainage from the oral cavity structures flows to the internal jugular vein via the facial vein and pterygoid plexus and to the external jugular vein via numerous smaller veins, including the facial vein and the maxillary vein.

Lymphatics

■ Lips: upper lip—preauricular, infraparotid, submandibular, and submental lymph nodes; relative absence of anastomotic channels results in ipsilateral drainage.
Lower lip, medial portion—submental lymph nodes.
Lower lip, lateral portion—submandibular lymph nodes.

■ Due to numerous anastomotic lymphatic vessels near the midline of the lower lip, lymphatic drainage occurs bilaterally.

■ Buccal mucosa: lymph nodes in the submental and submandibular triangles of the neck.

■ Alveolar ridges: buccal aspect—submental and submandibular lymph nodes.

■ Retromolar trigone: upper deep cervical lymph nodes.

■ Floor of mouth, anterior part—inferior lymph nodes of the upper deep cervical group via the submental lymph nodes; all other parts—submandibular and upper deep cervical lymph nodes.

■ Tongue: lymphatics arise from an extensive submucosal plexus, with ultimate drainage to the deep cervical lymph nodes.

■ Hard palate: upper deep cervical and retropharyngeal lymph nodes.

■ Gingiva, upper gums and lower posterior part—submandibular lymph nodes; lower anterior part—submental lymph nodes.

NASOPHARYNX AND OROPHARYNX

Embryology

■ The primitive pharynx is derived from the foregut, developing from both the branchial arches and pharyngeal pouches; the epithelium and glands are of endodermal derivation.
The tonsils develop from the second pharyngeal pouch.
The tubotympanic recess (which forms the eustachian tube and tympanic cavity) develops from the first pharyngeal pouch.

Innervation

■ Both motor and sensory innervation are primarily supplied from the pharyngeal plexus, formed by branches of cranial nerves IX (glossopharyngeal) and X (vagus).

Vascular Supply and Lymphatic Drainage

Arteries and Veins

■ Arterial supply comes from branches of the external carotid artery, including the ascending pharyngeal, facial, lingual, maxillary, and superior thyroid arteries.

■ The veins form a plexus that drains into the internal jugular and facial veins directly or via a communication with the pterygoid venous plexus.

Lymphatics

■ Nasopharynx: directly to the upper deep cervical lymph nodes.

■ Oropharynx, including the tonsil and base of tongue: upper deep cervical lymph nodes, particularly to the jugulodigastric and jugulo-omohyoid group of lymph nodes.

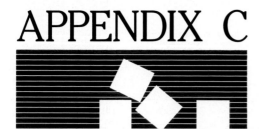

APPENDIX C

Larynx and Hypopharynx— Embryology and Anatomy

LARYNX

Embryology

- Epithelium and glands of the larynx arise from the endoderm lining the laryngotracheal groove.
- Cartilage, muscle, and other connective tissue elements develop from the mesenchyme around the foregut:

    Thyroid, cricoid, arytenoid, corniculate, and cuneiform cartilages derive from the fourth and sixth branchial arch.

    Greater cornu and inferior part of the body of the hyoid bone derive from the third branchial arch cartilage; lesser cornu and superior part of the body of the hyoid bone derive from the second branchial arch cartilage.

    Intrinsic muscles of the larynx derive from the fourth and sixth branchial arch.

    Superior laryngeal and recurrent laryngeal nerves (both branches of the vagus nerve) derive from the fourth and sixth branchial arch.

Innervation

- Innervation of the larynx is by two sets of nerves, both branches of the X (vagus) nerve:

    Superior laryngeal nerve: largely sensory.

    Inferior laryngeal nerve: largely motor, supplying the intrinsic muscles of the larynx.

Vascular Supply and Lymphatic Drainage

Arteries and Veins

- Arterial supply to the larynx consists of two pairs: superior and inferior laryngeal arteries, derived from the the superior and inferior thyroid artery branches of the carotid artery and the subclavian artery, respectively.
- Superior and inferior laryngeal veins parallel the arteries.

Lymphatics

- Divided into superior and inferior groups by the vocal fold.
- Superior group: drain to the upper portion of the deep cervical lymph nodes.
- Inferior group: drain to the lower deep cervical lymph nodes.

HYPOPHARYNX

Embryology

- The primitive pharynx is derived from the foregut, developing from both the branchial arches and pharyngeal pouches; the epithelium and glands are of endodermal derivation.
- Constrictor muscles of the pharynx derive from the fourth and sixth branchial arch.

Innervation

- Motor and most of the sensory supply to the pharynx is via the pharyngeal plexus formed by the pharyngeal branches of cranial nerves IX (glossopharyngeal) and X (vagus).

Vascular Supply and Lymphatic Drainage

Arteries and Veins

- Arterial supply to the hypopharynx is from branches of the superior and inferior thyroid artery and branches of the carotid artery and the subclavian artery, respectively.
- Venous plexus communicates with the pterygoid plexus above and the superior thyroid and lingual veins below, or directly with the facial vein or the internal jugular vein.

Lymphatics

- Drain to the lymph nodes of the deep cervical chain.

401

APPENDIX D

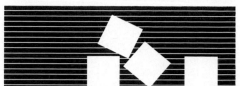

Salivary Glands — Embryology and Anatomy

EMBRYOLOGY

- All salivary glands develop as solid proliferations or buds from the epithelium of the stomodeum during the sixth to seventh weeks of gestation.
- Parotid glands:
  The first to form in humans.
  Arise from the ectodermal lining of the stomodeum, from which the ducts, lumina, and acini evolve.
  The capsule and connective tissue develop from the surrounding mesenchyme.
- Submandibular glands:
  Develop from buds of the endoderm in the floor of the stomodeum, from which the ducts, lumina, and acini evolve.
- Sublingual glands:
  Appear later than the other glands.
  Develop from buds of the endoderm in the paralingual sulcus, from which the ducts, lumina, and acini evolve.
- Minor salivary glands (seromucous glands):
  Develop later in gestational life (third month).
  Endodermally derived.

INNERVATION

Parotid Glands

- Auriculotemporal branch of the IX cranial nerve traverses the parotid gland and provides its sensory and secretomotor functions.
  Frey's syndrome or auriculomotor nerve syndrome: occurs following parotidectomy, when misdirected regeneration of the secretomotor fibers with innervation of the cutaneous sweat glands results in facial sweating during eating.
  The VII (facial) nerve passes through the deep and posterior aspects of the parotid gland prior to dividing into its branches to the face; any surgical procedure to remove portions of the parotid gland, unless it involves only the superficial part, carries the danger of damage to the nerve; maintaining the integrity and function of the facial nerve in a total parotidectomy is a difficult and delicate procedure.

Submandibular and Sublingual Glands

- Facial nerve (VII) provides the sensory and secretomotor function of these glands via the chorda tympani, accompanying the lingual nerve (a branch of the mandibular division of V nerve), which passes through the submandibular ganglion.

VASCULAR SUPPLY AND LYMPHATIC DRAINAGE

Arteries and Veins

Parotid Glands

- Arterial supply is via branches of the external carotid artery and includes the posterior auricular, maxillary, superficial temporal, and transverse facial arteries.
- Venous structures parallel those of the arteries and empty into the external jugular vein.

Lymphatics

- Lymphatic drainage is to the superficial and deep cervical lymph nodes via the superficial parotid lymph nodes.

Submandibular and Sublingual Glands

- Arterial supply to the submandibular gland is via branches of the external carotid artery and the facial and lingual arteries; arterial supply to the sublingual gland is by the sublingual and submental arteries, and branches of the lingual and facial arteries, respectively.

■ Venous structures parallel those of the arteries and empty into the external and internal jugular veins.

Lymphatics

■ To the superficial and deep cervical lymph nodes via submandibular and sublingual lymph nodes.

APPENDIX E

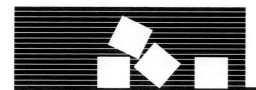

The Ear — Embryology and Anatomy

EMBRYOLOGY

External Ear

- The auricle (pinna) develops from the auricular hillocks, a group of six mesenchymal swellings, from the first and second branchial arches lying around the first branchial groove.
- The mesenchymal structures of the auricle arise from the mesoderm of the first and second branchial arches.
- The epithelium of the external auditory canal develops from the ectoderm at the dorsal end of the first branchial groove or cleft.
- The tympanic membrane develops from three sources:
  - Ectoderm of the first branchial groove gives rise to the epithelium on the external side.
  - Endoderm of the tubotympanic recess from the first pharyngeal pouch gives rise to the epithelium on the internal side.
  - Mesoderm of the first and second branchial arches gives rise to the connective tissue lying between the external and internal epithelial surfaces.

Middle Ear

- The endoderm of the tubotympanic recess, a derivative of the first pharyngeal pouch, gives rise from its distal portion to the epithelium of the tympanic cavity and the mastoid antrum, and from its proximal portion to the epithelium of the auditory tube (eustachian or pharyngotympanic tube).
- The middle ear ossicles have different derivations with the malleus and incus arising from the first branchial arch cartilage (Meckel's cartilage), and the stapes arising from the second branchial arch cartilage (Reichert's cartilage).
- The tensor tympani muscle, attached to the malleus, derives from the first branchial arch; the stapedius muscle attached to the stapes derives from the second branchial arch.

Internal Ear

- First of the three anatomic divisions of the ear to develop, beginning toward the end of the first month of gestation.
- The membranous labyrinth (utricle, saccule, semicircular ducts, cochlear duct) arises from the otic vesicle (otocyst), an invagination from the surface ectoderm that migrates into its position, losing its connection to the surface ectoderm.
- The bony labyrinth (vestibule, semicircular canals, cochlea) arises from the mesenchyme around the otic vesicle.

INNERVATION

External Ear

- Overlapping innervation, including auriculotemporal branch of the mandibular branch of trigeminal (V) nerve, cutaneous branches of the cervical plexus, primarily the greater auricular and lesser occipital nerves from C2 and C3, and the auricular branches of the vagus (X) (nerve of Arnold), glossopharyngeal (IX) and facial (VII) nerves.
- The external aspect of the tympanic membrane is innervated from the auriculotemporal branch of V nerve and the auricular branches of cranial nerves X, IX, and VII.

Middle Ear

- Nerve supply is chiefly from the tympanic plexus, formed by the tympanic branch of the glossopharyngeal nerve (nerve of Jacobson) and from the caroticotympanic nerves derived from the internal carotid plexus.

Internal Ear

- The nerve to the inner ear is the vestibulocochlear nerve or the VIII cranial nerve; these nerves run together in the internal auditory canal until the lateral end, at which point they separate into three parts, two vestibular and one cochlear.

■ The fibers of the vestibular nerve arise from Scarpa's ganglion.

VASCULAR SUPPLY AND LYMPHATIC DRAINAGE

Arteries and Veins

External Ear

■ The blood supply to the auricle comes from branches of the external carotid artery.
■ The blood supply to the external auditory canal is the same as that to the auricle and, in addition, receives blood from the deep auricular artery, a branch of the internal maxillary artery.
■ The veins from the auricle and external auditory canal are the superficial temporal and posterior auricular veins, which join with the jugular veins and sometimes to the sigmoid sinus.

Lymphatics

■ From the auricle and external auditory canal to the parotid lymph nodes, the superficial cervical nodes, and the retroauricular lymph nodes.

Middle Ear

■ Arterial supply to the middle ear is mostly derived from branches of the external carotid artery, including the internal maxillary, posterior auricular, and ascending pharyngeal arteries.
■ The veins of the middle ear parallel those of the arteries and empty into the pterygoid venous plexus and the superior petrosal sinus.

Lymphatics

■ To the retropharyngeal and parotid lymph nodes.

Internal Ear

■ The primary arterial supply to the internal ear is via the labyrinthine or internal auditory artery, a branch of the anterior inferior cerebellar artery, or from the basilar artery.
■ The veins parallel those of the arteries and empty into the superior petrosal sinus or the transverse sinus.

Lymphatics

■ The internal ear is not usually described.

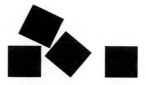

INDEX

Note: Numbers followed by an i indicate illustrations; those followed by a t indicate tables.

A

Acinic cell adenocarcinoma, 309–310, 310i, 311i
Acoustic neuroma, 371–372, 372i, 373i
Acoustic schwannoma, 371–372, 372i, 373i
Acquired immunodeficiency syndrome (AIDS), cytomegalovirus with, 132–133, 135i
  gonorrhea with, 134
  herpes with, 132–133, 135i
  infections with, 132–134, 135i–138i
  Kaposi's sarcoma with, 194–195, 195i, 196i
  lymphadenopathies with, 138–139, 139i–141i
  lymphomas with, 138, 175
  syphilis with, 134, 137i, 138i
Actinomycosis, cervicofacial, 103t, 129, 129i, 130i
Adamantinoma, 54–55, 56i
Adamantoblastoma, 54–55, 56i
Adenocarcinoma, acinic cell, 309–310, 310i, 311i
  basal cell, 328, 329i
  middle ear, 386–387, 387i
  not otherwise specified, 319–320, 321i
  papillary, 172–173, 174i
  polymorphous, 322–323, 323i–325i
  sinonasal, 5t, 61–63, 63i–66i
  temporal bone, 388, 389i–391i
Adenoid cystic carcinoma, 311–313, 313i, 314i
Adenolymphoma, of salivary glands, 286–287, 288i, 289i
Adenoma, basal cell, 292, 293i, 294i
  canalicular, 295, 296i
  ceruminal gland, 363–364, 364i, 365i, 381–382, 382i
  clear cell, 325–326, 327i
  middle ear, 365–366, 367i, 368i
  monomorphic, 286–288, 288i, 289i
  oxyphilic, 290–291, 291i
  pleomorphic, carcinoma ex, 315–316, 317i, 318i
  of salivary glands, 283–284, 285i, 286i
Adenosquamous carcinoma, 252–253, 253i, 254i
AIDS. See *Acquired immunodeficiency syndrome (AIDS).*
AIDS-related complex (ARC). See also *Acquired immunodeficiency syndrome (AIDS).*
  infections with, 132–134, 135i–138i
  lymphadenopathies with, 138–139, 139i–141i
ALHE. See *Angiolymphoid hyperplasia with eosinophilia (ALHE).*

Alveolar soft part sarcoma (ASPS), 151, 153i, 154i
Ameloblastoma, 54–55, 56i
Amyloidosis, laryngeal, 216–217, 217i
  lingual, 217i
Angiofibroma, juvenile, 145–146, 146i, 147i
  nasopharyngeal, 145–146, 146i, 147i
Angiolymphoid hyperplasia with eosinophilia (ALHE), 350, 351i
Angiosarcoma, 88, 89i
Aspergillosis, 16, 16i, 17i
ASPS. See *Alveolar soft part sarcoma (ASPS).*
Atypia, epithelial, 222t

B

Basal cell adenocarcinoma, of salivary glands, 328, 329i
Basal cell adenoma, of salivary glands, 292, 293i, 294i
Basal cell carcinoma, of external ear, 375–377, 377i, 378i
Basaloid squamous cell carcinoma, laryngeal, 250, 251i, 252i
Benign lymphoepithelial lesion (BLL), 278–279, 280i, 281i
Benign mixed tumor, of salivary glands, 283–284, 285i, 286i
BLL. See *Benign lymphoepithelial lesion (BLL).*
Branchial cleft, anomalies of, 103t, 105–107, 107i–109i
Burkitt's lymphoma, 175–176, 178i
  staging of, 176t

C

Canalicular adenoma, 295, 296i
Candidiasis, in AIDS patients, 133, 136i
Carcinoid tumor, 254–255, 256i, 257i
  atypical, 255, 258i, 259i
Carcinoma. See also specific types, e.g., *Adenocarcinoma.*
  adenosquamous, 252–253, 253i, 254i
  basal cell, of ear, 375–377, 377i, 378i
  clear cell, 325–326, 327i
  cystic, adenoid, 311–313, 313i, 314i
  epidermoid, of external ear, 379–380, 381i
  sinonasal, 57–58, 58i–60i
  epithelial-myoepithelial cell, 325–326, 327i